Hepatobiliary and Pancreatic Surgery

Other titles in the series:

Emergency Surgery and Critical Care
Simon Paterson-Brown

Upper Gastrointestinal Surgery
S. Michael Griffin and Stephen A. Raimes

Colorectal Surgery
Robin K. S. Phillips

Breast and Endocrine Surgery
John R. Farndon

Vascular and Endovascular Surgery
Jonathan D. Beard and Peter A. Gaines

Transplantation Surgery
John L. R. Forsythe

A COMPANION TO SPECIALIST SURGICAL PRACTICE

Series editors

Sir David Carter
O. James Garden
Simon Paterson-Brown

Hepatobiliary and Pancreatic Surgery

Edited by

O. James Garden

Professor of Hepatobiliary Surgery
at the Royal Infirmary
Director of Organ Transplantation
University Department of Surgery
Royal Infirmary
Edinburgh

W B Saunders Company Ltd
London · Philadelphia · Toronto · Sydney · Tokyo

W B Saunders Company Ltd 24–28 Oval Road
London NW1 7DX

The Curtis Center
Independence Square West
Philadelphia, PA 19106-3399, USA

Harcourt Brace & Company
55 Horner Avenue
Toronto, Ontario, M8Z 4X6, Canada

Harcourt Brace & Company, Australia
30–52 Smidmore Street
Marrickville, NSW 2204, Australia

Harcourt Brace & Company, Japan
Ichibancho Central Building, 22-1 Ichibancho
Chiyoda-ku, Tokyo 102, Japan

A catalogue record for this book is available from the British Library

ISBN 0-7020-2142-3

Typeset by Paston Press Ltd, Loddon, Norfolk
Printed and bound in Great Britain by The Bath Press, Bath

Contents

Contributors

Jacques Belghiti *MD*
Chef de Service, Service de Chirurgie Digestive, Hôpital Beaujon, Clichy, France

Irving S. Benjamin *BSc MD FRCS*
Professor of Surgery, Academic Department of Surgery, King's College School of Medicine & Dentistry, King's College Hospital, London, UK

Sir David C. Carter *MD FRCS(Ed) FRCS(Glas), FRCS(Eng), Hon FRCS(Ire), Hon FACS, FRCP(Ed), FRS(Ed)*
Chief Medical Officer in Scotland, Formerly Regius Professor of Clinical Surgery, University Department of Surgery, Royal Infirmary, Edinburgh, UK

James N. Crinnion *MB ChB FRCS*
Specialist Registrar in General Surgery, Hanwell, London, UK

Tom Diamond *BSc MD FRCS FRCSI*
Consultant Surgeon, Department of Surgery, Mater Hospital Trust, Belfast, Northern Ireland

Olivier Farges *MD*
Service de Chirurgie Digestive, Hôpital Beaujon, Clichy, France

O. James Garden
Professor of Hepatobiliary Surgery at the Royal Infirmary, Director of Organ Transplantation, University Department of Surgery, Royal Infirmary, Edinburgh, UK

Thomas J. Hugh *FRACS*
Research Fellow, Directorate of General Surgery, Royal Liverpool University Hospital NHS Trust, Liverpool, UK

Timothy G. John *FRCS Ed(Gen) MB ChB*
Senior Registrar, University Department of Surgery, Royal Infirmary, Edinburgh, UK

Donald Menzies *MS FRCS*
Consultant Surgeon, Department of Surgery, Colchester General Hospital, Colchester, UK

Roger W. Motson *MS FRCS*
Consultant Surgeon, Department of Surgery, Colchester General Hospital, Colchester, UK

Rowan W. Parks *FRCS*
Research Registrar, Department of Surgery, The Queen's University of
Belfast, Belfast, Northern Ireland

Graeme J. Poston *MS FRCS*
Consultant Surgeon, Hepato-Pancreato-Biliary Unit, Royal Liverpool
University Hospital, Liverpool, UK

Ib C. Rasmussen *MD, PhD*
Associate Professor of Surgery, Department of Surgery, University
Hospital, Uppsala, Sweden

Ajith Siriwardena *MD FRCS*
Senior Lecturer, University Department of Surgery, Royal Infirmary,
Edinburgh, UK

Robin C. N. Williamson *MA MD MChir FRCS*
Professor of Surgery, Royal Postgraduate Medical School, Hammersmith
Hospital, Department of Surgery, London, UK

Foreword

General surgery defies easy definition. Indeed, there are those who claim that it is dying, if not yet dead – a corpse being picked clean by the vulturine proclivities of the other specialties of surgery. Unfortunately for those who subscribe to this view, general surgery is not lying down, indeed it is rejoicing in a new enhanced vigour, as this new series demonstrates.

The general surgeon is the specialist who, along with his other colleagues, provides a 24-hour, 7-day, emergency surgical cover for his, or her, hospital. Also it is to general surgical clinics that patients are referred, unless their condition is manifestly related to one of the other surgical specialties, e.g. urology, cardiothoracic services, etc. Moreover, trainees in these specialities must, during their training, receive experience in general surgery, whose techniques underpin the whole of surgery. General surgery occupies a pivotal position in surgical training. The number of general surgeons required to serve a community, outstrips that required by any other surgical specialty.

General surgery is a specialty in its own right. Inevitably, there are those who wish to practice exclusively one of the sub-specialties of general surgery, e.g. vascular or colorectal surgery. This arrangement may be possible in a few large tertiary referral centres. Although the contribution of these surgeons to patient care and to advances in their discipline will be significant, their numbers are necessarily low. The bulk of surgical practice will be undertaken by the general surgeon who has developed a sub-specialty interest, so that, with his other colleagues in the hospital, comprehensive surgery services can be provided.

There is therefore a great need for a text which will provide comprehensively the theoretical knowledge of the entire specialty and act as a guide for the acquisition of the diagnostic and therapeutic skills required by the general surgeon. The unique contribution of this companion is that it comes as a series, each chapter fresh from the pen of a practising clinician and active surgeon. Each volume is right up to date and this is evidenced by the fact that the first volumes of the series are being published within 12 months from the start of the project. This is a series which has been tightly edited by a team from one of the foremost teaching hospitals in the United Kingdom.

Quite properly the series begins with a volume on emergency surgery and critical care – two of the greatest challenges confronting the practising surgeon. These are the areas that the examination candidate finds the greatest difficulty in acquiring theoretical knowledge and practical experience. Moreover, these are the areas in which advances are at present so rapid that they constantly test the experienced consultant surgeon.

This series not only provides both types of reader with the necessary up-to-date detail but also demonstrates that general surgery remains as challenging and vigorous as it ever has been.

Sir Robert Shields *DL, MD, DSc, FRCS(Ed, Eng, Glas, Ire),*
FRCPEd, FACS
President, Royal College of Surgeons of Edinburgh

Preface

A *Companion to Specialist Surgical Practice* was designed to meet the needs of the higher surgeon in training and busy practising surgeon who need access to up to date information on recent developments, research and data in the context of accepted surgical practice.

Many of the major surgery text books either cover the whole of what is termed 'general surgery' and therefore contain much which is not of interest to the specialist surgeon, or are very high level specialist texts which are outwith the reach of the trainee's finances, and though comprehensive are often out of date due to the lengthy writing and production times of such major works.

Each volume in this series therefore provides succinct summaries of all key topics within a specialty, concentrating on the most recent developments and current data. They are carefully constructed to be easily readable and provide key references.

A specialist surgeon, whether in training or in practice, need only purchase the volume relevant to his or her chosen specialist field plus the emergency surgery and critical care volume, if involved in emergency care.

The volumes have been written in a very short time frame, and produced equally quickly so that information is as up to date as possible. Each volume will be updated and published as a new edition at frequent intervals, to ensure that current information is always available.

We hope that our aim – of providing affordable up-to-date specialist texts – has been met and that all surgeons, in training or in practice will find the volumes to be a valuable resource.

Sir David C. Carter MD, FRCS(Ed), FRCS(Glas), FRCS(Eng), Hon FRCS(Ire), Hon FACS, FRCP(Ed), FRS(Ed)
Chief Medical Officer in Scotland, Formerly Regius Professor of Clinical Surgery, University Department of Surgery, Royal Infirmary, Edinburgh

O. James Garden BSc, MD, FRCS(Glas), FRCS(Ed)
Professor of Hepatobiliary Surgery at the Royal Infirmary, Director of Organ Transplantation, University Department of Surgery, Royal Infirmary, Edinburgh

Simon Paterson-Brown MS, MPhil, FRCS(Ed), FRCS(Eng), FCSHK
Consultant General and Upper Gastrointestinal Surgeon, University Department of Surgery, Royal Infirmary, Edinburgh

Acknowledgements

I am indebted to all the authors who have contributed to this Volume for their perseverance and expertise. I am grateful to my fellow editors for assistance and advice in the initial planning of this book. The series editors give special thanks to Rachael Stock and Linda Clark from W B Saunders for their initial persuasion, continuing enthusiasm and ongoing support. I would like to acknowledge Carole Tomlinson for her secretarial expertise. I thank my wife Amanda and Stephen and Katie for their tolerance.

O. J. GARDEN

1 Investigation of hepatobiliary and pancreatic malignancy

Timothy G. John

Introduction

The majority of patients who present with malignant hepatobiliary and pancreatic tumours have a poor prognosis, and it is the clinician's duty to try and achieve optimal palliation of symptoms and quality of life. The grave implications of such a diagnosis dictate that it should be established as safely, accurately and rapidly as possible so that the patient may be informed and treatment options discussed. Advances in surgical technique in recent years have meant that for some patients, resectional surgery offers the hope of prolonged survival, and perhaps even of 'cure' from an otherwise fatal disease. Careful patient selection is fundamental to the success of any attempt at 'curative' resection in patients with hepatobiliary and pancreatic malignancy. In this task, the surgeon is reliant on a variety of investigations which fulfil both diagnostic and staging roles.

Investigation of pancreatic malignancy

Ductal carcinoma of the pancreas ranks as the fifth most common cause of cancer death and the second most common cause of death from gastrointestinal malignancy in the Western world. Although the overall prognosis remains very poor, many surgeons would accept that 'curative' resection of the pancreatic head offers the only hope of prolonged survival providing that morbidity and mortality are minimised. Periampullary cancers, arising from the epithelium of the lower common bile duct, duodenum, pancreatic duct or the papilla itself, tend to present at an earlier stage and have a better prognosis.

The clinical features of biliary obstruction usually predominate in patients presenting with carcinoma of the pancreatic head and periampullary region. Accordingly, investigation of the patient presenting with 'malignant obstructive jaundice' or 'malignant low bile duct obstruction' is the scenario which will be emphasised in this section, also including patients with cholangiocarcinoma of the distal bile duct. Less commonly, a focal pancreatic mass detected radiologically presents a 'diagnostic dilemma' in a patient with vague symptoms. Early and accurate diagnosis is desirable to differentiate between peripancreatic malignancies and benign lesions such as common bile duct calculi, or an inflammatory pancreatic mass such as focal chronic pancreatitis or a pseudocyst.

Rationale for non-operative assessment of patients with malignant low bile duct obstruction

Having established a probable diagnosis of pancreatic and periampullary carcinoma, the aim of preoperative investigation is to identify those patients with potentially resectable lesions who would benefit from 'curative' resection. Conversely, the detection of those with factors indicative of a poor prognosis allows a less aggressive treatment strategy to be employed. The rationale for such preoperative patient selection is dependent on several assumptions which are summarised in Table 1.1. However, no consensus exists, and more liberal use of surgical intervention has been justified for reasons summarised in Table 1.2. Ultimately, it is the philosophy of the individual surgical team which determines what sort of investigative algorithm is used, as well as the question of what constitutes a 'resectable' tumour.

The incidence of 'laparotomy and biopsy' as a means of confirming a diagnosis, and assessing the resectability, of pancreatic malignancy has been reported in 15–40% of patients.[1–4] However, recognition that non-therapeutic laparotomy is associated with unnecessary morbidity in patients with an already abbreviated life expectancy, and the development of modern imaging modalities, has led to a widespread (though not universal) acceptance that diagnostic laparotomy is an unacceptable primary method of investigating suspected pancreatic malignancy.

Table 1.1 *Rationale for 'minimally invasive' investigation of suspected pancreatic malignancy*

1. Avoids unnecessary laparotomy with its associated morbidity in patients shown to have unresectable tumours

2. Effective non-operative palliation of obstructive jaundice may be achieved by endoscopic or percutaneous biliary stent insertion

3. Avoids inappropriate resectional surgery with early tumour recurrence in patients shown to have disseminated malignancy

4. Identifies candidates for preoperative cytoreductive/neo-adjuvant chemo/ radiotherapy

5. Potential cost savings

6. Potential for laparoscopic biliary and duodenal bypass

Table 1.2 *Rationale for surgical assessment of suspected pancreatic malignancy*

1. Identifies 'non-ductal' pancreatic tumours

2. Patients with false positive staging investigations are not denied surgical assessment of resectability

3. Palliative pancreatic resection is favoured by some surgeons

4. Better palliation of malignant obstructive jaundice may be achieved by surgical biliary bypass in some patients

5. Better palliation of malignant gastric outflow obstruction may be achieved by gastroenterostomy in some patients

Although no survival advantage for either surgical biliary bypass or biliary endoprosthesis insertion has been demonstrated by randomised comparison in patients with malignant obstructive jaundice,[5,6] there appears to be at least a subgroup of elderly, frail or unfit patients, and those with abbreviated life expectancy (i.e. less than six months) who should benefit from non-operative relief of biliary obstruction. Nevertheless, some surgeons still emphasise the importance of surgical exploration for fear of labelling as unresectable a better prognosis tumour of non-ductal origin, such as a neuroendocrine tumour, cystadenoma, cystadenocarcinoma, sarcoma or lymphoma.[7] Also, laparotomy provides the opportunity for surgical relief of established or impeding malignant gastric outlet obstruction, although evidence to support a role for prophylactic gastroenterostomy is lacking.[8] Such issues are discussed more fully in Chapter 10.

Staging conventions and definitions of resectability in patients with pancreatic and periampullary cancer

It is generally accepted that extra-abdominal metastases, metastases to the liver or serosal surfaces and tumour invasion of adjacent viscera such as the mesenteric root, stomach and colon are absolute contraindications to attempts at 'curative' pancreatic resection. Relative contraindications to resection include regional malignant lymphadenopathy, and tumour invasion or encasement of the portal–superior mesenteric vein, or the coeliac or superior mesenteric arteries. Some surgeons are increasingly prepared during pancreaticoduodenectomy to undertake vascular resection and extended lymphadenectomy. However, most surgeons would still regard evidence of malignant invasion of the major peripancreatic blood vessels or regional lymph nodes as contraindications to 'curative' resectional surgery. Accurate tumour staging is important for meaningful interpretation of the results of different treatment strategies, such as radical resectional surgery and adjuvant chemotherapy. The 1992 UICC (Union Internationale Contre Le Cancer) TNM classification for

Table 1.3 *Pancreatic cancer staging using the 1992 UICC TNM classification*[9,10]

T category	
T_1	Limited to the pancreas
	T_{1a} ($\leqslant 2$ cm) T_{1b} (>2 cm)
T_2	Extends directly to duodenum, bile duct, peripancreatic tissues
T_3	Extends directly to stomach, spleen, colon, adjacent large vessels
N category	
N_0	No regional lymph node metastasis
N_1	Regional lymph node metastasis
M category	
M_0	No distant metastases
M_1	Distant metastases
Stage grouping	
Stage I	T_{1-2}, N_0, M_0
Stage II	T_3, N_0, M_0
Stage III	T_{1-3}, N_1, M_0
Stage IV	T_{1-3}, N_{0-1}, M_1

pancreatic carcinoma is the current standard by which staging data should be documented[9,10] and is shown in Table 1.3.

General considerations in the diagnosis and staging of pancreatic malignancy

Any investigation used in the assessment of the patient presenting with suspected pancreatic malignancy should be sensitive enough to identify the presence of tumour, whilst retaining high specificity in excluding alternative (benign) causes. Having established a likely diagnosis, it is important to identify which patients have potentially resectable lesions. The ideal staging investigation should be sensitive enough to detect factors which render the tumour unresectable according to accepted criteria. More importantly, its specificity should approach 100% as false positive results may deny the patient surgical exploration and the chance of potentially curative operation.

Of more clinical value to the surgeon, however, is the predictive value, which answers the question 'when a test is positive, or negative, how often is it correct?' The positive predictive value is the proportion of positive investigations which are true positive. In the context of tumour staging, the positive predictive value directly reflects the 'odds' that positive imaging findings correctly identify unresectable tumour. The converse applies for the negative predictive value which indicates the probability that a negative investigation has correctly identified the tumour as being resectable.

Unlike sensitivity and specificity, predictive values may be markedly affected by differences in disease prevalence. Thus, study of a population containing a high disease prevalence, rather than a random sample of the general patient population, is liable to produce results biased in favour of the test's sensitivity to detect that disease. Conversely, as the proportion of all pancreatic cancer patients with resectable tumours is small, so the results of a staging test may misleadingly favour its sensitivity in identifying tumour unresectability, at the cost of its specificity in detecting patients with resectable disease. In practice, however, the investigation of pancreatic malignancy is often performed in selected patients following secondary or tertiary referral, and the influence of such 'verification' or 'workup' bias is inevitable.

General methods of investigation

The vague early symptoms and signs exhibited by patients with pancreatic cancer partly explain the late presentation with advanced disease of most patients. Nevertheless, 90% of patients with pancreatic cancer present with abdominal pain and/or jaundice.[11] An analysis of 1020 patients with suspected pancreatic cancer, in 80 of whom the diagnosis was confirmed, defined weight loss, recent onset diabetes and the presence of a palpable gall bladder or abdominal mass as clinical features which were significantly predictive of this diagnosis.[12] Serum biochemical and haematological tests confirm the diagnosis of 'obstructive jaundice' and identify any resultant coagulopathy.

Accurate serum tumour markers for pancreatic cancer remain elusive, despite evaluation of a variety of tumour antigens, hormones and enzymes. None are sensitive or specific enough for use in either population screening or for differentiating reliably between pancreatic cancer and chronic pancreatitis.[13–16] The tumour marker which has attracted most interest is the carbohydrate antigen CA 19-9, although its lack of satisfactory tumour or organ specificity has limited its clinical role to follow-up surveillance for tumour recurrence in patients in whom the serum concentration falls after tumour resection.[17,18]

A plain chest radiograph may demonstrate pulmonary metastases or malignant pleural effusions and should be performed in all patients with suspected pancreatic malignancy. There is no evidence that routine computed tomographic (CT) scanning of the thorax is cost beneficial in the preoperative staging of patients with pancreatic cancer. In the past, plain abdominal radiographs have been used to discriminate between patients with pancreatic cancer and chronic pancreatitis on the basis that calcifications may be associated with 90% of the latter cases. Enhanced radiographic techniques which have also played a role in the diagnosis of pancreatic malignancies include barium meal (infiltration of the posterior gastric wall ('pad sign') and medial duodenal wall ('inverted 3 sign')), pneumoperitoneum and pneumostratigraphy and hypotonic duodenography (i.e. double-contrast duodenography with administration of a spasmolytic agent). These methods have been superseded by more sophisticated diagnostic radiological techniques and are now of mainly historical interest.

Endoscopic cholangiography

Combined with the opportunity for endoscopic observation and biopsy of locally invasive tumour, as well as therapeutic intervention to achieve biliary decompression,[19] endoscopic retrograde cholangiopancreatography (ERCP) has become established as a primary modality in the management of patients with malignant biliary obstruction. Freeny and Ball[20] performed ERCP in 376 patients with malignant pancreatic disease for a sensitivity of 94% and a specificity of 97% in the diagnosis of pancreatic cancer. Obstruction ('blunt, tapering, irregular or meniscus' stenoses) of the main pancreatic duct and/or common bile duct were the most commonly observed criteria for the diagnosis of pancreatic cancer, and the 'double duct' sign (i.e. dilatation of both pancreatic and bile duct) was present in 27% of patients with pancreatic cancer.[20]

Nevertheless, such abnormalities of the bile and pancreatic ducts are not exclusive to pancreatic cancer[16,21] and the limitations of ERCP (in common with all available investigations) in differentiating malignancy from chronic pancreatitis should be emphasised. Furthermore, the continued development of abdominal CT scanning led some authors to challenge the role of ERCP within increasingly complex diagnostic algorithms for suspected pancreatic cancer, in which ERCP contributed little in addition to less invasive investigations such as CT, particularly with regard to tumour staging.[22] Silverstein et al.[23] used the technique of decision analysis to model and analyse diagnostic strategies in the diagnosis of suspected pancreatic cancer in terms of diagnostic accuracy, cost and invasiveness. Assuming a sensitivity of 90% and a specificity of 95% from previously published studies, it was estimated that ERCP would be indicated in just 8–11% of patients if transabdominal ultrasonography (USS) was used as the first investigative method, but that abandonment of ERCP altogether would substantially increase the subsequent requirement for diagnostic laparotomy.

Transabdominal ultrasonography

Transabdominal ultrasonography is a non-invasive, safe, repeatable and relatively inexpensive technique which has become established in the initial investigation of patients with suspected pancreatic cancer. In particular, it is widely regarded as the method of choice for demonstrating biliary dilatation and establishing the diagnosis of obstructive jaundice. Disadvantages of USS include its operator dependency and its vulnerability to image degradation caused by factors such as body wall tissues and bowel gas. This is reflected by the mixed results which have been reported for USS in the investigation of obstructive jaundice. Whereas USS has been used successfully to define both the level of biliary obstruction and the underlying lesion in 92–95% and 68–81% of cases respectively,[24–27] such good results have not been universally reproduced.[28,29] However, increasing expertise and technical refinements have established the utility of USS in the investigation of malignant obstructive jaundice. Lindsell[30] reported a sensitivity of 84% and specificity of 95% for USS in defining abnormalities of the pancreas and biliary tract, and recommended USS as a prelude to ERCP in the management of patients with suspected malignant biliary obstruction (Fig. 1.1).

The reported performance of diagnostic USS in identifying focal pancreatic tumours also varied widely. Gudjonsson[1] reviewed the results of 23 studies reported between 1977 and 1986, in which USS was used in the diagnosis of pancreatic cancer. There were marked variations in the design of these studies, in patient selection, in the exclusion of technically inadequate examinations and in the requirement for histological proof of the diagnosis, and comparison of results was therefore difficult. The reported sensitivities for USS in diagnosing pancreatic cancer ranged from 23% to 95%.[1]

The results of more recent studies evaluating the diagnostic accuracy of USS in this role are variable. Single-centre, single-modality studies of

Figure 1.1
'Conventional' algorithm for the evaluation of patients with suspected pancreatic cancer.

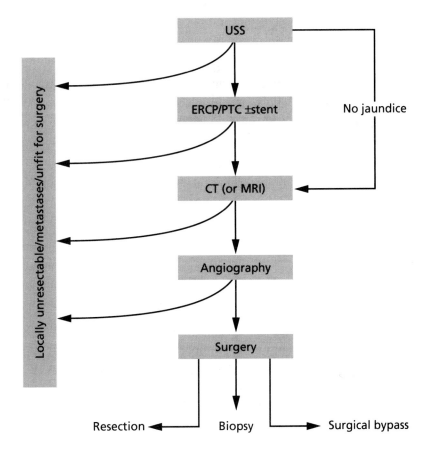

USS performed by enthusiasts yielded better results with sensitivities of 98%[31] and 83%.[12] Conversely, poorer results were reported from prospective studies where comparison with other newer modalities was performed (sensitivities 51%–65%).[28,32–37] Nevertheless, USS has been shown to be more sensitive than CT in the diagnosis of pancreatic cancer in two small comparative studies.[38,39]

Few studies have evaluated the role of transabdominal USS in the staging of pancreatic cancer (Table 1.4). The only study which has supported a primary role for transabdominal USS in the assessment of resectability of pancreatic cancer was reported by Campbell and Wilson.[31] Malignant lymphadenopathy, liver metastases and vascular invasion were correctly identified in 30%, 30% and 22% of cases. In terms of overall staging, no false positive examinations were reported (i.e. 100% specificity), and out of 38 patients 31 (82%) were identified as having unresectable tumours. However, not all these findings had been validated surgically.

Table 1.4 *Summary of studies evaluating transabdominal ultrasonography in the staging of peripancreatic and/or periampullary carcinoma*

Reference	Study design	Staging information	Sens (%)	Spec (%)	PPV (%)	NPV (%)
31	Retrospective USS only *n* = 51	Overall resectability	82	100	—	—
34	Retrospective vs. CT *n* = 24	Overall resectability	18	100	100	18
36	Prospective vs. CT/SVA *n* = 160	Overall resectability	16	98	95	29
35	Prospective vs. CT/EUS/SVA *n* = 40	PV invasion	9	72	11	68
		Node metastases	12	80	—	—
37	Prospective vs. CT/EUS *n* = 38	PV invasion	17	100	100	41
		Node metastases	8	100	100	33
39	Prospective vs. CT/EUS *n* = 29	Vascular invasion	Overall accuracy = 55%			

Sens = sensitivity; Spec = specificity; PPV = positive predictive value; NPV = negative predictive value; USS = transabdominal ultrasonography; CT = abdominal computed tomography; SVA = selective visceral angiography; EUS = endoscopic ultrasonography.

Four prospective, comparative studies (Table 1.4) have reported USS to have been insensitive in detecting criteria which contraindicated curative resection (sensitivities 8–16%), and poorly predictive of tumour resectability (predictive values of negative results 29–68%).[35–37,39] One study reported USS to have consistently overstaged the disease with respect to vascular invasion, citing the predictive value of a positive result as 11%.[35] However, this has not been the experience of others.[31,34,36,37]

Abdominal computed tomographic scanning (CT)

Computed tomographic scanning was introduced into clinical practice in 1975, and initial reports documented its ability to generate cross-sectional images of the abdominal organs, including the pancreas, and diagnose pancreatic cancer through the demonstration of focal pancreatic masses or contour abnormalities. Refinements in CT technology subsequently improved the quality of pancreatic imaging. The speed of data collation was increased, image resolution was improved by the use of thinner (5–10 mm) 'slices', and dynamic intravenous bolus contrast-enhanced CT protocols were developed.[40] These techniques maximised the density differences of normal and pathological tissues, achieving bright enhancement of the abdominal viscera with brilliant opacification of abdominal vessels. Thus, the development during the 1980s of rapid CT scanning techniques with 'dynamic incremental' table movements and high volume, high concentration bolus pump infusion of intravenous contrast enabled the detection of subtle, intraparenchymal lesions, pancreatic and/or bile duct dilatation as well as hepatic and/or nodal metastases. Oral contrast was also administered prior to scanning to opacify adjacent bowel loops. However, limitations associated with CT scanning were observed in patients with a history of allergy to contrast material, in uncooperative patients where respiratory movements or body motion prevents adequate scanning and in those with marked weight loss where the absence of retroperitoneal fat hindered the definition of tissue planes.

Gudjonsson[1] reviewed the results of 21 studies evaluating CT in the diagnosis of pancreatic cancer which had been reported between 1977 and 1986.[1] As before, methodological flaws and variations in CT technique and in the study designs confound valid comparison. This collective experience showed the proportion of positive CT examinations to vary in the range 63–100%.[1] Gudjonsson concluded that despite USS and CT having heralded a new era in diagnostic imaging, no changes in the duration of symptoms up to the time of diagnosis or in survival were apparent.[1] Nevertheless, CT rapidly became established as a prime method of investigation in the diagnosis and staging of pancreatic cancer (Fig. 1.1).

More recent studies evaluating the 'accuracy' of CT in the diagnosis of pancreatic cancer have yielded diagnostic sensitivities in the range 69–99%[28,32–44] (which is not at variance with the earlier experience reported by Gudjonsson[1]). That CT imaging alone is ultimately unable to differentiate reliably between pancreatic cancer and other focal lesions such as chronic pancreatitis is illustrated by the occurrence of false positive examinations, giving specificities of 53–69%, and positive predictive values of 83–92%.[41,43–45]

The results of abdominal CT in the staging of pancreatic and periampullary cancer in studies reported since 1984 are summarised in Table 1.5. Freeny et al.[41,42] have strongly recommended dynamic CT in the staging of pancreatic cancer. In their initial study of 161 patients with pancreatic cancer, no proven instances of tumour overstaging by CT or angiography were reported, the findings of angiography and CT were approximately comparable, and the abandonment of angiography in favour of CT was recommended.[41] The same group subsequently reported their updated experience over ten years.[42] The incidence of CT criteria indicating tumour unresectability were essentially the same as the previous study. As before, there were no false positive results pertaining to tumour resectability, and angiography again failed to contribute additional staging information over CT. However, it should be noted that surgical validation of positive findings was obtained in no more than one-third of all patients, and the prevalence of resectable pancreatic cancer was low (6%).[42]

Similarly, Fuhrman et al.[46] have recommended thin-section CT of the pancreas using 1.5 mm slice thickness at 5 mm intervals and report having correctly identified patients with resectable pancreatic carcinomas in 88% of cases. They contend that thin-section CT 'represents the only accurate method' for the preoperative evaluation of vascular invasion. However, their study should be regarded in the context of an aggressive surgical policy where portal vein resection was not necessarily considered a contraindication to curative resection, and mere *patency* of the superior mesenteric-portal vein was accepted as being indicative of resectability. Also, surgical validation of CT findings was achieved in only 42 of 145 patients.[46]

Other studies have reported a variable tendency to overstage pancreatic tumours (Table 1.5), as reflected by specificities of 50–98%, whereas the predictive value of a CT result indicating tumour unresectability varied from 70 to 97%.[34,36,43,47–49] In particular, the specificity of CT in demonstrating vascular invasion has been reported as 39–86%, and the positive predictive value as 50–89%.[35,37,43] Some authors therefore maintain that CT alone is not an adequate basis on which to determine the operability of patients with pancreatic or periampullary cancer.[43,47,48]

Despite a commonly held belief that CT is highly sensitive in identifying liver metastases,[40,50] several workers have recorded the failure of CT to detect small metastatic lesions of the liver and peritoneal surfaces.[34,43,47,49,51,52] Moreover, in their study of 88 consecutive patients with pancreatic or periampullary cancer, Warshaw et al.[48] reported CT to have missed such 'occult' metastases in 25 out of 27 patients, and have recommended routine preoperative laparoscopy to address this

Table 1.5 *Summary of studies evaluating CT scanning in the staging of pancreatic cancer*

Reference	Study design	Staging information	Sens (%)	Spec (%)	PPV (%)	NPV (%)
69	Retrospective vs. SVA n = 27	Overall staging	91	100	100	71
41	Retrospective vs. SVA n = 51	Overall staging	95	100	100	78
47	Retrospective CT only n = 66	Overall staging	72	75	93	38
		Local invasion	56	82	90	38
34	Retrospective vs. USS n = 26	Overall staging	50	50	85	15
48	Prospective vs. MRI/Lap/SVA n = 55	Overall staging	56	88	92	45
36	Prospective vs. USS/SVA n = 209	Overall staging	27	98	97	35
49	Retrospective CT only n = 67	Overall staging	91	76	89	80
35	Prospective vs. USS/EUS/SVA n = 60	PV Invasion	36	85	50	78
		N stage	36	80	—	—
42	Prospective vs. SVA n = 71	Overall staging	90	100	100	33
43	Retrospective CT only n = 52	Overall staging	68	67	70	64
		Vascular invasion	90	39	62	78
37	Prospective vs. USS/EUS n = 38	PV invasion	71	86	89	63
		N stage	19	92	83	34

Sens = sensitivity; Spec = specificity; PPV = positive predictive value; NPV = negative predictive value; USS = transabdominal ultrasonography; CT = abdominal computed tomography; SVA = selective visceral angiography; EUS = endoscopic ultrasonography.

deficiency. However, not all surgeons accept these findings as representative of their practice.[53]

A significant recent advance in CT technology was the development of spiral (or helical) CT.[54,55] This technique enables faster acquisition of truly volumetric CT data, and was made possible because of technical refinements such as the slip-ring gantry, improved detector efficiency and greater tube cooling efficiency. A pilot study of spiral CT of the pancreas has reported far superior vascular opacification with reduced respiratory artefact compared with conventional CT, whereas the capability for rapid imaging permits the acquisition of thin ($\leqslant 5$ mm) sections with correspondingly increased resolution.[54] Also, retrospective reconstruction of overlapping slices has enabled three-dimensional images of the portal venous system to be created.[56]

Gmeinwieser et al.[57] have reported the first results of 'state of the art' helical CT in the evaluation of vascular invasion in 38 patients with pancreatic cancer. Although the technique performed well in its assessment of portal vein involvement (sensitivity 91%, specificity 94%), complete avoidance of both false negative and false positive examinations proved elusive.[57] Also, liver metastases were proven in 13 patients (37%), in five of whom (38%) helical CT failed to detect such lesions '... owing to their small size (between 1–3 mm) and only proved intraoperatively or laparoscopically'.[57] Notwithstanding the excellent images obtained using contrast-enhanced spiral CT, further studies validating this new technology are obviously required.

Magnetic resonance imaging

The role of magnetic resonance imaging (MRI) in the diagnosis and staging of patients with pancreatic and periampullary carcinoma is unclear. Several comparative studies have reported no discernible advantage for MRI over CT in identifying tumour unresectability due to extrapancreatic tumour spread.[44,48,58,59] The results of an American multicentre study comparing CT and MRI in the staging of pancreatic cancer are awaited.[40]

Selective visceral angiography (SVA)

The rationale for performing angiography in patients with suspected pancreatic malignancy is threefold: (1) to establish the diagnosis of pancreatic cancer; (2) to assess tumour resectability and (3) to define the arterial anatomy of peripancreatic region.

The diagnostic sensitivity of angiography in demonstrating pancreatic cancer is 54–72% at best.[60–63] Experience has not supported earlier observations[64] that a normal angiogram 'nearly excluded' pancreatic cancer, and no angiographic criteria have been identified which are specific enough to differentiate between pancreatic cancer and chronic pancreatitis.[21,65] The advent of less-invasive imaging techniques such as USS, CT and ERCP have replaced angiography as a diagnostic modality in patients with suspected pancreatic pathology, with recommendations that it should be reserved for investigation of rare vascular neoplasms, for instances where the results of other investigations were equivocal and for the preoperative assessment of tumour resectability[65] (Fig. 1.1).

The use of angiography in the preoperative staging and assessment of resectability of pancreatic and periampullary cancer is controversial. The role of angiography in the detection of hepatic metastases has now been abandoned because of poor sensitivities (33–46%), and frequent false positive findings.[21,66,67] In the assessment of vascular invasion, it is recognised that portal-superior mesenteric venous invasion is inevitably present in patients with involvement of the coeliac and/or mesenteric arteries due to cancer of the pancreatic head.[48] Indeed, Buranasiri and Baum[68] emphasised the importance of the portal venous phase of selective visceral angiography in identifying portal vein invasion in their report of 1972, and portal venous occlusion, stenosis, encasement or displacement during the portal venous phase of SVA became established as criteria indicating tumour unresectability.

The results of studies evaluating the ability of angiography to predict tumour resectability, and validating the findings by surgical exploration, vary and are summarised in Table 1.6. It is clear that SVA commonly understages pancreatic cancer, inasmuch as its reported sensitivity in demonstrating tumour unresectability ranges from 41–91%, and the predictive value of negative findings ranges from 44 to 83%.[35,36,48,63,67,69,70] Therefore, the absence of angiographic abnormal-

Table 1.6 *Summary of studies of selective visceral angiography in the staging of pancreatic cancer*

Reference	Study design	Number of patients	Sens (%)	Spec (%)	PPV (%)	NPV (%)
69	Retrospective vs. CT	27	91	100	100	71
63	Retrospective SVA alone	43	58	88	88	58
48	Prospective vs. CT/MRI/Lap	54	66	94	95	54
70	SVA alone	90	—	—	79	77
36	Prospective vs. USS/CT	72	44	88	88	44
35	Prospective vs. CT/EUS/SVA	40	45	100	100	83
67	Prospective SVA alone	46	41	90	85	52

Sens = sensitivity; Spec = specificity; PPV = positive predictive value; NPV = negative predictive value; USS = transabdominal ultrasonography; CT = abdominal computed tomography; SVA = selective visceral angiography; EUS = endoscopic ultrasonography.

ities neither excludes the diagnosis of pancreatic cancer, nor the presence of malignant vascular invasion.

Of more concern is the incidence of false positive angiographic findings (Table 1.6). This reality is reflected by reported specificities of 88–94%, whereas the predictive values of positive results have been cited in the range 79–95%.[36,48,63,67,70] However, not all studies report tumour overstaging with SVA.[35,69] Explanations for false positive findings include 'notching' in the vicinity of the portal-superior mesenteric venous junction which has been labelled a 'normal variant',[70] spasm of the superior mesenteric artery mimicking tumour encasement[70] and coiling of the hepatic artery causing indentation of the portal vein.[71] Detractors from angiography therefore cite its unreliability in tumour staging and the availability of effective alternative modalities.[62,65,67,71,72]

Finally, the rationale for obtaining a preoperative 'anatomical roadmap' has been justified by the reported high incidence of anomalies of the peripancreatic arterial anatomy (Fig. 1.1). In particular, an accessory or replaced common or right hepatic artery arising from the aorta or superior mesenteric artery (SMA) has been reported with an incidence of 14–27% in angiographic series[62,63,67,69,70,73,74] and is at increased risk of injury during surgical dissection, particularly after previous surgery, and during transection of the retropancreatic fascia during resection of the pancreatic head. Injury to such an artery may result in ischaemia of the biliary anastomosis causing dehiscence, stenosis and/or hepatic ischaemia. Nevertheless, it may be possible to identify anomalous hepatic arterial anatomy using other modalities such as dynamic CT[42,46] (and laparoscopic ultrasonography, see below), and angiography can itself fail to identify important vascular anomalies.[53] Moreover, the detection and safeguarding of arterial anomalies during surgery for pancreatic cancer can be accomplished by experienced pancreatic surgeons without resort to angiography.[71]

Laparoscopy

The highly resolved and magnified view of the peritoneal cavity obtained using modern optics and light sources has rendered laparoscopy a sensitive technique in the detection of intraperitoneal tumours, as well as small quantities of malignant ascites, and tiny metastatic lesions involving the serosal surfaces of the peritoneal cavity, omentum and liver. Staging laparoscopy has therefore come to be regarded as a mandatory prelude to laparotomy by many surgeons (Fig. 1.2), although this view is not held universally.

Ishida[75] performed laparoscopy in 71 patients with pancreatic cancer and detected intra-abdominal metastatic disease in 43% of examinations. Cuschieri and colleagues performed laparoscopy immediately prior to a proposed laparotomy in 73 patients with pancreatic cancer.[76,77] They visualised omental deposits, peritoneal seedlings, hepatic metastases and/or direct tumour invasion of adjacent organs in the majority of patients examined and achieved an overall histological/cytological

Figure 1.2
Algorithm for the preoperative evaluation of pancreatic cancer using laparoscopy with laparoscopic ultrasonography.

Based on John *et al.* (1995)[80]

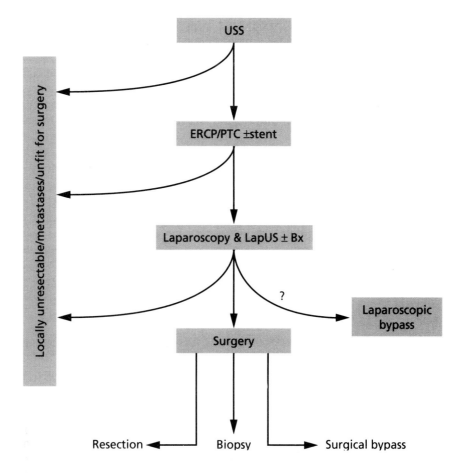

diagnosis of pancreatic malignancy in 61/65 patients (92%). Warshaw and co-workers performed staging laparoscopy to assess tumour resectability in 88 patients between 1982 and 1989.[48,78,79] Laparoscopy detected intra-abdominal metastases in a total of 35 patients (41%). The sensitivity of laparoscopy in detecting such lesions was 96% (22/23), whereas intravenous contrast-enhanced CT failed to detect these in all but two cases. Stepwise discriminant analysis confirmed the unique role played by staging laparoscopy in this context.[48] These findings have been reproduced in The Royal Infirmary, Edinburgh, where staging laparoscopy demonstrated occult intra-abdominal metastases in 14 out of 40 patients (35%) considered, on the basis of ultrasonography and CT, to have potentially resectable lesions.[52,80] Similarly, workers in the University of Amsterdam performed staging laparoscopy in 73 patients with carcinoma of the pancreatic head or periampullary region who were considered to have stage 1 disease on the basis of ERCP and Doppler USS.[81] The incidence of unsuspected metastases was 24% and these were identified laparoscopically in 16 of 21 patients (76%). Conlon *et al.*[82] also performed preoperative laparoscopy in 115 patients with 'radiologically resectable' pancreatic cancer between 1992 and 1994, defining liver metastases in 17%, peritoneal carcinomatosis in 14% and/or visible malignant lymphadenopathy in 7%. These reports thus corroborate the observation that in patients with pancreatic or periampullary cancer, 'occult' intra-abdominal metastases are encountered commonly despite imaging with contemporary radiological techniques, and that staging laparoscopy is a sensitive method for their detection.

However, laparoscopic assessment of primary pancreatic malignancies is hindered by the retroperitoneal location of the gland, and the diagnosis of pancreatic malignancy was usually inferred from the observation or 'palpation' of a retrogastric mass, and secondary signs such as the features of obstructive jaundice, ascites or metastases, and portal hypertension or splenomegaly in the presence of portal vein invasion. Although the feasibility of direct laparoscopic inspection (and biopsy) of the pancreas via the lesser sac using the approaches of 'supragastric pancreoscopy', 'supragastric bursoscopy' and 'infragastric bursoscopy' have been described, such invasive laparoscopic techniques are generally considered unnecessary, especially with the advent of laparoscopic ultrasonography.

Laparoscopic (and intraoperative) ultrasonography

Laparoscopic intraoperative ultrasonography (LapUS) utilises the principles of intraoperative contact ultrasonography (IOUS) during laparoscopy. The fundamental advantage of IOUS compared with conventional transabdominal USS derives from the placement of the ultrasound transducer in direct apposition with the intra-abdominal tissues. This manoeuvre permits the use of relatively high frequency transducers (7.5–10 MHz) which achieve correspondingly high image resolution, while avoiding the image degradation experienced when scanning from outside the body wall during transabdominal USS.

Intraoperative ultrasonography (IOUS) has been shown to aid the operative decision making process during operations for both benign and malignant pancreatic disease, by localising and characterising impalpable abnormalities and providing information which would otherwise require extensive dissection. In particular, IOUS may help establish the diagnosis of pancreatic carcinoma, and define the local resectability of the lesion with regards to its involvement of the adjacent peripancreatic blood vessels.[83–85] Nevertheless, many pancreatic surgeons have preferred to undertake a trial dissection or mobilisation of the pancreas at open operation, and the adoption of IOUS in this role has remained confined to a relatively small number of enthusiasts.

Laparoscopic ultrasonography is now possible using commercially available ultracompact, sterilisable probes with similar imaging specifications as contemporary high resolution IOUS systems, and which may be introduced through standard 10/11 mm diameter laparoscopic ports. Initial reports have validated the accuracy of LapUS in the T staging of pancreatic and periampullary carcinoma, and have established its ability to enhance the sensitivity of laparoscopy in detecting occult intrahepatic metastases.[52,80,81] The combination of laparoscopy with LapUS represents a potent method for detecting intra-abdominal metastases and local tumour invasion, and obtaining a tissue diagnosis (Fig. 1.2). Proponents therefore justify the performance of LapUS as a general anaesthetic procedure separate from a planned laparotomy according to the principles stated in Table 1.1. However, the technique is operator dependent with an inherent learning curve, and, as with endoscopic ultrasonography, accurate staging of regional lymph node status has proved elusive (see below). Although morbidity is negligible, anecdotal reports of malignant port site seeding have aroused concern.[86,87]

Prospective comparative studies of LapUS with spiral CT scanning and endoscopic ultrasonography in the evaluation of pancreatic cancer are awaited.

Endoscopic ultrasonography

Endoscopic ultrasonography (EUS) permits high resolution, real-time B-mode scanning of the pancreas and neighbouring tissues from within the lumen of the stomach and duodenum using an 'echoendoscope'. The echoendoscope incorporates a small, high-frequency ultrasound transducer at its distal end, and high resolution images of the adjacent tissues are generated using similar principles of contact ultrasonography as those exploited during IOUS and LapUS. Studies evaluating EUS in the diagnosis of pancreatic and periampullary cancer have reported excellent results, with EUS demonstrating superior sensitivities (85–100%) compared with ERCP, USS, CT and/or SVA.[33,35,37,39,44,88] However, there is substantial overlap in the sonographic appearances of malignant and benign lesions, and no reliable criteria have been defined which allow accurate differentiation between focal pancreatic lesions due to neoplasia and those due to chronic pancreatitis.[89]

In the staging of pancreatic and periampullary cancer, and in the hands of experts, EUS has been shown reproducibly to be highly accurate in determining resectability according to the T stage.[33,35,37,39,88,90,91] In particular, prospective comparison with USS, CT and/or SVA has shown EUS to be superior in determining malignant vascular invasion.[33,35,37,39,91]

However, EUS seems to be less performant in the diagnosis of regional malignant lymphadenopathy.[89,92] Having adopted an arbitrary node size of $\geqslant 5$ mm in diameter to represent malignant involvement, reported positive and negative predictive values vary from 47 to 100% and from 55 to 71%, respectively.[35,37,90] Although significantly better than corresponding results of USS and CT (see Tables 1.4 and 1.5), the incidence of false positives due to reactive hyperplasia, and false negatives due to nodal micrometastases has limited the clinical utility of EUS in lymph node staging.[89]

The procedure is also technically difficult, requiring ultrasound and endoscopic expertise, and has been slow to gain widespread acceptance.

Several other limitations have emerged in the use of EUS. These include difficulties in intubating the pylorus and duodenum with large calibre echoendoscopes, especially in patients with locally invading tumours of the pancreatic head or periampullary region. Imaging of the distal pancreas from within the stomach may also be impeded by interposed bowel gas, and these factors have accounted for technical failure rates of 5–14%.[89] The optimal focal range of the transducer is usually 2–4 cm, which restricts imaging of the majority of the right hemiliver, and of the peripancreatic vasculature when tumours larger than 4 cm are encountered. For this reason, EUS is insensitive in detecting distant metastases during tumour staging in patients with pancreatic and periampullary cancer.

Percutaneous needle biopsy

The inability of the aforementioned imaging modalities to discriminate accurately between malignant and benign abnormalities of the pancreas established the requirements for a tissue diagnosis without resort to laparotomy and intraoperative biopsy. This may be achieved by percutaneous fine-needle aspiration cytology (FNAC) using 'skinny' needles <1 mm in diameter, or by core-cutting needle biopsy (⩾1 mm in diameter). The FNAC technique may be sufficient to prove the presence of malignancy, whereas histological examination of a core biopsy is required to classify the type of tumour. Percutaneous needle biopsy is usually performed under local anaesthesia using USS or CT guidance (although ERCP and percutaneous transhepatic cholangiography (PTC) guided techniques have been described).

The indications for percutaneous needle biopsy vary according to the philosophy of the clinical team, although most surgeons practise a selective policy. Needle biopsy is usually reserved for patients who are deemed unsuitable for surgery because of age, infirmity or unequivocal evidence of tumour unresectability, and in whom a tissue diagnosis is desirable. It should be emphasised that most experienced pancreatic surgeons do not practise biopsy of potentially resectable lesions prior to surgery when clinical and/or radiological evidence supports a diagnosis of malignancy. Although the reported mortality and morbidity is negligible in experienced hands,[93,94] malignant needle-track seeding of pancreatic cancer has been reported.[94–97]

Furthermore, concern was aroused by the observations that peritoneal washings obtained during laparoscopy or laparotomy were cytologically malignant in 30% of patients examined, and that there was a significant association between positive peritoneal cytology and prior percutaneous tumour biopsy.[98] However, subsequent studies[99–101] (including the authors' own experience[102]) have indicated that positive peritoneal cytology is a rarer event than originally thought, and that the case for extrapancreatic dissemination of malignancy by needle biopsy may have been overstated. Nevertheless, it is also clear that positive peritoneal cytology, when present, indicates an appalling prognosis, and it would seem prudent to avoid a policy of liberal pancreatic biopsy, especially in patients in whom surgical intervention seems likely.

The results of percutaneous FNAC and biopsy of the pancreas vary, reflecting operator-dependency both in obtaining a representative tissue sample, and in its cytopathological interpretation. In general, however, both techniques are regarded as virtually 100% specific and predictive of malignancy, although there have been anecdotal reports of false positive results. The main problem lies with the interpretation of negative or equivocal findings, as false negative rates of 9–51% are a practical reality.[103–105] Although immunocytochemical studies may be helpful in distinguishing neuroendocrine tumours from exocrine cancers, differentiating the epithelial atypia of chronic pancreatitis from that of a well-differentiated pancreatic cancer is a recognised pitfall. A negative percutaneous pancreatic FNAC or biopsy does not, therefore, exclude the presence of malignancy. The same conclusions also apply to brush cytology samples obtained during ERCP.[105]

Investigation of biliary malignancy

Introduction

The investigation of biliary malignancy usually stems from the assessment of the patient presenting with obstructive jaundice. Having confirmed the suspicion of extrahepatic biliary tract obstruction, the aim of the diagnostic algorithm is to define the level of obstruction and the nature of the obstructing lesion. Staging investigations aim to select patients for appropriate treatment, which may involve tumour resection or surgical bypass, palliation by interventional radiological or endoscopic methods, or no further intervention.

The management of malignant low biliary obstruction due to distal cholangiocarcinoma has already been considered in the section on 'Investigation of pancreatic malignancy'. The challenge faced in the evaluation of hilar cholangiocarcinoma and gall bladder cancer are emphasised in this section. As with most malignancies, definitions of resectability vary. However, most biliary surgeons would concur with the following criteria contraindicating 'curative' resection in patients with hilar cholangiocarcinoma: bilateral invasion of the second-order bile ducts, invasion of more than three hepatic segments, invasion of the main portal vein or both right and left portal veins, invasion of the common hepatic artery or both right and left hepatic arteries and local or distant dissemination of tumour beyond the liver or biliary tree (including regional lymph nodes).[106] Thus, complete excision of a resectable hilar tumour would be expected to preserve an adequate volume of non-atrophic and tumour-free liver retaining an intact portal venous and hepatic arterial circulation.

General methods of investigation

Routine biochemical and haematological studies should always be performed to identify obstructive jaundice, hepatobiliary and renal dysfunction, and coagulation and nutritional deficiencies. Plain abdominal radiographs are usually non-specific, although they may occasionally identify gallstones, a distended or calcified gall bladder (gall bladder cancer) and pneumobilia (biliary fistula, papillotomy etc.).

USS, CT and MRI

As discussed earlier, USS is a rapid, safe and non-invasive method which confirms biliary dilatation and defines the level of obstruction in the majority of cases.[24–27,30] However, obstructive jaundice without biliary dilatation may occur in 16% of cases,[106] especially in the context of concomitant hepatic disease such as cirrhosis or fibrosis. Also, difficulties in imaging the distal common bile duct in some patients may fail to resolve an underlying diagnosis such as malignant low biliary obstruction or choledocholithiasis. In a direct comparison of USS, CT and cholangiography (ERCP or PTC) in the diagnosis of cholangiocarcinoma sensitivities of 47%, 69% and 97%, respectively, were reported.[107] Conversely, in the diagnosis of hilar tumours the corresponding results for USS and CT were 90% and 71%.[26] The apparent fallibility of CT in the evaluation of intrahepatic bile duct dilatation has also been highlighted by Teefey et al.[108] who observed that the distribution and extent of intrahepatic duct dilatation at CT could not differentiate between malignant and benign lesions, and that of primary sclerosing cholangitis. Thus in comparison with CT scanning, USS appears to be at least as accurate and more cost effective in the primary evaluation of such patients[30] (Fig. 1.3).

The role of the various scanning techniques in the staging of locally invasive bile duct cancer is less clear-cut. Gibson et al.[26] reported that both USS and CT had failed to identify malignant invasion by hilar tumours of second-order bile ducts in the majority of cases, and that this deficiency was maximal in the left hepatic lobe. However, both modalities performed better in demonstrating intrahepatic tumour spread and hepatic lobar atrophy in this study,[26] although understaging of portal vein invasion was also identified as a weakness for each technique. Doppler ultrasound techniques (with colour flow imaging) have been used to improve the detection of vascular invasion by hilar tumours, with the correct identification of portal venous occlusion in four out of four patients and vein wall infiltration in 15 out of 18 (83%) cases with 100% specificity being reported.[109] Nevertheless, USS failed to accurately stage involvement of the hepatic artery, hepatic parenchyma or regional lymph node metastases in a substantial proportion of patients in the same study. Nesbit et al.[107] have also reported poor sensitivities for USS (19%) and CT (44%) in the overall staging of

Figure 1.3
Algorithm for the preoperative evaluation of suspected biliary malignancy.

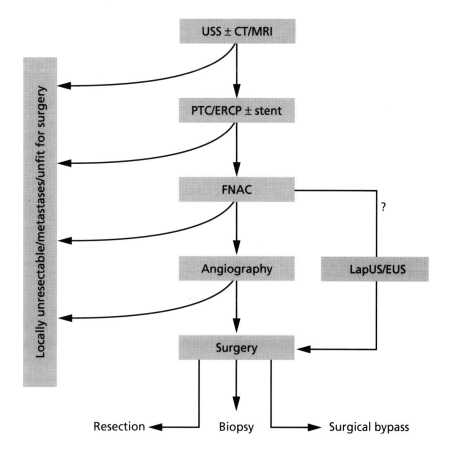

cholangiocarcinoma, and it is clear that additional investigations are required to achieve adequate patient selection for surgery (Fig. 1.3).

MR cholangiography is a recent innovation for demonstration of the biliary tree, although there is no evidence yet to support its role in the diagnosis and staging of biliary malignancy over conventional cholangiography. Similarly, MR angiography is a novel technique which appears promising in the evaluation of tumour invasion of the portal veins and hepatic arteries. Prospective validation in comparison with established techniques is awaited before these newer techniques can be adopted in routine practice.

Cholangiography

The need for complete imaging of the biliary tree and definitive imaging of the level of biliary obstruction in patients with suspected biliary malignancy requires direct cholangiography by means of ERCP or PTC. In the majority of patients with suspected distal bile duct obstruction, ERCP tends to be favoured, and as discussed before, usually differentiates patients with malignant strictures from those with choledocholithiasis and other benign lesions. Conversely, PTC tends to be reserved for instances where proximal biliary malignancy is suspected, in which case ERCP may be unable to delineate the intrahepatic biliary tree despite the use of balloon catheters. Local expertise may influence which of these techniques is favoured, and their complementary roles should be stressed. However, many biliary surgeons regard PTC as the mainstay of investigation in patients with suspected hilar cholangiocarcinoma, reserving ERCP for instances where imaging of the distal bile duct is required in cases of complete hilar occlusion (Fig. 1.3).

The pattern of involvement of the second-order intrahepatic bile ducts has important implications for tumour resectability[106,110] (Fig. 1.4), although as discussed earlier, USS and CT tend to understage this aspect of local tumour assessment.[26,107,109,111] PTC will define the extent of intrahepatic biliary invasion, and provides an 'anatomical roadmap' for the biliary surgeon. Multiple separate puncture PTC may be required in patients in whom there is separation of the right and left duct systems. However, it should be borne in mind that invasive attempts at defining the biliary anatomy may risk introducing infection into obstructed biliary tree. If surgical decompression by segment III cholangioenteric anastomosis is proposed for the patient with unresectable malignancy, contamination of the right duct system may compromise long-term palliation through the development of biliary sepsis and abscess formation.[112] Close consultation between radiologist and surgeon are important at each stage, and it may be preferable to delay PTC until

Figure 1.4
Classification of tumour invasion of the proximal biliary tree in patients with hilar cholangiocarcinoma.

After Bismuth and Corlette[110].

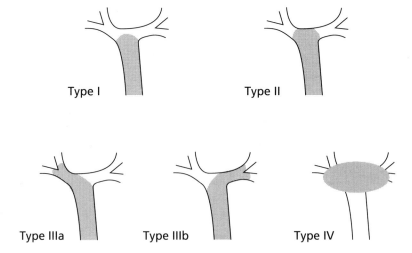

Type I: hilar tumour with sparing of the confluence, Type II: hilar tumour invading the confluence but sparing the left and right hepatic ducts, Type III: hilar tumour invading the confluence with unilateral involvement of the right (Type IIIa) or left (Type IIIb) segmental ducts, Type IV: hilar tumour invading the confluence with bilateral or multicentric involvement of the segmental ducts.

immediately before operation to minimise possible side effects such as cholangitis or biliary peritonitis. Percutaneous biliary stent insertion may be deemed appropriate, either as a temporising measure, or as a definitive palliative measure in patients who are not considered candidates for major surgery or who have advanced disease, and this approach may best be avoided in other patients for whom planned surgery is imminent. Although a preference for endoscopic biliary stent insertion may be appropriate in patients with low malignant biliary obstruction, this is not necessarily so with hilar lesions where more than one stent may be required, and where a period of percutaneous transhepatic biliary drainage (PTBD) may be desirable. It is also important to obtain bile for cytological examination during such manoeuvres, and it is important that rapid transport of fresh bile samples for immediate chilling is performed. However, although the specificity of this technique appears to be 100%, its poor sensitivity may only detect malignant cells in a third of cases.[113]

A remarkable approach to the preoperative assessment of patients with proximal cholangiocarcinoma involves the combination of transhepatic biliary drainage (PTBD) with percutaneous cholangioscopy to achieve diagnosis and staging of biliary malignancy. In particular, multiple segment PTBD and cholangioscopy with sequential biopsy is used in patients with hilar cholangiocarcinoma to establish a 'map' for guidance of radical central resections of the liver and intrahepatic biliary tree.[114]

Tissue diagnosis

Just as cross-sectional imaging and cholangiography fail to differentiate accurately between malignant distal biliary strictures and benign lesions (e.g. chronic pancreatitis), so it may also prove impossible to distinguish proximal bile duct malignancies from inflammatory causes such a focal sclerosing cholangitis using these modalities. A preoperative cytodiagnosis of malignancy is therefore frequently desirable, and this may be achieved by exfoliative cytology of bile (see above), brush cytology and FNAC or needle biopsy guided by USS or PTC. The use of endobiliary brush cytology during ERCP has been reported to be more sensitive than exfoliative bile cytology, with a diagnostic yield of over 60% which may be improved with repeated sampling.[115] The diagnostic yield of percutaneous FNAC tends to be limited by the small size and poor cellularity of bile duct cancers, and results vary. Desa et al.[116] cite a sensitivity of 61% for percutaneous FNAC in the diagnosis of cholangiocarcinoma (with unsatisfactory samples in 15%), although they also report a rare false positive for a specificity of 98%.[116] Although other workers have generally reported slightly inferior sensitivities as low as 44%, and notwithstanding the aforementioned concerns regarding needle tract seeding, percutaneous FNAC remains an important part of the investigative algorithm for patients with malignant biliary strictures (Fig. 1.3).

A further development which may facilitate a tissue diagnosis in patients in whom the diagnosis of biliary malignancy proves elusive is endobiliary biopsy and endobiliary fine needle aspiration cytology.[117] Respectively, these techniques employ an endoluminal biopsy forceps via the endoscopic route, and an endoscopically or percutaneously introduced fine needle. Preliminary studies suggest that these methods may be particularly suited to obtaining positive cytology in patients with biliary malignancy causing extrinsic compression but with intact biliary epithelium.[117]

Selective visceral angiography

Notwithstanding the modest success cited for Doppler USS,[109] the shortcomings of various scanning techniques and cholangiography in the evaluation of vascular invasion by bile duct cancer have established selective visceral angiography with portal phase venography as an important staging investigation in the armamentarium of the biliary surgeon[118] (Fig. 1.3). However, false positive results are a recognised pitfall, and some surgeons have recommended that caution should be exercised in attributing unresectability to the signs of vascular 'encasement' unless unequivocal invasion of the common hepatic artery or bilateral portal vein involvement is shown.[119]

An alternative approach is direct percutaneous transhepatic portography (see below), although this is an invasive procedure which provides no information regarding arterial invasion, and has failed to find widespread popularity.

Contact sonography

Several novel techniques which exploit the concept of high resolution contact sonography are currently under evaluation in the staging of biliary malignancy. Although the utility of endoscopic ultrasonography (EUS) in the staging of low malignant biliary lesions has already been discussed, its role in evaluation of hilar malignancy is less well established. Tio *et al.*[120] evaluated EUS in 40 patients with 'common hepatic duct carcinoma' and validated the findings against the pTNM stage derived from histopathological examination of the resection specimen. They showed accurate estimation of the depth of tumour invasion (pT stage) in 34/40 patients (85%), with three false positives (vascular invasion) and three false negatives. Also, a tendency to overstage nodal metastases were reported, although distant metastases were missed in all five such patients (12%).

The latter observation again lends support to the rationale for staging laparoscopy prior to surgery in patients with potentially resectable hilar cancers, although no studies have specifically examined this issue. The role of LapUS in the assessment of resectability of such patients is currently under investigation.

Intraportal endovascular ultrasound requires the insertion of a high resolution (20 MHz) intravascular ultrasound catheter into the portal vein by the percutaneous transhepatic route preoperatively, or by cannulation of the superior mesenteric vein intraoperatively. Kaneko *et al.*[121] have performed these procedures in a small series of patients with cholangiocarcinoma of the proximal bile duct and gall bladder (and pancreatic cancer), validating the findings surgically and pathologically. Precise information was obtained regarding malignant invasion of the portal vein wall, with superior sensitivity and specificity (100% and 93%) compared with percutaneous transhepatic portography (80% and 68%) and dynamic CT (53% and 80%).

Diagnosis and staging of gall bladder carcinoma

Gall bladder carcinoma is often difficult to distinguish from hilar cholangiocarcinoma, and its evaluation involves the same principles as for the investigation of proximal bile duct cancer. The poor sensitivity of both USS and CT in defining a gall bladder mass is well recognised, although a combination of both methods may demonstrate diffuse thickening of the wall or a mass in a half of all patients.[122] Cholangiography is again mandatory, and ERCP may be particularly useful in demonstrating a patent cystic duct, a finding which virtually excludes the diagnosis of established gall bladder cancer as this usually obliterates the cystic duct.[118] However, the role of PTC is complementary in ensuring visualisation of the intrahepatic ducts, particularly in showing the specific sign of distortion of the segment V ducts.[122] However, the elusive nature of this tumour is reflected in its frequent discovery during or after cholecystectomy for presumed benign disease.

Investigation of hepatic malignancy

Introduction

Confirmation or exclusion of an intrahepatic mass is required in patients presenting with clinical, biochemical or radiological features suggesting hepatic malignancy. Staging investigations should identify patients with potentially resectable primary or secondary liver tumours for whom hepatic resection with curative attempt (or liver transplantation) may be appropriate. In contrast with some patients with unresectable pancreatic/biliary malignancy, there is little evidence that palliative surgery has anything to offer those with unresectable hepatic tumours, and avoidance of unnecessary laparotomy is fundamental to the management of hepatic malignancy.

The investigation of hepatic malignancy is also important in the context of the staging of primary malignant tumours affecting other organs. Liver metastases are often a common manifestation of such diseases, with profound implications for the choice of treatment for the primary lesion, and the prognosis. Much interest has focused on the detection of liver metastases of colorectal origin, with emphasis on the selection of suitable patients with colorectal liver metastases for hepatic resection.

General methods of investigation

Full clinical assessment may reveal the stigmata of chronic liver disease, portal hypertension and/or a palpable abdominal mass in patients with suspected hepatic malignancy. A biochemical and haematological screen (including coagulation) is mandatory, and viral serology for hepatitis B and C and an autoantibody screen should be performed when cirrhosis/hepatocellular carcinoma is suspected. Tumour markers include carcinoembryonic antigen (CEA) (particularly for colorectal metastases) and alphafetoprotein (AFP) for hepatocellular carcinoma, although the sensitivity and specificity of each falls short of the ideal.

In patients with suspected hepatic malignancy under consideration for curative liver resection, a plain chest radiograph should be obtained, and thoracic CT performed in those suspected of harbouring extrahepatic disease in the thorax. Radioisotope bone scanning is usually reserved for patients with symptoms suggestive of bony metastases.

Segmental anatomy of the liver

An understanding of the hepatic segmental anatomy is fundamental to modern radiological investigation and surgical management of hepatic malignancy (Fig. 1.5). The classification described by the French surgical anatomist Couinaud, and later popularised by Bismuth[123–125] is recognised globally,[126] although the essentially similar American system differs in its nomenclature. The eight hepatic segments are divided into those constituting the right hemiliver (V–VIII), the left hemiliver (II–IV) and caudate lobe (segment I). The right and left hemilivers are separated in the functional midline by the plane of the principal fissure between the gall bladder fossa and the inferior vena cava. This plane is defined by the

Figure 1.5
Segmental anatomy of the liver.

Reproduced with permission from Garden and Bismuth.[217]

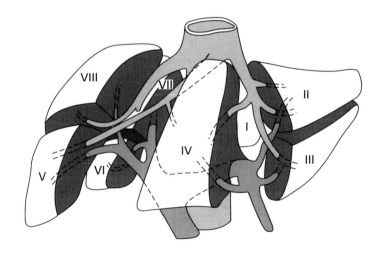

course of the middle hepatic vein, and in common with most aspects of the hepatic segmental anatomy, has no external markings.

Principles of hepatic contrast enhancement for CT

Unenhanced CT

The type, the route and the timing of contrast administration and scan acquisition are variables which are vitally important for the optimal visualisation of malignant hepatic lesions.[127] A difference in CT appearance between the focal lesion and the background liver parenchyma must be established if the lesion is to be detected. Unenhanced CT scans may identify tumours characterised by differences in vascularity, cystic change, necrosis and fluid content because their density differs from background parenchyma. The higher soft tissue discrimination of CT scanning compared with plain radiographs permits the visualisation of a large proportion of liver tumours on unenhanced scans, which are usually performed as a prelude to contrast-enhanced scans. They are useful in screening for the majority of (hypovascular) liver metastases which may be discovered during routine abdominal CT, or when calcification or haemorrhage within lesions is suspected, and in patients with hepatic cirrhosis where portal venous inflow is poor.

Intravenous contrast-enhanced CT

The mechanisms whereby the intravenous injection of iodinated contrast facilitates the demonstration of liver tumours during hepatic CT scanning depends on the dual blood supply of the liver (the hepatic artery delivering 20–25% of blood flow), and the different phases of contrast delivery.[127] During the 'bolus phase', the dilutional effect of the predominant portal venous blood supply to the normal hepatic parenchyma renders it relatively unenhanced compared with the 'arterialised' solid abdominal organs (e.g. spleen, kidneys and pancreas). Similarly, hypervascular liver tumours receive relatively concentrated contrast enhancement from their hepatic arterial supply and are rendered hyperdense and maximally conspicuous relative to the normal hepatic parenchyma (Fig. 1.6a–b). This principle is exploited further in CT angiography, where selective angiographic injection of contrast via the hepatic artery causes selective enhancement of malignant liver tumours relative to the background parenchyma, even when relatively hypovascular.

During the 'portal venous phase', hypovascular tumours (i.e. the majority of liver metastases) appear poorly enhanced and hypodense relative to the normal liver (Fig. 1.6c). However, vascular enhancement rapidly declines with recirculation and diffusion of contrast into the interstitial spaces until the 'equilibrium phase' is reached and any differential disappears. The kinetics of contrast delivery are therefore crucial to the CT detectability of liver tumours, and dynamic incremental bolus contrast-enhanced CT has become the 'gold standard' technique for the routine detection of hepatic neoplasms during abdominal CT compared with slower methods of intravenous contrast delivery (e.g.

Figure 1.6
Schematic diagrams of various methods of CT contrast enhancement for the demonstration of focal hepatic tumours.

After Baron (1994).[127]

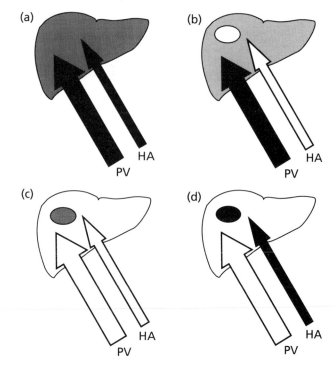

(a) Unenhanced scans showing predominant blood supply to the liver from the portal vein (PV) compared with the hepatic artery (HA) (as indicated by arrow size). (b) Hepatic arterial enhancement (white arrow) of a hypervascular tumour following intravenous contrast administration. (c) Portal venous enhancement phase following intravenous contrast injection. (d) Hypovascular tumours appear markedly hypodense relative to the normal parenchyma during the portal venous phase of CT angioportography.

drip infusion).[127,128] Fast scanning times are possible with modern CT machines (in particular spiral CT), and CT protocols are tailored for maximal enhancement of the hepatic parenchyma and demonstration of hypovascular liver metastases during the portal venous phase of enhancement (Fig. 1.6c).

Delayed CT

The delayed CT technique involves the administration of a large dose of intravenous iodine and scanning the liver between four and six hours later. As 1–2% of iodinated contrast is being excreted into the bile by normal hepatocytes at this time (but not by neoplastic lesions), tumours appear hypodense and conspicuous. However, small tumours may appear similar to central blood vessels in the absence of circulating contrast at this time, and the technique is consequently dependent on conventional contrast-enhanced CT as an adjunct. The logistics of the technique render it rather cumbersome, and it has found little popularity in European countries.

CT angioportography ('Portoscanner')

CT angioportography (CTAP) involves the selective angiographic delivery of contrast to the splenic or superior mesenteric arteries, thus achieving enhancement of the hepatic parenchyma via the portal venous system while bypassing the hepatic arterial circulation. As most liver neoplasms receive an exclusive hepatic arterial blood supply and no portal venous blood supply, they appear hypodense (or 'lucent') relative to the densely enhanced normal liver (Fig. 1.6d). This technique is highly sensitive in detecting lesions even several millimetres in size because the tumour/liver attenuation difference is maximised.

Apart from the potential for morbidity associated with the angiographic technique, the main disadvantage of CTAP lies with the occurrence of perfusion defects which mimic metastases and can cause false positive results in up to 40% of cases.[129–132] Some perfusion defects may be caused by benign hepatic lesions (e.g. cysts, haemangiomas and focal nodular hyperplasia), but the majority are due to areas of laminar intrahepatic blood flow caused by incomplete mixing of contrast-enhanced blood from the splenic and superior mesenteric veins. However, most of the larger benign lesions may be characterised by techniques such as USS, careful angiographic technique may diminish the incidence of perfusion defects and typical perfusion defects may be correctly identified by experienced observers. Nevertheless, the high sensitivity of CTAP must still be balanced against the risk of denying potentially curative resectional surgery to patients who are 'overstaged'.

CT angiography (and 'Lipiodol CT')

Conventional CT angiography, whereby dilute contrast is selectively injected via the hepatic artery, is prone to imaging artefacts and has been superseded by CTAP in the investigation of metastatic liver disease (see above). However, iodised poppy seed oil may be delivered by the hepatic arterial route using this technique ('Lipiodol CT'), and its retention within hepatocellular carcinoma nodules causes dense enhancement of these areas. Lipiodol CT is ideally performed one or two weeks after the initial injection, by which time the reticuloendothelial system of the surrounding hepatic parenchyma will have cleared the contrast material. Lipiodol CT has high sensitivity for detecting hepatocellular carcinoma, and is especially useful for detecting small foci within cirrhotic livers.[133]

Liver biopsy

Biopsy of a solid liver lesion is indicated to resolve instances of diagnostic doubt (e.g. liver metastases from a primary of unknown origin), during the staging of hepatic malignancy when clinical management may be affected by the resultant information and in the context of clinical trials where confirmation of diagnosis is mandatory. Also, the presence of diffuse parenchymal liver diseases such as steatosis, hepatitis and cirrhosis may be documented through representative sampling of the liver adjacent to focal liver abnormalities. The confirmation of such findings may establish a relative contraindication to hepatic resection, especially in patients with hepatocellular carcinoma.

Conversely, the importance of exercising restraint when contemplating biopsy of focal liver lesions must be emphasised. Percutaneous (or laparoscopic) biopsy of potentially resectable liver tumour is contraindicated in such circumstances because of the risk of malignant seeding into the peritoneal cavity, to the port site or to the needle track. This is a well-described complication and should be regarded as an avoidable catastrophe.[134–139] When investigations demonstrate focal liver tumour in an anatomically resectable location, exploratory laparotomy is warranted with a view to liver resection. Histological proof of malignancy is rarely, if ever, required under these circumstances, as the biochemical, radiological and/or laparoscopic findings and the clinical context of the case are usually sufficient to establish the likely diagnosis.

The optimal method for performing needle biopsy of suspected malignant liver lesions has long been a controversial issue among proponents of blind percutaneous biopsy, radiologically guided percutaneous biopsy, laparoscopically guided biopsy, and the use of fine needle aspiration cytology (FNAC) or core-cutting (BX) techniques. The benefits of laparoscopic liver biopsy over blind percutaneous biopsy in patients with hepatic malignancy are well established, the positive yield of a single random percutaneous liver biopsy being less than 50%. More recently, the evolution of non-invasive radiological imaging techniques such as USS, CT and MRI has challenged the role of laparoscopy in the assessment of suspected liver disease, and as a means of obtaining guided-biopsy specimens,[140] and studies have failed to show a significant advantage for laparoscopy compared with scan-guided biopsy in diagnosing overt focal hepatic lesions. A comparison of USS-guided FNAC against laparoscopic biopsy using core-cutting needles in 63 patients[141] found no significant differences with respect to sensitivity and accuracy (76% versus 74%, and 84% versus 83%, respectively). Nevertheless, these results do not detract from the role of laparoscopy in providing additional information which may alter the surgical decision making process (see below).

When the debate between blind percutaneous needle biopsy or USS-guided needle biopsy of the liver is examined, it appears that there is no difference in safety between the techniques, despite the theoretical reduced risk of gall bladder puncture with the latter.[142] Nor is there any advantage for guided biopsy in patients with diffuse non-malignant liver disease. However, it has been established beyond doubt that guided percutaneous needle biopsy is indicated when hepatic malignancy is suspected, or when a focal intrahepatic lesion has already been identified.[142]

Smith has documented an overall mortality of 0.006–0.0311% for all percutaneous needle biopsies of abdominal organs, haemorrhage from hypervascular lesions being the usual cause of death following percutaneous liver biopsy.[143] There is, therefore, a general assumption that percutaneous FNAC is safer than core-cutting needle biopsy, and the latter tends to be reserved for instances where the former technique is uninformative, or where formal histolopathological evaluation is required to evaluate the presence of a background diffuse liver disease.

Laparoscopy with laparoscopic ultrasonography

Radiological imaging techniques are limited in their ability to define subtle changes associated with diffuse parenchymal abnormalities such as cirrhosis, and despite continuing refinements in the various cross-sectional imaging modalities, small hepatic lesions measuring less than 1 cm in diameter, especially those situated superficially or on the liver capsule, may be missed. Also, extrahepatic tumour dissemination, in the form of serosal seedlings in the subphrenic spaces in particular, may go undetected until the time of exploratory laparotomy. Lefor et al.[144] documented unexpected intra-abdominal extrahepatic disease at laparotomy in 28 out of 107 patients (26%) considered to have potentially resectable colorectal hepatic metastases on the basis of negative staging investigations (i.e. abdominal CT).[144]

Such limitations may be addressed by laparoscopy which is unrivalled in its ability to detect minimal volume extrahepatic tumour spread and small superficial bilobar lesions. Laparoscopic identification of hepatic malignancy requires that the tumour encroaches upon the liver surface, or that the liver contour be distorted by the intrahepatic lesion. In the absence of adhesions, much of the liver surface is available for laparoscopic inspection, and approximately two-thirds of liver metastases may be detected laparoscopically and are amenable to laparoscopically directed needle biopsy.

Staging laparoscopy is of proven benefit in the detection of the small liver (and peritoneal) metastases which characterise a variety of primary malignancies. The laparoscopic discovery of distant metastases may preclude an unnecessary exploratory laparotomy in a significant proportion of patients in whom a curative or palliative operation may no longer be appropriate. The sensitivity of laparoscopy in the detection of occult hepatic metastases has been demonstrated for a variety of primary malignancies, including gastric and oesophageal carcinoma,[145-149] gall bladder carcinoma,[150] and ovarian tumours,[151] bronchogenic carcinoma,[152] carcinoma of the breast,[153] malignant melanoma[154] and lymphoma.[155,156]

Nevertheless, the use of laparoscopy as a prelude to liver resection in patients with known hepatic malignancy has not found popularity, despite evidence supporting its role in the staging of both primary and secondary liver tumours in patients considered candidates for surgery. Lightdale reported findings contraindicating operation in 13 out of 16 patients with hepatocellular carcinoma (multifocal tumour, peritoneal dissemination and/or severe cirrhosis).[157] Jeffers et al.[158] documented unresectability in all 27 patients with hepatocellular carcinoma for similar reasons. Brady et al.[159] performed laparoscopy in 25 CT scan-negative patients with suspected liver disease, documenting hepatic and/or peritoneal malignancy in 12 patients, and unsuspected cirrhosis in three. Similarly, Babineau *et al.*[160] demonstrated tumour unresectability at staging laparoscopy in 14 out of 29 patients (48%). In Edinburgh, staging laparoscopy was performed in 50 patients with a variety of primary and secondary liver tumours (56% with colorectal metastases), thought to be potentially resectable on the basis of preceding USS, dynamic CT and/or CTAP scans.[161] Factors precluding laparotomy were confirmed in 23 cases (46%), due to extrahepatic dissemination in 18 patients and/or bilobar spread in 11 patients.

A deficiency of laparoscopy in the evaluation of hepatic malignancy is its inability to detect intrahepatic liver tumours situated away from the visible organ surface in approximately one third of patients. As discussed before, exploitation of the principles of IOUS during LapUS may address this limitation, also permitting evaluation of the relationships of intrahepatic liver tumours with the intrahepatic vascular structures. Thus the site, size and number of liver tumours, and their pattern of involvement with respect to the segmental hepatic anatomy may be defined at the time of staging laparoscopy.

Several reports testify to the utility of LapUS in this role,[161–163] including the application of LapUS-guided needle biopsy of small intrahepatic tumours which were not visible laparoscopically[164,165] and the detection of tumour invasion of the portal vein in patients with hepatocellular carcinoma.[161,166] Initial work in Edinburgh indicated that LapUS provided additional staging information in 18 out of 43 patients examined (42%) (bilobar or multifocal liver tumour, hilar lymphadenopathy and main portal or hepatic venous invasion). In seven patients, LapUS was the only investigation to demonstrate tumour unresectability, so averting unnecessary laparotomy.[161] When compared with historical control patients in whom no attempt at laparoscopic staging had been made, a significant increase in tumour resectability was observed for those evaluated laparoscopically (58% versus 93%).[161]

Detection of occult hepatic metastases from colorectal cancer

Up to 50% of patients with a diagnosis of colorectal carcinoma will at some stage develop liver metastases with profound implications for survival.[167] Although synchronous liver metastases discovered at the time of the primary colorectal surgery have been reported with an incidence of 15–20%,[167,168] a further group of patients are known to harbour 'occult' liver metastases which may not be apparent until their metachronous discovery in the postoperative period.[169] Finlay and McCardle reported the discovery of 'occult hepatic metastases' by USS, CT and radioisotope scintigraphy in 24–29% of the patients in whom a curative colorectal resection had been anticipated.[170,171] The crude five-year survival of patients with occult tumour dissemination was 6%, whereas the disease-related five-year survival rates for patients with 'corrected Dukes' stage A, B and C tumours but without evidence for occult metastases were 100%, 76% and 59%, respectively.[171]

Early detection of occult liver metastases is therefore important for informed decisions regarding the appropriateness of additional regional or systemic adjuvant therapies. Prompt detection of localised liver lesions may identify patients suitable for hepatic resection with curative intent, which represents the only realistic chance of achieving long-term survival, while the validity of the results of clinical trials of surgery and regimens of adjuvant therapy are dependent on accurate disease staging.

Preoperative investigations contribute little to the detection of colorectal liver metastases in patients for whom an exploratory laparotomy is already inevitable. Prospective comparative studies evaluating the diagnostic accuracy of liver function tests (LFTs), serum tumour markers, transabdominal USS, radioisotope scintigraphy, abdominal CT, and/or MRI have shown little benefit over intraoperative assessment in detecting hepatic metastases in advance of exploratory laparotomy.[172–176] The most sensitive method for detecting space-occupying lesions within the liver during exploratory laparotomy is the combination of careful bimanual palpation of the organ and intraoperative contact ultrasound scanning.

Intraoperative ultrasonography

Careful bimanual palpation of the liver during exploratory laparotomy was the only method available for the detection of hepatic metastases prior to the development of modern radiological techniques, and seemed remarkably sensitive. Nevertheless, the concept of occult liver metastases stimulated the search for more sensitive screening methods.

As described earlier, IOUS using high resolution ($\geqslant 5$ MHz), linear array contact ultrasound probes in direct apposition with the smooth moist capsule of the liver yields B-mode ultrasound images of exceptional resolution and quality. Studies have demonstrated that IOUS is the most sensitive available method for the detection of liver metastases at the time of primary colorectal cancer surgery. Comparisons performed on a 'lesion-by-lesion' basis reported superior sensitivities for IOUS compared with preoperative USS, CT and intraoperative palpation[85,177–180] and despite careful exploratory laparotomy, IOUS has been reported to be the only method sensitive enough to detect impalpable lesions in 14–24% of patients.[178,181–184] Machi and colleagues prospectively compared IOUS with operative inspection and palpation of the liver, preoperative USS and CT in detecting hepatic metastases on a 'lesion-by-lesion' basis in patients undergoing colorectal cancer resections with follow-up of 18–52 months.[85,177] Significantly superior results for IOUS were demonstrated with respect to sensitivity, negative predictive value and overall accuracy. Others have emphasised the utility of IOUS in excluding metastases in patients with false positive preoperative USS or CT scans.[180,185]

However, the benefit to the individual patient and the cost effectiveness of IOUS in the detection of occult hepatic metastases has been challenged.[180,184,186,187] Stone et al.[184] reported that IOUS was the sole modality in detecting occult hepatic metastases in 5% of patients, although its incremental benefit over other methods increased to 10% (rising to 12.5% for $T_3 N_0$ lesions) when patients with T3 and T4 primary tumours only were considered. It was also evident that repeated palpation of the liver with the benefit of the knowledge of the IOUS findings had led to the discovery of intrahepatic metastases which had not been previously emphasised, thus confirming the mutual benefit of these manoeuvres.

Doppler perfusion index

An exciting concept in the detection of occult hepatic metastases and recurrent disease after apparently curative colorectal resection has been developed in Glasgow Royal Infirmary. Liver metastases acquire a predominant blood supply from the hepatic artery, and the resultant subtle changes in haemodynamics may be detected by hepatic scintigraphy[188,189] or Doppler ultrasonography.[190] Leen et al.[190] measured the relative blood flow in the hepatic artery and portal vein, and calculated the Doppler perfusion index (DPI) according to the equation:

$$\mathrm{DPI} = \frac{\text{Hepatic arterial flow}}{\text{Hepatic arterial flow} + \text{portal venous flow}}$$

In their hands, and after 2 years of follow-up, an abnormally elevated DPI (>0.3) was shown to be remarkably predictive in identifying patients who died or developed recurrent disease, whereas a normal DPI (<0.26) identified patients with disease-free survival following apparently curative colorectal cancer resection.[190]

However, the technique is inherently operator dependent, relying on the calculation of blood flows within relatively small vessels from the product of time-averaged cross-sectional area of the vessel and the time-averaged velocity of blood within that vessel. The potential for error is therefore large. It remains to be seen whether this attractive concept will be reproducible enough to acquire widespread use.

Diagnosis and staging of colorectal liver metastases

Radiological imaging techniques continue to evolve, although radiological expertise and the prevailing philosophy as to what constitutes resectable disease vary widely. Such institutional variables hinder generalisations regarding the optimal diagnostic and staging algorithm for patients presenting with suspected colorectal hepatic metastases. However, most liver surgeons would accept the following factors as relative or absolute contraindications to hepatic resection with 'curative' intent: extrahepatic tumour (including malignant regional lymphadenopathy), multifocal intrahepatic lesions (> four deposits), bilobar tumour, vascular involvement (invasion or thrombosis of the main portal vein, hepatic artery or hepatic venous confluence). Also, a tumour-free resection margin of at least 1 cm is desirable, and the volume and functional reserve of the residual liver should be adequate following planned liver resection. Close liaison between radiologist and surgeon is therefore critical.

Although recognising the aforementioned limitations, a proposed algorithm for the management of patients presenting with confirmed or suspected colorectal hepatic metastases is shown in Fig. 1.7. Adequate measures should be taken to exclude extrahepatic tumour due to local recurrence[191] or extra-abdominal spread, and patients are assessed regarding their fitness to undergo major surgery.

CT angioportography and magnetic resonance imaging

The diagnostic sensitivities of dynamic bolus-enhanced CT (38–80%) and delayed CT (52–82%) in the detection of metastatic lesions have been surpassed by those of CTAP (78–94%) and MRI (63–95%) which currently represent the mainstay of diagnosis and staging of such patients[192] (Fig. 1.7). Ward *et al.*[176] showed no advantage for CTAP over MRI in this context, and Soyer *et al.*[193] investigated the diagnostic

Figure 1.7
Algorithm for the selection of patients for resection of liver metastases of colorectal origin.

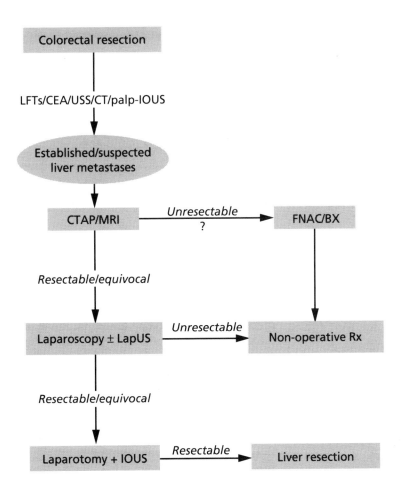

accuracy of arterial portography performed during both CT and MRI and reported no advantage for either technique. However, other studies have suggested that CTAP is probably more sensitive than MRI in detecting intrahepatic metastases,[194–196] although MRI may have an advantage in evaluating vascular invasion.[192] Although the current roles of CTAP and MRI in the staging of colorectal liver metastases may be considered complementary, in practice the choice is usually determined by availability and local expertise.

The sensitivity of CTAP in detecting hepatic tumours has been further validated by comparison with IOUS and pathological examination of the liver resection specimen in studies by Soyer et al.[196] and Moran et al.[197], both groups reporting similarly high sensitivities for CTAP and IOUS (91% versus 96%, and 95% versus 98%, respectively). The latter study was noteworthy inasmuch as the false positive rate for CTAP was remarkably low (5%),[197] and Moran et al. emphasised the importance of radiological experience in interpreting correctly the perfusion defects which plague this technique. In particular, they recommended delayed-phase scanning to overcome the problems posed by areas of hypoperfusion in hepatic segment IV adjacent to the porta hepatis and at the base of the falciform ligament, and the 'straight line sign' caused by a large area of hypodensity due to compression of the portal venous supply by tumour.[197,198] The importance of the recognition of such pitfalls is illustrated by a report which observed that CTAP had predicted unresectability in six (15%) out of 40 patients with resectable lesions.[199]

It is noteworthy that the technique of iodised oil emulsion (IOE) enhanced CT, which initially showed great promise as a sensitive modality for the detection of colorectal liver metastases, had not been shown to be significantly superior to CTAP or MRI.[176] The intravenous administration of lipid contrast material was also associated with systemic side effects, and the technique failed to become established in routine clinical practice.

Novel techniques of contrast-enhanced MRI have been developed which utilise agents with specific affinity for normal liver tissue. This has obvious attractions such as the avoidance of angiography, easier timing with avoidance of precontrast scans and improved sensitivity and specificity for focal liver lesions. The use of superparamagnetic iron oxide particles (which targets reticuloendothelial cells) for MR enhancement, although initially encouraging, has been superseded by hepatobiliary contrast agents which are taken up by hepatocytes and excreted into bile.[200] In particular, the use of Mn-DPDP enhanced MRI has shown great promise in improving lesion conspicuity, and different enhancement patterns have been observed for benign lesions, hepatocellular carcinomas and metastases.[200] In particular, the observation of peripheral accumulation of contrast ('rim-enhancement') on delayed images seems to be specific to metastases, the peripheral retention of Mn-DPDP reflecting malignant infiltration and impaired local drainage of hepatic parenchyma. Whether such techniques will prove to be more sensitive and specific than CTAP in the detection of liver metastases remains to be seen.

Laparoscopy, laparoscopic ultrasonography and intraoperative ultrasonography

The rationale for staging laparoscopy as a prelude to laparotomy in patients thought to have potentially resectable liver metastases has already been discussed.[160,161] The role of LapUS in this context was recently investigated by direct comparison with CTAP in 37 patients with colorectal liver metastases.[201] Although staging laparoscopy was useful in detecting extrahepatic and bilobar tumour spread in 10 patients (27%), the actual benefit attributable to LapUS was more marginal inasmuch as upstaging of disease occurred in just three out of 37 patients (8%). False positive CTAP findings ('bilobar lesions and portal vein invasion') occurred in 6/37 patients (16%), all of which were refuted by laparoscopy with LapUS.

Exploratory laparotomy and operative assessment of resectability is the ultimate arbiter of operability, and IOUS may contribute a unique role in this. Several studies have testified to the superior sensitivity of IOUS compared with conventional preoperative investigations in detecting established hepatic metastases in patients under consideration for liver resection,[185,202,203] including a comparison with CTAP.[204] Its ability to demonstrate precisely the pattern of intrahepatic disease and so facilitate operative decision making has rendered IOUS indispensable to many surgeons performing liver resection.[85,204–208]

Investigation of hepatocellular carcinoma

Hepatocellular carcinoma (HCC) is one of the commonest malignancies worldwide, although it is encountered less commonly in Europe and the United States. Hepatocellular carcinomas are unresectable in the majority of patients at presentation due to multifocality, large tumour size, extrahepatic and vascular spread, distant metastases and coexisting cirrhosis with poor heptic reserve. Ideally, the investigation of HCC should be sensitive in the early detection of small tumours (i.e. <3 cm) and specific in differentiating hepatomas from benign lesions such as the regenerating nodules of cirrhosis. The selection of patients for curative hepatic resection requires the detection of small intrahepatic metastases and portal vein invasion in particular.

In areas of the world where HCC is endemic such as the Far East, the principles of population screening have been employed with surveillance of patients with chronic liver disease by serum α-fetoprotein measurement and USS. The results of various modalities in the detection of HCC vary widely, with sensitivities for the investigation of small HCCs in the range 55–84% for USS, 46–84% for CT, 61–81% for angiography, 82% for CT angiography, 86–91% for CTAP, 71–96% for Lipiodol CT and 94–96% for IOUS.[209] The results of comparative studies

Figure 1.8
Algorithm for the investigation of patients with hepatocellular carcinoma.

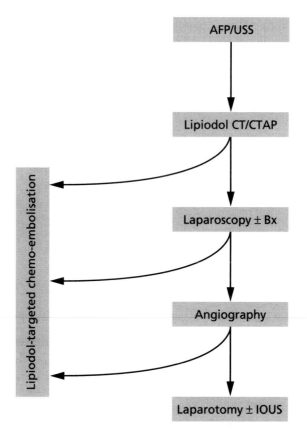

are reflected in the preferred choice of Lipiodol CT, CTAP and IOUS in the diagnosis and staging of patients with suspected HCC (Fig. 1.8). Therapeutic options such as Lipiodol-based cytotoxic-embolic regimens and Lipiodol-targeted radiotherapy further support the use of Lipiodol CT as an important component in the investigative algorithm.[210] Selective visceral angiography with portal phase venography tends to be reserved for patients with potentially resectable lesions, in whom the patency of the main portal vein and hepatic artery should be confirmed (Fig. 1.8). No advantage for MRI has been demonstrated to date, although preliminary work with Mn-DPDP enhanced MRI suggests a possible important role in differentiating HCC from metastases and benign lesions[200] (as discussed before). The limitations of current staging investigations (USS, CT, CTAP, angiography, MRI) in detecting multifocal intrahepatic daughter nodules of HCC have been highlighted, CTAP proving to be the least insensitive modality.[211]

The rationale for diagnostic and staging laparoscopy is supported by the propensity for occult extrahepatic and multifocal bilobar tumour dissemination of HCC as previously discussed.[157–161] The value of IOUS during operations for HCC should be emphasised, as the operator's tactile ability to localise intrahepatic tumour may be impaired by a rigid and nodular liver in patients with cirrhosis (Fig. 1.8). Thus, small tumours may be distinguished from cirrhotic nodules,[212] and precise parenchyma-sparing anatomical resections may be facilitated by IOUS, thus diminishing operative blood loss and preserving postoperative hepatic function.[213–216]

References

1. Gudjonsson B. Cancer of the pancreas. Cancer 1987; 60: 2284–303.
2. de Rooij PD, Rogatko A, Brennan MF. Evaluation of palliative surgical procedures in unresectable pancreatic cancer. Br J Surg 1991; 78: 1053–8.
3. Watanapa P, Williamson RCN. Surgical palliation for pancreatic cancer: developments during the past two decades. Br J Surg 1992; 79: 8–20.
4. Bramhall SR, Allum WH, Jones AG, Allwood A, Cummins C, Neoptolemos JP. Treatment and survival in 13 560 patients with pancreatic cancer, and incidence of the disease, in the West Midlands: an epidemiological study. Br J Surg 1995; 82: 111–15.
5. Andersen JR, Sorensen SM, Kruse A, Rollaer M, Matzen P. Randomised trial of endoscopic endoprosthesis versus operative bypass in malignant obstructive jaundice. Gut 1989; 30: 1132–5.
6. Smith AC, Dowsett JF, Russell RCG, Hatfield ARW, Cotton PB. Randomised trial of endoscopic stenting versus surgical bypass in malignant low bile duct obstruction. Lancet 1994; 344: 1655–60.
7. De Jong SA, Pickleman J, Rainsford K. Nonductal tumors of the pancreas. The importance of laparotomy. Arch Surg 1993; 114: 730–6.
8. van der Schelling GP, van den Bosch RP, Klinkenbijl JHG, Mulder PGH, Jeekel J. Is there a place for gastroenterostomy in patients with advanced cancer of the head of the pancreas? World J Surg 1993; 17: 128–33.
9. Hermanek P, Sobin LH. UICC: TNM classification of malignant tumors, 4th edn. Berlin: Springer-Verlag, 1992.
10. Wittekind C, Hermanek P. UICC classification of pancreatic cancer. Int J Pancreatol 1994; 16: 99–101.
11. Kalser MH, Barkin J, MacIntyre JM. Pancreatic cancer. Assessment of prognosis by clinical presentation. Cancer 1985; 56: 397–402.
12. Maringhini A, Ciambra M, Raimondo M *et al.* Clinical presentation and ultrasonography in the diagnosis of pancreatic cancer. Pancreas 1993; 8: 146–50.
13. Fabris C, Del Favero G, Basso D, *et al.* Serum markers and clinical data in diagnosing pancreatic cancer: a contrastive approach. Am J Gastroenterol 1988; 83: 549–53.
14. Carter DC. Cancer of the pancreas. Gut 1990; 31: 494–6.
15. Warshaw AL, Fernández-del Castillo C. Pancreatic carcinoma. N Engl J Med 1992; 326: 455–65.
16. Carter DC. Cancer of the head of the pancreas or chronic pancreatitis? A diagnostic dilemma. Surgery 1992; 111: 602–3.
17. Steinberg W. The clinical utility of the CA 19-9 tumor-associated antigen. Am J Gastroenterol 1990; 85: 350–5.
18. Glenn J, Steinberg W, Kurtzman SH, Steinberg SM, Sindelar WF. Evaluation of the utility of a radioimmunoassay for serum CA 19-9 levels in patients before and after treatment of carcinoma of the pancreas. J Clin Oncol 1988; 6: 462–8.
19. Soehendra N, Reynders-Frederix V. Palliative bile duct drainage – a new endoscopic method of introducing a transpapillary drain. Endoscopy 1980; 12: 8–11.
20. Freeny PC, Ball TJ. Endoscopic retrograde cholangiopancreatography (ERCP) and percutaneous transhepatic cholangiography (PTC) in the evaluation of suspected pancreatic carcinoma: diagnostic limitations and contemporary roles. Cancer 1981; 47: 1666–78.
21. Mackie CR, Cooper MJ, Lewis MH, Moossa AR. Non-operative differentiation between

pancreatic cancer and chronic pancreatitis. Ann Surg 1979; 189: 480–7.

22. Mackie CR, Dhorajiwala J, Blackstone MO, Bowie J, Moossa AR. Value of new diagnostic aids in relation to the disease process in pancreatic cancer. Lancet 1979; ii: 385–8.

23. Silverstein MD, Richter JM, Podolsky DK, Warshaw AL. Suspected pancreatic cancer presenting as pain or weight loss: analysis of diagnostic strategies. World J Surg 1984; 8: 839–45.

24. Koenigsberg M, Wiener SN, Walzer A. The accuracy of sonography in the differential diagnosis of obstructive jaundice: a comparison with cholangiography. Radiology 1979; 133: 157–65.

25. Haubek A, Pederson JH, Burcharth F, Gamelgaard J, Hancke S, Willumsen L. Dynamic sonography in the evaluation of jaundice. Am J Roentgenol 1981; 136: 1071–4.

26. Gibson RN, Yeung E, Thompson JN et al. Bile duct obstruction: radiologic evaluation of level, cause, and tumor resectability. Radiology 1986; 160: 43–7.

27. Laing FC, Jeffrey RB, Wing VW, Nyberg DA. Biliary dilatation: defining the level and cause by real-time US. Radiology 1986; 160: 39–42.

28. Baron RL, Stanley RJ, Lee JKT et al. A prospective comparison of the evaluation of biliary obstruction using computed tomography and ultrasonography. Radiology 1982; 145: 91–8.

29. Honickman SP, Mueller PR, Wittenberg J et al. Ultrasound in obstructive jaundice: prospective evaluation of site and cause. Radiology 1983; 147: 511–15.

30. Lindsell DRM. Ultrasound imaging of pancreas and biliary tract. Lancet 1990; i: 390–4.

31. Campbell JP, Wilson SR. Pancreatic neoplasms: how useful is evaluation with ultrasound? Radiology 1988; 167: 341–4.

32. Hessel SJ, Siegelman SS, McNeil BJ et al. A prospective evaluation of computed tomography and ultrasound of the pancreas. Radiology 1982; 143: 129–33.

33. Yasuda K, Mukai H, Jujimoto S, Nakajima M, Kawai K. The diagnosis of pancreatic cancer by endoscopic ultrasonography. Gastrointest Endosc 1988; 34: 1–8.

34. de Roos WK, Welvaart K, Bloem JL, Hermans J. Assessment of resectability of carcinoma of the pancreatic head by ultrasonography and computed tomography. A retrospective analysis. Eur J Surg Oncol 1990; 16: 411–16.

35. Rösch T, Braig C, Gain T et al. Staging of pancreatic and ampullary carcinoma by endoscopic ultrasonography. Comparison with conventional sonography, computed tomography, and angiography. Gastroenterology 1992; 102: 188–99.

36. Bakkevold KE, Arnesjø B, Kambestad B. Carcinoma of the pancreas and papilla of Vater – assessment of resectability and factors influencing resectability in stage I carcinomas. A prospective multicentre trial in 472 patients. Eur J Surg Oncol 1992; 18: 494–507.

37. Palazzo L, Roseau G, Gayet B et al. Endoscopic ultrasonography in the diagnosis and staging of pancreatic adenocarcinoma: results of a prospective study with comparison to ultrasonography and CT scan. Endoscopy 1993; 25: 143–50.

38. Päivansalo M, Lähde S. Ultrasonography and CT in pancreatic malignancy. Acta Radiol (Diagn) 1988; 29: 343–4.

39. Yasuda K, Mukai M, Nakajima M, Kawai K. Staging of pancreatic carcinoma by endoscopic ultrasonography. Endoscopy 1993; 25: 151–5.

40. Megibow AJ. Pancreatic adenocarcinoma: designing the examination to evaluate the clinical questions. Radiology 1992; 183: 297–303.

41. Freeny PC, Marks WM, Ryan JA, Traverso LW. Pancreatic ductal adenocarcinoma: diagnosis and staging with dynamic CT. Radiology 1988; 166: 125–33.

42. Freeny PC, Traverso LW, Ryan JA. Diagnosis and staging of pancreatic adenocarcinoma with dynamic computed tomography. Am J Surg 1993; 165: 600–6.

43. Bryde Andersen H, Effersoe H, Tjalve E, Burcharth F. CT for assessment of pancreatic and periampullary cancer. Acta Radiol 1993; 34: 569–72.

44. Müller MF, Meyenberger C, Bertschinger P, Schaer R, Marincek B. Pancreatic tumors: evaluation with endoscopic US, CT and MR imaging. Radiology 1994; 190: 745–51.

45. Palazzo L, Roseau G, Salmeron M. Endoscopic ultrasonography in the preoperative localization of pancreatic endocrine tumors. Endoscopy 1992; 24 (Suppl 1): 350–3.

46. Fuhrman GM, Charnsangavej C, Abbruzzese JL *et al.* Thin-section contrast-enhanced computed tomography accurately predicts the resectability of malignant pancreatic neoplasms. Am J Surg 1994; 167: 104–13.
47. Ross CB, Sharp KW, Kaufman AJ, Andrews T, Williams LF. Efficacy of computerized tomography in the preoperative staging of pancreatic carcinoma. Am Surg 1988; 54: 221–6.
48. Warshaw AL, Gu ZY, Wittenberg J, Waltman AC. Preoperative staging and assessment of resectability of pancreatic cancer. Arch Surg 1990; 125: 230–3.
49. Gulliver DJ, Baker ME, Cheng CA, Meyers WC, Pappas TN. Malignant biliary obstruction: efficacy of thin-section dynamic CT in determining resectability. Am J Roentgenol 1992; 159: 503–7.
50. Freeny PC. Radiology of the pancreas: two decades of progress in imaging and intervention. Am J Roentgenol 1988; 150: 975–81.
51. Vellet AD, Romano W, Bach DB, Passi RB, Taves DH, Munk PL. Adenocarcinoma of the pancreatic ducts: comparative evaluation with CT and MR imaging at 1.5T. Radiology 1992; 183: 87–95.
52. Murugiah M, Paterson-Brown S, Windsor JA, Miles WFA, Garden OJ. Early experience of laparoscopic ultrasonography in the management of pancreatic carcinoma. Surg Endosc 1993; 7: 177–81.
53. Trede M. Commentary on the role of selective visceral angiography in the management of pancreatic and periampullary cancer. World J Surg 1993; 17: 800.
54. Dupuy DE, Costello P, Ecker CP. Spiral CT of the pancreas. Radiology 1992; 183: 815–18.
55. Zeman RK, Fox SH, Silverman PM *et al.* Helical (spiral) CT of the abdomen. Am J Roentgenol 1993; 160: 719–25.
56. Rubin GD, Dake MD, Napel SA, McDonnell CH, Jeffrey RB. Three-dimensional spiral CT angiography of the abdomen: initial clinical experience. Radiology 1993; 186: 147–52.
57. Gmeinwieser J, Feuerbach S, Hohenberger W *et al.* Spiral-CT in diagnosis of vascular involvement in pancreatic cancer. Hepatogastroenterology 1995; 42: 418–22.
58. Steiner E, Stark DD, Hahn PF *et al.* Imaging of pancreatic neoplasms: comparison of MR and CT. Am J Roentgenol 1989; 152: 487–91.
59. Pavone P, Occhiato R, Michelini O *et al.* Magnetic resonance imaging of pancreatic carcinoma. Eur Radiol 1991; 1: 124–30.
60. Tylén U, Arnesjö B. Resectability and prognosis of carcinoma of the pancreas evaluated by angiography. Scand J Gastroenterol 1973; 8: 691–7.
61. Freeny PC, Ball TJ, Ryan J. Impact of new diagnostic imaging methods on pancreatic angiography. Am J Roentgenol 1979; 133: 619–24.
62. Mackie CR, Noble HG, Cooper MJ, Collins P, Block GE, Moossa GR. Prospective evaluation of angiography in the diagnosis and management of patients suspected of having pancreatic cancer. Ann Surg 1979; 189: 11–17.
63. Appleton GVN, Cooper MJ, Bathurst NCG, Williamson RCN, Virjee J. The value of angiography in the surgical management of pancreatic disease. Ann R Coll Surg Engl 1989; 71: 92–6.
64. Bookstein JJ, Reuter SR, Martel W. Angiographic evaluation of pancreatic cancer. Radiology 1969; 93: 757.
65. Stanley RJ, Sagel SS, Evens RG. The impact of new imaging methods on pancreatic arteriography. Radiology 1980; 136: 251–3.
66. Fredens M, Egeblad M, Holst-Nielsen F. The value of selective angiography in the diagnosis of tumors in pancreas and liver. Radiology 1969; 93: 765.
67. Murugiah M, Windsor JA, Redhead D *et al.* The role of selective visceral angiography in the management of pancreatic and periampullary cancer. World J Surg 1993; 17: 796–800.
68. Buranasiri S, Baum S. The significance of the venous phase of celiac and superior mesenteric angiography in evaluating pancreatic carcinoma. Radiology 1972; 102: 11–20.
69. Jafri SZH, Aisen AM, Glazer G, Weiss CA. Comparison of CT and angiography in assessing resectability of pancreatic carcinoma. Am J Roentgenol 1984; 142: 525–9.
70. Dooley WC, Cameron JL, Pitt HA, Lillemoe KD, Yue NC, Venbbrux AC. Is preoperative angiography useful in patients with periampullary tumors? Ann Surg 1990; 211: 649–55.
71. Trede M, Schwall G, Saeger HD. Survival after pancreatoduodenectomy. 118 consecu-

tive resections without an operative mortality. Ann Surg 1990; 211: 447–58.

72. Ferrucci JT, Wittenberg J. A comprehensive approach for diagnosing pancreatic disease. Radiology 1980; 136: 255–6.

73. Rong GH, Sindelar WF. Aberrant peripancreatic arterial anatomy. Considerations in performing pancreatectomy for malignant neoplasms. Am Surg 1987; 12: 726–9.

74. Biehl TR, Traverso LW, Hauptmann E, Ryan JA. Preoperative visceral angiography alters intraoperative strategy during the Whipple procedure. Am J Surg 1993; 165: 607–12.

75. Ishida H. Peritoneoscopy and pancreas biopsy in the diagnosis of pancreatic diseases. Gastrointest Endosc 1983; 29: 211–18.

76. Cuschieri A, Hall AW, Clark J. Value of laparoscopy in the diagnosis and management of pancreatic carcinoma. Gut 1978; 19: 672–7.

77. Cuschieri A. Laparoscopy for pancreatic cancer: does it benefit the patient? Eur J Surg Oncol 1988; 14: 41–4.

78. Warshaw AL, Tepper JE, Shipley WU. Laparoscopy in the staging and planning of therapy for pancreatic cancer. Am J Surg 1986; 151: 76–80.

79. Fernández-del Castillo C, Warshaw AL. Laparoscopy for staging in pancreatic carcinoma. Surg Oncol 1993; 2: 25–9.

80. John TG, Greig JD, Carter DC, Garden OJ. Carcinoma of the pancreatic head and peri-ampullary region: tumor staging with laparoscopy and laparoscopic ultrasonography. Ann Surg 1995; 221: 156–64.

81. Bemelman WA, de Wit LT, van Delden OM et al. Diagnostic laparoscopy combined with laparoscopic ultrasonography in staging cancer of the pancreatic head region. Br J Surg 1995; 82: 820–4.

82. Conlon KC, Dougherty E, Klimstra DS, Coit DG, Turnbull ADM, Brennan MF. The value of minimal access surgery in the staging of patients with potentially resectable peripancreatic malignancy. Ann Surg 1996; 223: 134–40.

83. Plainfosse MC, Bouillot JL, Rivaton F, Vaucamps P, Hernigou A, Alexandre JH. The use of operative sonography in carcinoma of the pancreas. World J Surg 1987; 11: 654–8.

84. Serio G, Fugazzola C, Iacono C et al. Intra-operative ultrasonography in pancreatic cancer. Int J Pancreatol 1992; 11: 31–41.

85. Machi J, Sigel B, Zaren HA, Kurohiji T, Yamashita Y. Operative ultrasonography during hepatobiliary and pancreatic surgery. World J Surg 1993; 17: 640–6.

86. Siriwardena A, Samarji WN. Cutaneous tumour seeding from a previously undiagnosed pancreatic carcinoma after laparoscopic cholecystectomy. Ann R Coll Surg Engl 1993; 75: 199–200.

87. Jorgensen JO, McCall JL, Morris DL. Port site seeding after laparoscopic ultrasonographic staging of pancreatic carcinoma. Surgery 1995; 117: 118–19.

88. Snady H, Cooperman A, Siegel J. Endoscopic ultrasonography compared with computed tomography with ERCP in patients with obstructive jaundice or small peripancreatic mass. Gastrointest Endosc 1992; 38: 27–34.

89. Kelsey PJ, Warshaw AL. EUS: an added test or a replacement for several? Endoscopy 1993; 25: 179–81.

90. Tio TL, Tytgat GNJ, Cikot RJLM, Houthoff HJ, Sars PRA. Ampullopancreatic carcinoma: preoperative TNM classification with endosonography. Radiology 1990; 175: 455–61.

91. Snady H, Bruckner H, Siegel J, Cooperman A, Neff R, Kiefer L. Endoscopic ultrasonographic criteria of vascular invasion by potentially resectable pancreatic tumors. Gastrointest Endosc 1994; 40: 326–33.

92. Grimm H, Hamper K, Binmoeller KF, Soehendra N. Enlarged lymph nodes: malignant or not? Endoscopy 1992; 24 (Suppl 1): 320–3.

93. Livraghi T, Damascelli B, Lombardi C, Spagnoli J. Risk in fine-needle abdominal biopsy. J Clin Ultrasound 1983; 11: 77–81.

94. Fornari F, Civardi G, Cavanna L et al. The Cooperative Italian Study Group. Complication of ultrasonically guided fine-needle abdominal biopsy. Scand J Gastroenterol 1989; 24: 949–55.

95. Ihse I, Isaksson G. Preoperative and operative diagnosis of pancreatic cancer. World J Surg 1984; 8: 846–53.

96. Rashleigh-Belcher HJC, Russell RCG, Lees WR. Cutaneous seeding of pancreatic carcinoma by fine-needle aspiration biopsy. Br J Radiol 1986; 59: 182–3.

97. Bergenfeldt M, Genell S, Lindholm K, Ekberg O, Aspelin P. Needle-tract seeding after

percutaneous fine-needle biopsy of pancreatic carcinoma. Acta Chir Scand 1988; 154: 77–9.

98. Warshaw AL. Implications of peritoneal cytology for staging of early pancreatic cancer. Am J Surg 1991; 161: 26–30.

99. Lei S, Kini J, Kim K, Howard JM. Pancreatic cancer. Cytologic study of peritoneal washings. Arch Surg 1994; 129: 639–42.

100. Fernández-del Castillo C, Rattner DW, Warshaw AL. Further experience with laparoscopy and peritoneal cytology in the staging of pancreatic cancer. Br J Surg 1995; 82: 1127–9.

101. Leach SD, Rose JA, Lowy AM et al. Significance of peritoneal cytology in patients with potentially resectable adenocarcinoma of the pancreatic head. Surgery 1995; 118: 472–8.

102. John TG, McGoogan E, Wigmore SJ, Paterson-Brown S, Carter DC, Garden OJ. Laparoscopic peritoneal cytology in the staging of pancreatic cancer. Gut 1995; 37(2): A3.

103. Ihse I, Andrèn-Sandberg A. Percutaneous fine-needle aspiration cytology. In: Trede M, Carter DC (eds) Surgery of the pancreas. Edinburgh: Churchill Livingstone, 1993:

104. Karlson B-M, Forsman CA, Wilander E et al. Efficiency of percutaneous core biopsy in pancreatic tumor diagnosis. Surgery 1996; 120; 75–9.

105. Enayati PG, Traverso LW, Galagan K et al. The meaning of equivocal pancreatic cytology in patients thought to have pancreatic cancer. Am J Surg 1996; 171: 525–8.

106. Blumgart LH, Hadjis NS, Benjamin IS, Beasley R. Surgical approaches to cholangiocarcinoma at the confluence of hepatic ducts. Lancet 1984; i: 66–70.

107. Nesbit GM, Johnson CD, James EM, Mac-Carty RL, Nagorney DM, Bender CE. Cholangiocarcinoma: diagnosis and evaluation of resectability by CT and sonography as procedures complementary to cholangiography. Am J Roentgenol 1988; 151: 933–8.

108. Teefey SA, Baron RL, Schulte SJ, Patten RM, Molloy MH. Patterns of intrahepatic bile duct dilatation at CT: correlation with obstructive disease processes. Radiology 1992; 182: 139–42.

109. Neumaier CE, Bertolotto M, Perrone R, Martinoli C, Loria F, Silvestri E. Staging of hilar cholangiocarcinoma with ultrasound. J Clin Ultrasound 1995; 23: 173–8.

110. Bismuth H, Corlette MB. Intrahepatic cholangioenteric anastamosis in carcinoma of the hilus of the liver. Surg Gynecol Obstet 1975; 140: 170–8.

111. Looser C, Stain SC, Baer HU, Friller J, Blumgart LH. Staging of hilar cholangiocarcinoma by ultrasound and duplex sonography: a comparison with angiography and operative findings. Br J Radiol 1993; 65: 871–7.

112. Guthrie CM, Banting SW, Garden OJ, Carter DC. Segment III cholangiojejunostomy for palliation of malignant hilar obstruction. Br J Surg 1994; 81: 1639–41.

113. Davidson B, Varsamidakis N, Dooley J et al. The value of exfoliative cytology for investigating bile duct strictures. Gut 1992; 33: 1408–11.

114. Nimura Y. Staging of biliary carcinoma: cholangiography and cholangioscopy. Endoscopy 1993; 25: 76–80.

115. Rabinowitz M, Zajko AB, Hassanein T et al. Diagnostic value of brush cytology in the diagnosis of bile duct carcinoma: a study of 65 patients with bile duct strictures. Hepatology 1990; 12: 747–52.

116. Desa LA, Akosa AB, Lazzara S, Domizio P, Krausz T, Benjamin IS. Cytodiagnosis in the management of extrahepatic biliary stricture. Gut 1991; 32: 1188–91.

117. Davidson BR. Progress in determining the nature of bile duct strictures. Gut 1993; 34: 725–6.

118. Wetter LA, Ring EJ, Pellegrini CA, Way LW. Differential diagnosis of sclerosing cholangiocarcinoma of the common hepatic duct (Klatskin tumors). Am J Surg 1991; 161: 57–62.

119. Bismuth H, Castaing D, Traynor O. Resection or palliation: priority of surgery in the treatment of hilar cancer. World J Surg 1988; 12: 39–47.

120. Tio TL, Cheng J, Wijers OB, Sars PRA, Tytgat GNJ. Endosonographic TNM staging of extrahepatic bile duct cancer: comparison with pathological staging. Gastroenterology 1991; 100: 1351–61.

121. Kaneko T, Nakao A, Inoue S et al. Intraportal endovascular ultrasonography in the diagnosis of portal vein invasion by pancreatobiliary carcinoma. Ann Surg 1995; 222: 711–18.

122. Collier NA, Carr D, Hemmingway A, Blum-

gart LH. Preoperative diagnosis and its effect on the treatment of carcinoma of the gallbladder. Surg Gynecol Obstet 1984; 159: 465–70.

123. Bismuth H. Surgical anatomy and anatomical surgery of the liver. World J Surg 1982; 6: 3–9.

124. Bismuth H, Houssin D, Castaing D. Major and minor segmentectomies 'réglées' in liver surgery. World J Surg 1982; 6: 10–24.

125. Bismuth H, Kuntslinger F, Castaing D. Intraoperative ultrasound and liver surgery. In: Bismuth H, Kuntslinger F, Castaing D (eds). A text and atlas of liver ultrasound. London: Chapman and Hall, 1991, pp. 113–23.

126. Soyer P. Segmental anatomy of the liver: utility of nomenclature accepted worldwide. Am J Roentgenol 1993; 161: 572–3.

127. Baron RL. Understanding and optimizing use of contrast material for CT of the liver. Am J Roentgenol 1994; 163: 323–31.

128. Paushter DM, Zeman RK, Scheibler ML, Choyke PL, Jaffe MH, Clark LR. CT evaluation of suspected hepatic metastases: comparison of techniques for IV contrast enhancement. Am J Roentgenol 1989; 152: 267–71.

129. Freeny PC, Marks WM. Hepatic perfusion abnormalities during CT angiography. Radiology 1986; 159: 685–91.

130. Miller DL, Simmons JT, Chang R et al. Hepatic metastasis detection: comparison of 3 CT contrast enhancement methods. Radiology 1987; 165: 785–90.

131. Peterson MS, Baron RL, Dodd GD et al. Hepatic parenchymal perfusion defects detected with CTAP: imaging-pathologic correlation. Radiology 1992; 185: 149–55.

132. Soyer P, Lacheheb D, Levesque M. False-positive CT portography: correlation with pathologic findings. Am J Roentgenol 1993; 160: 285–9.

133. Merine D, Takayasue K, Wakao F. Detection of hepatocellular carcinoma: comparison of CT during arterial portography with CT after intraarterial injection of iodized oil. Radiology 1990; 175: 707–10.

134. Keate RF, Shaffer R. Seeding of hepatocellular carcinoma to peritoneoscopy insertion site. Gastrointest Endosc 1992; 38: 203–4.

135. John TG, Garden OJ. Needle track seeding of primary and secondary liver carcinoma after percutaneous liver biopsy. Hepatobiliary Surgery 1993; 6: 199–204.

136. Nduka CC, Monson JRT, Menzies-Gow N, Darzi A. Abdominal wall metastasis following laparoscopy. Br J Surg 1994; 81: 648–52.

137. Yamada N, Shinzawa H, Ukai K et al. Subcutaneous seeding of small hepatocellular carcinoma after fine needle aspiration biopsy. J Gastroenterol Hepatol 1993; 8: 195–8.

138. Russi EG, Pergolizzi S, Mesiti M et al. Unusual relapse of hepatocellular carcinoma. Cancer 1992; 70: 1483–7.

139. Ishida H, Dohzono T, Furukawa Y, Kobayashi M, Tsuneoka K. Laparoscopy and biopsy in the diagnosis of malignant intra-abdominal tumors. Endoscopy 1984; 16: 140–2.

140. Leuschner M, Leuschner U. Diagnostic laparoscopy in focal parenchymal disease of the liver. Endoscopy 1992; 24: 689–92.

141. Fornari F, Rapaccini GL, Cavanna L et al. Diagnosis of hepatic lesions: ultrasonically guided fine needle biopsy or laparoscopy? Gastrointest Endosc 1988; 34: 231–4.

142. Vautier G, Scott B, Jenkins D. Liver biopsy: blind or guided? Br Med J 1994; 309: 1455–6.

143. Smith EH. Complications of percutaneous abdominal fine-needle biopsy. Radiology 1991; 178: 253–8.

144. Lefor AT, Hughes KS, Shiloni E et al. Intra-abdominal extrahepatic disease in patients with colorectal hepatic metastases. Dis Colon Rectum 1988; 31: 100–3.

145. Possik RA, Franco EL, Pires DR, Wohnrath DR, Fereira EB. Sensitivity, specificity, and predictive value of laparoscopy for the staging of gastric cancer and for the detection of liver metastases. Cancer 1986; 58: 1–6.

146. Shandall A, Johnson C. Laparoscopy or scanning in oesophageal and gastric carcinoma. Br J Surg 1985; 72: 449–51.

147. Watt I, Stewart I, Anderson D, Bell G, Anderson JR. Laparoscopy, ultrasound and computed tomography in cancer of the oesophagus and gastric cardia: a prospective comparison for detecting intra-abdominal metastases. Br J Surg 1989; 76: 1036–9.

148. Gross E, Bancewicz J, Ingram G. Assessment of gastric carcinoma by laparoscopy. Br Med J 1984; 288: 1577.

149. Molloy RG, McCourtney JS, Anderson JR. Laparoscopy in the management of patients with cancer of the gastric cardia and oesophagus. Br J Surg 1995; 82: 352–4.

150. Dagnini G, Marin G, Patella M, Zotti S. Laparoscopy in the diagnosis of primary carcinoma of the gallbladder. A study of 98 cases. Gastrointest Endosc 1984; 30: 289–91.

151. Rosenhoff SH, Young RC, Anderson TC et al. Peritoneoscopy: a valuable staging tool in ovarian carcinoma. Ann Intern Med 1975; 83: 37–41.

152. Margolis R, Hansen H, Muggia F, Kanhouwa S. Diagnosis of liver metastases in bronchogenic carcinoma. A comparative study of liver scans, function tests, and peritoneoscopy with liver biopsy in 111 patients. Cancer 1974; 34: 1825–9.

153. Van der Spuy S, Levin W, Smit BJ, Graham T, McQuaide JR. Peritoneoscopy in the management of breast cancer. S Afr Med J 1978; 54: 402–3.

154. Bleiberg H, La Meir E, Lejeune F. Laparoscopy in the diagnosis of liver metastases in 80 cases of malignant melanoma. Endoscopy 1980; 12: 215–18.

155. Huberman M, Bunn P, Matthews M et al. Hepatic involvement in the cutaneous T-cell lymphomas. Results of percutaneous biopsy and peritoneoscopy. Cancer 1980; 45: 1683–8.

156. Bagley C, Thomas L, Johnson R, Chretien P, DeVita V. Diagnosis of liver involvement by lymphoma: results in 96 consecutive peritoneoscopies. Cancer 1973; 31: 840–7.

157. Lightdale CJ. Laparoscopy and biopsy in malignant liver disease. Cancer 1982; 50: 2672–5.

158. Jeffers L, Spieglman G, Reddy R et al. Laparoscopically directed fine needle aspiration for the diagnosis of hepatocellular carcinoma: a safe and accurate technique. Gastrointest Endosc 1988; 34: 235–7.

159. Brady PG, Peebles M, Goldschmid S. Role of laparoscopy in the evaluation of patients with suspected hepatic or peritoneal malignancy. Gastrointest Endosc 1991; 37: 27–30.

160. Babineau TJ, Lewis WD, Jenkins RL, Bleday R, Steele GD, Forse RA. Role of staging laparoscopy in the treatment of hepatic malignancy. Am J Surg 1994; 167: 151–5.

161. John TG, Greig JD, Crosbie JL, Miles WFA, Garden OJ. Superior staging of liver tumors with laparoscopy and laparoscopic ultrasound. Ann Surg 1994; 220: 711–19.

162. Miles WFA, Paterson-Brown S, Garden OJ. Laparoscopic contact hepatic ultrasonography. Br J Surg 1992; 79: 419–20.

163. Cuesta MA, Meijer S, Borgstein PJ, Sibinga Mulder L, Sikkenk AC. Laparoscopic ultrasonography for hepatobiliary and pancreatic malignancy. Br J Surg 1993; 80: 1571–4.

164. Fukuda M, Mima S, Tanabe T, Suzuki Y, Hirata K, Terada S. Endoscopic sonography of the liver – diagnostic application of the echolaparoscope to localize intrahepatic lesions. Scand J Gastroenterol 1984; 19 (suppl 102): 24–8.

165. Bönhof JA, Linhart P, Bettendorf U, Holper H. Liver biopsy guided by laparoscopic sonography. A case report demonstrating a new technique. Endoscopy 1984; 16: 237–9.

166. Okita K, Kodama T, Oda M, Takemoto T. Laparoscopic ultrasonography. Diagnosis of liver and pancreatic cancer. Scand J Gastroenterol 1984; 19 (suppl 94): 91–100.

167. Bengtsson G, Carlsson G, Hafström L, Jonsson P-E. Natural history of patients with untreated liver metastases from colorectal cancer. Am J Surg 1981; 141: 586–9.

168. Oxley EM, Ellis H. Prognosis of carcinoma of the large bowel in the presence of liver metastases. Br J Surg 1969; 56: 149–52.

169. Goligher JC. The operability of carcinoma of the rectum. Br Med J 1941; ii: 393–7.

170. Finlay IG, Meek DR, Gray HW, Duncan JG, McArdle CS. Incidence and detection of occult hepatic metastases in colorectal carcinoma. Br Med J 1982; 248: 803–9.

171. Finlay IG, McArdle CS. Occult hepatic metastases in colorectal carcinoma. Br J Surg 1986; 73: 732–5.

172. de Brauuw LM, van de Velde CJH, Pauwels EKJ et al. Prospective comparative study of ultrasound, CT scan, scintigraphy and laboratory tests to detect hepatic metastases. J Nucl Biol Med 1991; 35: 131–4.

173. Kemeny MM, Ganteaume L, Goldberg DA, Hogan JM. Preoperative staging with computerized axial tomography and biochemical laboratory tests in patients with hepatic metastases. Ann Surg 1986; 203: 169–72.

174. Schreve RH, Terpesta OT, Ausema L, Lameris JS, van Seijen AJ, Jeekel J. Detection of liver metastases. A prospective study comparing liver enzymes, scintigraphy, ultrasonography and computed tomography. Br J Surg 1984; 71: 947–9.

175. Smith T, Kemeny M, Sugarbaker P *et al.* A prospective study of hepatic imaging in the detection of metastatic disease. Ann Surg 1982; 195: 486–91.

176. Ward B, Miller D, Frank J *et al.* Prospective evaluation of hepatic imaging studies in the detection of colorectal metastases: correlation with surgical findings. Surgery 1989; 105: 180–7.

177. Machi J, Isomoto H, Kurohiji T *et al.* Accuracy of intraoperative ultrasound in diagnosing liver metastasis from colorectal cancer: evaluation with postoperative follow-up results. World J Surg 1991; 15: 551–7.

178. Stadler J, Hölscher AH, Adolf J. Intraoperative ultrasonographic detection of occult liver metastases in colorectal cancer. Surg Endosc 1991; 5: 36–40.

179. Olsen AK. Intraoperative ultrasonography and the detection of liver metastases in patients with colorectal cancer. Br J Surg 1990; 77: 998–9.

180. Paul MA, Siblinga Mulder L, Cuesta MA, Sikkenk AC, Lyesen GKS, Meijer S. Impact of intraoperative ultrasonography on treatment strategy for colorectal cancer. Br J Surg 1994; 81: 1660–3.

181. Boldrini G, de Gaetano AM, Giovannini I, Castagneto M, Colagrande C, Castiglioni G. The systematic use of operative ultrasound for detection of liver metastases during colorectal surgery. World J Surg 1987; 11: 622–7.

182. Charnley RM, Morris DL, Dennison AR, Amar SS, Hardcastle JD. Detection of colorectal liver metastases using intraoperative ultrasonography. Br J Surg 1991; 78: 45–8.

183. Stewart PJ, Chu JM, Kos SC, Chapuis PH, Bokey EL. Intra-operative ultrasound for the detection of hepatic metastases from colorectal cancer. Aust NZ J Surg 1993; 63: 530–4.

184. Stone MD, Kane R, Bothe A, Jessup JM, Cady B, Steele GD. Intraoperative ultrasound imaging of the liver at the time of colorectal cancer resection. Arch Surg 1994; 129: 431–6.

185. Knol JA, Marn CS, Francis IR, Rubin JM, Bromberg J, Chang AE. Comparison of dynamic infusion and delayed computed tomography, intraoperative ultrasound, and palpation in the diagnosis of liver metastases. Am J Surg 1993; 165: 81–7.

186. Gozzetti G. Operative ultrasonography during hepatobiliary and pancreatic surgery: (Invited commentary). World J Surg 1991; 17: 645–6.

187. Leen E, Angerson WJ, O'Gorman P, Cooke TG, McArdle CS. Intraoperative ultrasound in colorectal cancer patients undergoing apparently curative surgery: correlation with two year follow-up. Clin Radiol 1996; 51: 157–9.

188. Leveson SH, Wiggins PA, Giles GR, Parkin A, Robinson PJ. Deranged liver blood flow patterns in the detection of liver metastases. Br J Surg 1985; 72: 128–30.

189. Huguier M, Maheswari S, Toussaint P, Houry S, Mauban S, Mensch B. Hepatic flow scintigraphy in evaluation of hepatic metastases in patients with gastrointestinal malignancy. Arch Surg 1993; 128: 1057–9.

190. Leen E, Angerson WJ, Cooke TG, McArdle CS. Prognostic power of Doppler perfusion index in colorectal cancer. Ann Surg 1996; 223: 199–203.

191. Freeny PC, Marks WM, Ryan JA, Bolen JW. Colorectal carcinoma evaluation with CT: preoperative staging and detection of postoperative recurrence. Radiology 1986; 158: 347–53.

192. Tubiana JM, Deutsch JP, Taboury J, Martin B. Imaging of hepatic colorectal metastases. Diagnosis and resectability. In: Nordlinger B, Jaeck D (eds) Treatment of hepatic metastases of colorectal cancer. Paris: Springer-Verlag, 1992; pp. 55–69.

193. Soyer P, Laissy J-P, Sibert A *et al.* Focal hepatic masses: comparison of detection during arterial portography with MR imaging and CT. Radiology 1994; 190: 737–40.

194. Nelson RC, Chezmar JL, Sugarbaker PH, Bernardino ME. Hepatic tumours: comparison of CT during arterial portography, delayed CT, and MR imaging for preoperative evaluation. Radiology 1989; 172: 27–34.

195. Heiken JP, Weyman PJ, Lee JKT, Balfe DM, Picus D, Brunt EM, Flye MW. Detection of focal hepatic masses: prospective evaluation with CT, delayed CT, CT during portography, and MR imaging. Radiology 1989; 171: 47–51.

196. Soyer P, Levesque M, Elias D, Zeitoun G, Roche A. Detection of liver metastases from

colorectal cancer: comparison of intraoperative US and CT during arterial portography. Radiology 1992; 183: 541–4.

197. Moran BJ, O'Rourke N, Plant GR, Rees M. Computed tomographic portography in preoperative imaging of hepatic neoplasms. Br J Surg 1995; 82: 669–71.

198. Nazarian LN, Wechsler RJ, Grady CK *et al.* CT done 4–6 hr after CT arterial portography: value in detecting hepatic tumors and differentiating from other hepatic perfusion defects. Am J Roentgenol 1994; 163: 851–5.

199. Vogel SB, Drane WE, Ros PR, Kerns SR, Bland KI. Prediction of surgical resectability in patients with hepatic colorectal metastases. Ann Surg 1994; 219: 508–16.

200. Mitchell DG. Hepatobiliary contrast material: a magic bullet for sensitivity and specificity? Radiology 1993; 188: 21–2.

201. John TG, Madhavan KK, Redhead DN, Crosbie JL, Garden OJ. Laparoscopic ultrasonography in the staging of colorectal liver metastases: a prospective comparison with CT arterioportography. Br J Surg 1996; 83: 31.

202. Clarke MP, Kane RA, Steele G Jr *et al.* Prospective comparison of preoperative imaging and intraoperative ultrasonography in the detection of liver tumours. Surgery 1989; 106: 849–55.

203. Parker GA, Lawrence W, Horsley SJ *et al.* Intraoperative ultrasound of the liver affects operative decision making. Ann Surg 1989; 209: 569–77.

204. Solomon MJ, Stephen MS, Gallinger S, White GH. Does intraoperative hepatic ultrasonography change surgical decision making during liver resection? Am J Surg 1994; 168: 307–10.

205. Rifkin MD, Rosato FE, Branch HM *et al.* Intraoperative ultrasound of the liver. An important adjunctive tool for decision making in the operating room. Ann Surg 1987; 466–72.

206. Soyer P, Elias D, Zeitoun G, Roche A, Levesque M. Surgical treatment of hepatic metastases: impact of intraoperative sonography. Am J Roentgenol 1993; 160: 511–14.

207. Traynor O, Castaing D, Bismuth H. Peroperative ultrasonography in the surgery of hepatic tumours. Br J Surg 1988; 75: 197–202.

208. Gozzetti G, Mazziotti A, Bolondi L *et al.* Intraoperative ultrasonography in surgery for liver tumours. Surgery 1986; 99: 523–9.

209. Choi BI, Takayasu K, Han MC. Small hepatocellular carcinomas and associated nodular lesions of the liver: pathology, pathogenesis, and imaging findings. Am J Roentgenol 1993; 160: 1177–87.

210. Bhattacharya S, Novell JR, Winslett MC, Hobbs KEF. Iodized oil in the treatment of hepatocellular carcinoma. Br J Surg 1994; 81: 1563–71.

211. Utsunomiya T, Matsumata T, Adachi E, Honda H, Sugimachi K. Limitations of current preoperative liver imaging techniques for intrahepatic metastatic nodules of hepatocellular carcinoma. Hepatology 1992; 16: 694–701.

212. Sheu J-C, Lee C-S, Sung J-L, Chen D-S, Yang P-M, Lin T-Y. Intraoperative hepatic ultrasonography – An indispensable procedure in resection of small hepatocellular carcinomas. Surgery 1985; 97: 97–103.

213. Castaing D, Garden OJ, Bismuth H. Segmental liver resection using ultrasound-guided selective portal venous occlusion. Ann Surg 1989; 210: 20–3.

214. Bismuth H, Castaing D, Garden OJ. The use of operative ultrasound in surgery of primary liver tumors. World J Surg 1987; 11: 610–14.

215. Makuuchi M, Hasegwa H, Yamazaki S, Takayasu K, Moriyama N. The use of operative ultrasound as an aid to liver resection in patients with hepatocellular carcinoma. World J Surg 1987; 11: 615–21.

216. Makuuchi M, Hasegwa H, Yamazaki S. Ultrasonically guided subsegmentectomy. Surg Gynecol Obstet 1985; 161: 346–50.

217. Garden OJ, Bismuth H. Anatomy of the liver. In: Carter DC, Russell RCG, Pitt HA, Bismuth H (eds) Operative surgery: hepatobiliary and pancreatic surgery. London: Chapman and Hall, 1996, pp. 1–4.

2 Benign liver lesions

Ib C. Rasmussen
O. James Garden

Introduction Benign lesions of the liver are not uncommon and may be difficult to differentiate from primary and secondary hepatic tumours. Solid lesions may be identified as an incidental finding when radiological investigation is undertaken for unrelated intra-abdominal disease. Similarly, such lesions may be identified when co-existent hepatic pathology is present and give rise to problems of management. Although these lesions may be of congenital origin, most are of unknown aetiology. They generally do not give rise to any symptoms but, since they are often slow growing, they may produce symptoms caused by mass effect. Such lesions may give rise to acute symptoms because of necrosis, thrombosis, haemorrhage or rupture.

Routine liver function tests are invariably within normal limits in patients with benign hepatic pathology and are therefore of value in guiding the clinician towards a diagnosis of benign disease. Nonetheless, complications such as secondary haemorrhage and necrosis may be associated with increases in serum transaminase levels. Elevation in tumour markers such as carcinoembryonic antigen (CEA) or alpha-fetoprotein (AFP) and the development of paraneoplastic syndromes such as erythrocytosis, hyperglycaemia and hypercalcaemia are rarely observed with such benign pathology.

Characterisation of hepatic lesions is provided by imaging tests of the liver. Ultrasonography (US) and computed tomography (CT) are the cornerstone of diagnosis and often complement one another. More recently, magnetic resonance imaging has shown promising results in the imaging of hepatic lesions. Abdominal ultrasonography will differentiate cystic forms from solid lesions, whereas computed tomography using intravenous contrast and delayed imaging may detect the number and size of the lesions. Although hepatic angiography has been used in the past, it is not routinely employed in modern clinical practice to provide a specific diagnosis.

None of these tests will provide definitive histological diagnosis but the role of needle biopsy or aspiration of suspected hepatic lesions remains much debated. A biopsy is absolutely contraindicated for patients with suspected haemangioma, haemangioendothelioma and cysts suspected of being echinococcal in origin. In addition, it may be dangerous in patients with suspected hypervascular solid tumours to undertake either needle biopsy or fine needle aspiration cytology. Such invasive investigation may be associated with haemorrhage, sampling error, misdiagnosis and needle-tract tumour seeding. Tissue from a haemangioma may resemble fibrosis and focal nodular hyperplasia may resemble cirrhosis. Needle samples of hepatic adenoma may be interpreted as normal tissue and may be difficult to differentiate from hepatocellular carcinoma. Percutaneous biopsy should only be performed in those patients who are not considered candidates for surgical intervention and only where the results of biopsy might influence further management. Despite extensive radiological imaging in an attempt to characterise the lesion, the final diagnosis may not be made until the lesion has been resected and the pathologist can undertake definitive examination of the resected lesion.

It is therefore apparent that the general surgeon should have a working knowledge of the management of patients with benign liver tumours. It is of vital importance that the surgeon is thoroughly familiar with the gross appearance, clinical significance and natural history of these benign lesions and the multidisciplinary approach with medical and surgical gastroenterologist and radiologist should be maintained when such a patient presents for investigation.

Classification

Although a variety of benign liver tumours have been described, by far the majority are sufficiently rare that they can easily be labelled medical curiosities. A detailed description of these various pathological lesions is beyond the scope of the current text[1-3] but the various benign pathological lesions are listed, based on cell lines, in Table 2.1. The majority of benign hepatic lesions encountered in clinical practice include hepatic cyst, haemangioma, bile duct hamartoma, focal nodular hyperplasia and liver cell adenoma. For completeness, a brief resumé is provided of less common and miscellaneous lesions, including hepatic abscess, since these may give rise to diagnostic dilemma.

Haemangioma

Haemangiomas are the most common benign hepatic tumour of mesenchymal origin. Small capillary haemangiomas of the liver are more common than the larger cavernous haemangiomas and are often multiple, always incidental findings. These may give rise to diagnostic difficulty in patients undergoing investigation for other hepatic pathology. Small lesions are almost always asymptomatic and once accurate diagnosis has been made no further therapy is needed. Haemangiomas are probably of congenital origin rather than neoplastic and they do not undergo malignant transformation. The incidence of cavernous haemangioma of the liver in autopsy series varies considerably but has been

Table 2.1 *Classification of benign tumours of the liver*[a]

Epithelial tumours
    Hepatocellular
        Nodular transformation
        Focal nodular hyperplasia
        Hepatocellular adenoma
    Cholangiocellular
        Bile duct adenoma
        Biliary cystadenoma

Mesenchymal tumours
    Tumours of adipose tissue
        Lipoma
        Myelolipoma
        Angiomyolipoma
    Tumours of muscle tissue
        Leiomyoma
    Tumours of blood vessels
        Infantile haemangioendothelioma
        Haemangioma
            hereditary haemorrhagic telangiectasia
            peliosis hepatis
    Tumours of mesothelial tissue
        Benign mesothelioma

Mixed mesenchymal and epithelial tumours
    Mesenchymal hamartoma
    Benign teratoma

Miscellaneous
    Adrenal rest tumour
    Pancreatic heterotopia
    Inflammatory pseudotumour

---

[a] From Ishak KG, Goodman ZD. Benign tumours of the liver. In: Berk JE (ed) Bockus Gastroenterology, 4th edn, Philadelphia: WB Saunders, 1985, pp. 3302.

reported as high as 8%. These lesions are considered the second most common hepatic tumour in the United States, exceeded only by hepatic metastases.[2] With the more widespread use of sensitive imaging studies of the upper abdomen, the identification of cavernous haemangiomas as an incidental finding will undoubtedly be more common. Cavernous haemangiomas may reach enormous size and lesions weighing up to 6 kg are well documented. Giant haemangiomas are defined as those 4 cm in diameter or greater.[4] Such haemangiomas are usually solitary, but multiple lesions have been described in about 10% of cases. They may be associated with similar lesions in the skin and other organs. Lesions are usually evenly distributed throughout the liver and within the liver substance but large lesions situated peripherally may form a pedicle.

Pathology

Cavernous haemangiomas occur in all age groups but are most frequently seen in patients in the third to fifth decades of life. They are more common and more likely to become clinically manifest at a younger age in women and are more common with increasing parity and may enlarge during pregnancy.[5–7] This indicates a possible role of female sex hormones in the development of hepatic haemangiomas, although an association with the oral contraceptive pill has not been proven. The aetiology of liver haemangiomas is still unclear but it is considered that they represent benign congenital hamartomas. These lesions appear to grow by progressive ectasia rather than hyperplasia or hypertrophy. At operation they may be multilobulated or smooth surfaced and large surface vessels may be evident. There is a dissectable plane between the lesion and the normal liver parenchyma. When sectioned, the lesion will partially collapse due to the escape of blood and has a honeycombed cut surface. There may be gross evidence of thrombosis, fibrosis or calcification. Microscopically, the haemangiomas are composed of cystically dilated vascular spaces, characteristic of cavernous haemangiomas. The lining consists of endothelial cells. The septic walls consist of fibrous tissue and the septae are relatively thin. The cavernous spaces may contain clotted blood.

Clinical presentation

Most haemangiomas are asymptomatic until they exceed a diameter of 10 cm. Symptoms are often non-specific and include vague abdominal pain, abdominal fullness, early satiety, nausea, vomiting or fever. Rare presentations include obstructive jaundice, biliary colic, gastric outlet obstruction and spontaneous rupture. Pain is most likely due to stretching of Glisson's capsule. Intra-abdominal haemorrhage due to spontaneous rupture of the lesion is a rare complication.[7] Thrombocytopenia and hypofibrinogenaemia have also been associated with cavernous haemangiomas of the liver and this effect may be related to consumption of coagulation factors.[2]

When a large haemangioma is present, the liver edge or a non-tender mass which descends with inspiration may be palpable. It is difficult to differentiate the consistency of a haemangioma from normal liver through the abdominal wall unless it has calcified or undergone thrombosis or fibrosis. Occasionally, a bruit is heard over a haemangioma, but this is a relatively non-specific finding. Liver function tests are normal in the patient presenting without complication.

Such lesions are generally hyperechoic on ultrasound examination. Farges et al.[8] found the diagnosis established by ultrasonography alone in 80% of the patients with haemangiomas smaller than 6 cm. However, this investigation alone cannot differentiate a haemangioma from hepatocellular carcinoma, liver cell adenoma, focal nodular hyperplasia, or a solitary metastasis. Computed tomography has proven most useful in the diagnosis of haemangiomas.[9] Prior to intravenous contrast infusion, computed tomography scan shows the haemangioma to consist of a well-demarcated hypodense mass. After the intravenous injection of contrast medium, serial scans will reveal a zone of progressive enhancement peripherally that varies in thickness and often demonstrates an irregular margin. The centre of the haemangioma remains hypodense and the overall lesion size does not change. Selective hepatic angiography shows a characteristic pattern consisting of normal-sized hepatic arteries without neovascularity or 'corkscrewing'. Typically there is rapid filling of the large blood-filled spaces of the haemangioma with contrast medium, producing the so-called 'cottonwool' appearance surrounding the feeding hepatic arteries. The computed tomography findings are often sufficiently characteristic that the role for angiography in the diagnosis of cavernous haemangiomas is limited.[9] Magnetic resonance imaging has been shown to have a high degree of specificity in the diagnosis of hepatic haemangiomas[10] and in a recent study,[8] it had a greater than 90% sensitivity.

Needle biopsy of vascular liver lesions should not be performed. Diagnostic uncertainty is seldom a problem with cavernous haemangiomas except where lesions not large enough to show cavernous characteristics may necessitate diagnostic removal.

Management

A wide range of management strategies from observation to resection have been advocated for such lesions. The therapeutic modalities of hepatic arterial ligation, radiation therapy and corticosteroids have also been reported with limited success. Clearly, in patients in whom such lesions have been detected as an incidental finding, simple reassurance should be given to the patient. For larger cavernous haemangiomas, consideration should be given between the risk of operation and the natural history of untreated lesions. In a study assessing the natural history, Trastek *et al.*[7] followed-up 34 untreated patients who were observed for a maximum of 15 years. No patient had a lesion which bled, none reported abdominal symptoms, and no patient had compromise of quality of life.

In a further report from the same group, two patients were subsequently lost to follow-up, and the observation period had been extended to 21 years with a mean follow-up of 12.5 years. Twenty-five patients remained asymptomatic and two patients with symptomatic lesions that were large and of questionable resectability at initial presentation remained symptomatic but with little documented growth of the haemangioma. There was no instance of rupture.[11]

Nichols *et al.*[11] reported the results of the resection of 41 cavernous haemangiomas of the liver. Twenty-five resections were in symptomatic patients and 21 of these had giant haemangiomas. There were no operative deaths and the single postoperative complication was a wound infection. Fifteen patients had resection of haemangiomas less than 4 cm in diameter. Only four of these patients were symptomatic. The remaining 11 patients had resection because of uncertainty in the diagnosis, to rule out metastatic disease while undergoing some other cancer operation, or when a haemangioma was found in a specimen that was resected for metastatic disease. Although safe resection of cavernous haemangiomas is possible, there is no evidence that asymptomatic patients should undergo resection since the risk of rupture is minimal.[8] The indications for resection are therefore symptomatic lesions in patients with an acceptable surgical risk and cases where the nature of the lesion is not established despite preoperative investigation.

When treatment is indicated, surgical excision provides the only effective therapy. Reports of the effectiveness of hepatic arterial ligation are anecdotal. Arterial ligation or embolisation may, however, be considered for the temporary control of haemorrhage in exceptional circumstances in order to allow time for definitive management in a specialist centre. The benefits of radiation in the treatment of cavernous haemangiomas have not been well documented and are inconsistent. Similarly, the effectiveness of corticosteroids in the treatment of haemangiomas is not well documented. It is possible that the success of non-resective therapy which has been ascribed to steroids, radiation and hepatic arterial ligation may well be largely due to the naturally occurring spontaneous involution of such lesions in children.

The choice of resection requires consideration of the size of the lesion, the anatomic location and the experience of the surgeon. Although no margin of normal liver tissue is required, it may in some cases be wiser and safer to perform a formal anatomic hepatectomy or extended hepatectomy in preference to enucleation or local wedge resection. At enucleation, a plane between the lesion and the liver is easily found and this can be developed by blunt dissection. This can be facilitated by the use of the Cavitron ultrasonic surgical aspirator (CUSA) with concomitant temporary control of the inflow vessels.

Liver cell adenoma

Although liver cell adenoma requires differentiation from any solid hepatic lesion, it is often considered alongside focal nodular hyperplasia.[12,13] Hepatic adenomas arise in otherwise normal liver and present as a focal abnormality or mass. The true incidence of the disease is difficult to assess. These were rarely reported before 1960, but it is recognised as an increasing cause of hepatic tumour in both males and females, although 90% develop in women in the third to fifth decades of life.[14,15] The introduction of oral contraceptives in 1960 and the apparent increase in frequency of hepatic adenomas in young women, strongly suggests that oral ingestion of oestrogens plays an important role in its development.[16] 90% of patients with hepatic adenomas have used oral contraceptives and the annual incidence among oral contraceptive users has been reported to be 3–4 per 100 000 in users for more than two years. The risk of development increases with its duration of use and strength of preparation. The introduction of low oestrogen-containing contraceptive preparations may result in a reduction in incidence, although adenomas are also associated with non-contraceptive oestrogen use, adrogenic steroid use, diabetes, glycogen storage disease, galactosaemia and iron overload. This association implicates non-aligned metabolic alteration in carbohydrate in the formation of liver cell adenomas.[17]

Pathology

Hepatic adenomas are usually solitary, round and occasionally encapsulated. Lesions are soft and smooth surfaced, but occasionally may be pedunculated. The cut surface has a pale yellow fleshy appearance and central degeneration and discoloration from haemorrhage are often seen. They are sharply demarcated from normal liver, although no fibrous capsule is present. Multiple lesions may be present in liver adenomatosis and one case of spontaneous transformation to cancer has been reported.[17]

Microscopically, the diagnosis is based on the findings of uniform masses of benign-appearing hepatocytes without ducts or portal triads. The hepatocytes appear paler than normal because of increased glycogen or fat content. Venous lakes (peliosis hepatis) are often seen. About 10% of surgically excised hepatic adenomas harbour foci of hepatocellular carcinoma.

Clinical presentation

Adenomas are typically seen in women over the age of 30 years with a history of oral contraceptive use. More than 35% of the patients will present with abdominal pain caused by haemorrhage into the tumour or adjacent liver. In 10–30% of patients, pain may be due to rupture and haemoperitoneum which may be associated with hypovolaemic shock. Up to one-third of patients sense the presence of an abdominal mass.[18] The remainder of adenomas are discovered incidentally at autopsy, laparotomy or during radiological assessment for another problem.

Although the clinical presentation may be suggestive of liver cell adenoma, definitive preoperative diagnosis may be difficult. Liver function tests are generally only abnormal in patients with associated tumour necrosis or haemorrhage. Anaemia may be present because of the tendency of these tumours to bleed. Ultrasound scan can detect small adenomas which characteristically display a lesion of mixed echoity and heterogeneous texture. Computed tomography may show evidence of recent haemorrhage or necrosis. Lesions are generally hypodense prior to infusion of contrast medium and demonstrate a wide range of densities after intravenous contrast administration. If undertaken, selective visceral angiography shows a hypervascular tumour with irregular areas of hypovascularity secondary to haemorrhage or necrosis. Hepatic adenomas generally exhibit a peripheral blood supply.[19] In the young female, the differential diagnosis is normally with that of fibronodular hyperplasia. An isotope scan may be helpful in pointing towards a diagnosis of adenoma which does not take up any isotope and therefore appears as a filling defect.

Our own experience has shown that percutaneous needle biopsy or fine needle aspiration cytology undertaken prior to referral is often misleading. Biopsy of these vascular tumours risks precipitating haemorrhage and even an experienced histopathologist may experience difficulty in differentiating between adenoma and a well-differentiated hepatocellular carcinoma.

Management

In the symptomatic patient, surgical intervention will be required. A minority of patients will present with intraperitoneal bleeding, the cause of which might only be identified at laparotomy. If ultrasound has been undertaken preoperatively, the presence of a hepatic mass may give a clue as to the underlying pathology. Hepatic arterial embolisation or packing might be considered to facilitate transfer of the patient to a specialist centre. Definitive control of bleeding is best achieved by formal hepatic resection. In some patients, haemorrhage may be contained within the liver or subcapsularly. If the patient remains haemodynamically stable, it may be prudent to defer elective surgical intervention to enable resolution of the haematoma, thereby enabling a more limited hepatic resection (Fig. 2.1).

For the asymptomatic patient, surgical intervention should still be considered. Non-operative discrimination between hepatic adenoma and hepatocellular carcinoma is difficult. Hepatic adenomas are known to harbour foci of tumour and may be premalignant lesions. Hepatic adenomas more commonly produce symptoms and may result in life-threatening haemorrhage. Several case reports document regression of liver cell tumours following cessation of oral contraceptives, although development of hepatocellular carcinoma in the site of adenoma regression has been reported. Patients must be individually evaluated and the risk of hepatic resection weighed against future morbidity and risk of mortality.

Most deaths from liver cell adenomas are secondary to haemorrhage, with intraperitoneal bleeding carrying a 20% mortality rate in one reported series.[14]

Focal nodular hyperplasia

Focal nodular hyperplasia (FNH) is often difficult to differentiate from adenoma and for this reason represents a substantial proportion of benign lesions submitted to hepatic resection (Table 2.2). The incidence of focal nodular hyperplasia has been increasing, although this is more likely to be related to improvements in abdominal imaging rather than a true increase in incidence. Many lesions are still found incidentally at laparotomy or autopsy. About 90% of cases occur in women, primarily in the second and third decades, although the condition may also afflict older women and a small number of men and children.

The incidence does not appear to have increased since the introduction of oral contraceptives and in a review by Kerlin et al.[15] the patient had used oral contraceptives in only 58% of cases. However, oral contra-

Figure 2.1 (a) *CT scan showing extensive subcapsular haematoma resulting from spontaneous haemorrhage into the liver.*

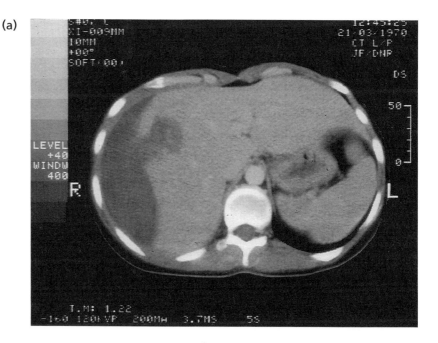

(b) *CT scan taken two months later showing a reduction in the size of the haematoma. Contrast is now present within a small adenoma lying adjacent to the haematoma.*

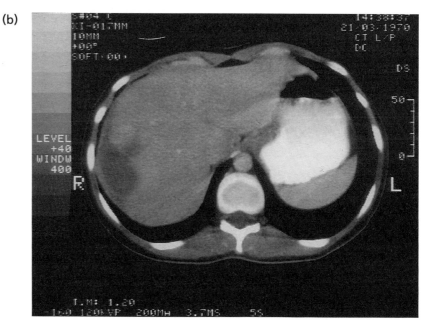

ceptives may foster growth or increased vascularity of focal nodular hyperplasia and have been implicated in the few cases which present with haemorrhage. Haemorrhage is therefore rare and, unlike adenoma, malignant transformation does not occur.

Table 2.2 *Indications for 29 hepatic resections for benign disease of liver in the Hepatobiliary Unit, Royal Infirmary, Edinburgh, October 1988–August 1996*

Diagnosis	Resection	
	Classical	Segmental
Focal nodular hyperplasia	5	1
Adenoma	1	0
Inflammatory mass (pseudotumour)	4	0
Cysts	6	0
Cystadenoma	1	0
Haemangioma	2	0
Biliary stricture	2	0
Primary sclerosing cholangitis	2	0
Trauma	3	1
Intrahepatic stones	1	0
Total	27	2

Pathology

Focal nodular hyperplasia has many similarities to liver cell adenoma and distinguishing between the two may be difficult. It consists of a firm lobulated localised lesion in an otherwise normal liver. These nodules are generally several centimetres in size and occasionally can grow much larger. Lesions are well circumscribed but have no capsule. On sectioning, there is generally a central scar with fibrous radiations which account for the nodular and sometimes umbilicated appearance. Lesions are usually lighter in colour than surrounding normal hepatic parenchyma since its vascularity is prominent.

Microscopically, focal nodular hyperplasia looks similar to cirrhosis with regenerating nodules and connective tissue septae. The lesions consist of many normal hepatic cells mixed with bile ducts or ductules and divided by fibrous bands of septae. The septae contain numerous bile ducts and a moderate predominantly lymphocytic infiltration and there is usually some evidence of mild cholestasis.

Clinical features

FNH is a benign process that does not cause symptoms but the main difficulty lies in differentiating this process from other hepatic lesions. Less than 10% of patients with focal nodular hyperplasia have symptoms which usually consist of mild chronic or intermittent abdominal pain. Acute symptoms due to haemorrhage are exceptional.

Most imaging techniques cannot reliably establish the diagnosis of focal nodular hyperplasia. The appearances on ultrasound and compu-

Figure 2.2 (a)
Iodised oil emulsion enhanced CT scan showing a mass lesion in segments V and VI of the liver but not previously evident on intravenous contrast enhanced CT scan. Percutaneous fine needle aspiration cytology undertaken under US guidance had suggested the diagnosis of adenoma.

(a)

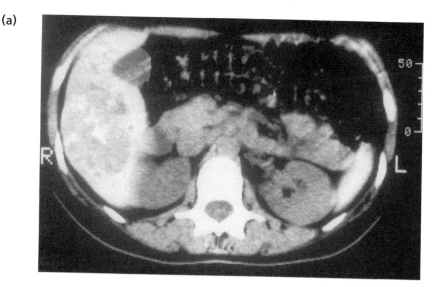

(b) *Selective hepatic angiogram of the same patient demonstrating a hypervascular lesion with an apparent tumour circulation arising from the right hepatic artery. The lesion was subsequently excised and confirmed on histology to be focal nodular hyperplasia.*

(b)

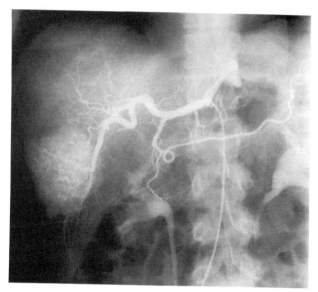

ter tomographic scans are non-specific. The lesion may not be evident on a CT scan. A more invasive investigation, such as arteriography is highly sensitive but lacks specificity (Fig. 2.2). The majority of arteriograms show a sharply delineated hypervascular mass with a single central artery and centrifugal filling of the vessels. Magnetic resonance imaging may aid in diagnosis of focal nodular hyperplasia but its reliability requires to be evaluated.

Management

Treatment of a patient with focal nodular hyperplasia depends essentially on the certainty of the diagnosis. Many surgeons believe that patients should be submitted to open biopsy because of the difficulty in establishing a diagnosis preoperatively and because of the dangers of needle biopsy.[20] Resection should be undertaken if it can be performed with minimal morbidity for any lesion that is increasing in size, bleeding or unequivocally symptomatic.

Recent data on the natural history of focal nodular hyperplasia have been gathered by Kerlin et al.[15] Of 41 patients studied, 11 had lesions found incidentally at autopsy. Sixteen patients had open surgical biopsies of clinically apparent lesions with the bulk of the lesions left in situ. These patients were observed for up to 15 years, during which time none of the lesions bled or increased in size. Although it could be claimed that such lesions are best managed conservatively, a balanced approach is best adopted, with surgical excision being undertaken if this can be undertaken with minimal morbidity and mortality. Observation in selected patients may be considered if there is a significant risk of morbidity with surgical intervention.

Bile duct adenoma

The surgeon requires to be aware of bile duct adenoma since they are common and may be mistaken on operative examination of the liver for metastatic disease.

Bile duct hamartomas do not manifest clinically but are incidental findings at laparotomy or autopsy.[21] They rarely exceed 1 cm in diameter and appear as raised greyish-white areas on the liver capsule and are composed of mature bile ducts and surrounding fibrous stroma. When they are found singly, they are often referred to as adenomas, but when multiple, as hamartomas even though the microscopic morphology is identical. At histological examination, these lesions are non-encapsulated but have a fibrous stroma which blends indistinctly into the adjacent liver. They require to be distinguished from the nests of hyerplastic bile ducts which occur in focal nodular hyperplasia and also undifferentiated adenocarcinomas of the biliary tract type. The only clinical significance of the bile duct adenoma is its possible confusion at laparotomy with metastatic carcinoma, cholangiocarcinoma or other focal hepatic lesions.

Hepatic pseudotumour

Hepatic pseudotumours may be considerable in size and can occur in any age group. These lesions are essentially overgrowths of chronic inflammatory tissue but may be mistaken for sarcomas. Some pseudotumours may result from healed abscesses. The pseudotumour appears as a hypodense lesion on computed tomography and may be either hyperechoic or hypoechoic on ultrasonography. Arteriography reveals a hypervascular mass.

Such pseudotumours may require resection to prevent reactivation of infection. The clinical history and presentation are likely to point towards a diagnosis of pseudotumour.

Miscellaneous benign tumours

Mesenchymal hamartomas are exceptional and probably of congenital origin. Such lesions are, therefore, most commonly described in infants under 12 months,[22] although a few have been described in adults.[23] Although such lesions are entirely benign, hamartomas can compromise the liver and the individual by progressive enlargement and should therefore be resected. A recurrence following excision has not been reported. Primary myxoma in the adult is exceptional.[24] Primary lipomas are rarely described in life but have been identified incidentally at post-mortem.[2] Other solid tumours include leiomyoma, mesothelioma and fibroma.[2] Benign teratoma of the liver has been reported but these generally occur in children.[2,22]

Liver abscess

The incidence of pyogenic liver abscess has remained relatively constant during this century despite earlier diagnosis and treatment of underlying causes and more aggressive antibiotic therapies.[25–28] In recent years, the decrease in cases resulting from haematogenous spread from infected foci has been mirrored by an increase in cases secondary to hepatobiliary pathology. In almost half the patients reviewed in our own centre over a four-year period, biliary sepsis was the major predisposing factor. In 20% of patients, the presumed source of infection was from the portal route but few cases were thought to have arisen from systemic infection.[28]

In most patients, the diagnosis will be evident and the patients present with symptoms of abdominal pain, fever and jaundice. Pyrexia is present in 75% of cases. The alkaline phosphatase is always abnormal in hepatic sepsis and 74% of patients demonstrate elevation in serum alanine aminotransferase levels.[28] On ultrasound scan it is invariably diagnostic and will demonstrate a fluid-filled cavity which will appear as a hypoechoic lesion. There may be a hyperechioc wall, the presence of which is dependent on the clinicity of the abscess. Computed tomography may be useful to exclude the presence of other abscesses and to identify a primary source within the abdomen.

Management includes percutaneous aspiration of pus for bacteriological analysis. Percutaneous drainage may be required for large chronic abscesses and decompression of the biliary tree may be required where obstruction of the bile duct has contributed to the development of hepatic abscess. The key to successful management is the administration of appropriate antibiotic therapy which is determined by the results of culture of aspirated pus and blood.

In our experience, one third of patients will not survive admission to hospital, although this reflects the high proportion of patients developing hepatic abscess related to underlying malignancy and biliary obstruction.

Amoebic abscess

This form of abscess is sufficiently common that it should be considered in the differential diagnosis of hepatic lesions. Liver abscess is the most common extra-intestinal manifestation of amoebiasis and is reported in 3–10% of affected patients. Males are more commonly affected than females and the highest incidence is in the 20–50-year-old age group.[29]

The diagnosis is likely to be straightforward in areas where amoebiasis is endemic. It should be recognised, however, that the liver abscess may present many years after previous intestinal infection. Some 75–90% of abscesses are in the right lobe and involvement of the left lobe usually indicates more advanced disease. Rupture occurs in less than 5% of cases. Signs and symptoms of the amoebic liver abscess are the same as for pyogenic abscess. On ultrasound and CT scanning, the boundaries of the abscess are generally poorly defined.

A preliminary diagnosis can be made on the basis of a dramatic clinical response to metranidozole. If clinical symptoms do not resolve within 48 hours of treatment, an incorrect diagnosis or a secondary bacterial infection should be suspected. Percutaneous aspiration produces a sterile and odourless fluid which is described as having the appearance of anchovy paste.

Hydatid cysts

Echinococcus is a cestode that can give rise to liver abscess. These collections are better classified as cysts rather than abscesses because the organism is almost entirely determined by the hepatic environment and little host inflammatory reaction is present. An intense fibrous reaction around the lesion is characteristic but there is no epithelial lining to the cyst. The incidence of *Echinococcus granulosis* is in decline but sporadic cases are reported in Europe, Australia, New Zealand, South America, Asia and Africa. The prevalence of human echinococcus is directly related to contact with dogs and sheep. *Echinococcus multilocularis* or alveolar hydatid disease is much less common, although it is a much more dangerous condition. It pursues a more invasive course than the more conventional form of the disease but is fortunately confined to specific areas of the United States and Europe.

Hydatid cysts are most commonly unilocular and may grow as large as 20 cm. The cyst wall is about 1 mm thick and consists of an external laminated hilar membrane and an internal enucleated general layer. The cyst is colourless or light yellow and contains daughter cysts, small replicas of the mother. In addition, there are numerous protocoscolices within the fluid, free or grouped in small capsules of germinal layers, known as brood capsules. They may resemble sand, leading to the term 'hydatid sand'. About 75% of lesions are in the right lobe and 25% in the left, although both lobes are involved in approximately 30% of cases.

Clinical presentation

Clinical symptoms of echinococcal cystic disease are often insidious but there is usually a history of contact with dogs or sheep. Distension of the liver capsule may produce right upper quadrant pain. Jaundice is infrequent but may be due to extrinsic biliary compression or direct communication with obstruction by cystic debris. Liver function tests are generally abnormal and eosinophilia is present in up to one-third of patients.

Echinococcal disease may occasionally mimic a primary liver tumour and metastatic disease. Serology may be helpful in establishing a diagnosis. Plain abdominal radiographs may reveal a calcified cyst wall. Ultrasound and CT scanning may demonstrate septae or sand within the cyst. A cyst wall is generally evident. Percutaneous aspiration and drainage should be avoided because of the risk of dissemination or anaphylaxis. Several cases resembling sclerosing cholangitis have been reported after the percutaneous instillation of scolicidal agents.

Management

Once the diagnosis has been established, surgery is generally required. Heavy calcification may be suggestive of old past infection and in the more elderly, frail patient, surgery might best be avoided. Treatment with mebendazole has been advocated by some, although there remains considerable doubt as to its efficacy. This drug is best given prophylactically before surgical intervention to minimise the risks of hydatid spread.[30–32]

At operation, the operating field is generally packed off with swabs soaked in hypertonic saline. Some surgeons would advocate that scolicidal agents such as hypertonic saline, 0.5% silver nitrate, chlorhexidine, formalin and alcohol be avoided because of anaphylactic reaction, and peritoneal irritation. Aspiration and instillation of scolicidal agents have been abandoned because of the risks of biliary contamination and sclerosing cholangitis. Pericystectomy is generally recommended but should preserve only those portions of the cyst wall which come into contact with major blood vessels which can be identified by means of intraoperative ultrasonography. For smaller, more peripheral lesions, formal hepatic resection may be considered and has been advocated by some where a diagnostic dilemma remains.

Cysts

Non-parasitic cystic disease of the liver can result from a congenital malformation of the intrahepatic bile ducts. These cysts are normally categorised to one of two types.

Simple cysts of the liver

Simple cysts contain serous fluid and do not communicate with the intrahepatic biliary tree. They may also be referred to as non-parasitic cysts of the liver, benign hepatic cysts, congenital hepatic cysts, unilocular cysts of the liver and solitary cysts of the liver, although this latter categorisation is inappropriate since simple cysts are invariably multiple. Small cysts are surrounded by normal liver tissue, although as these enlarge, there may be displacement and atrophy of adjacent hepatic tissue. A large cyst may occupy an entire lobe of the liver and result in compensatory hypertrophy of the residual liver. Such simple cysts have no septae and are unilocular. These cysts have no wall and are lined by a single layer of cuboid or columnar epithelial cells which resemble those of the biliary epithelium. Such simple cysts have previously been considered to be rare, with a prevalence of about 1%.[33] Although it is true that symptomatic or complicated simple cysts are rare, asymptomatic cysts are extremely common and are frequently detected as an incidental finding during radiological imaging of the liver (O.J. Garden, personal observation). Interestingly, female to male ratio is 1.5:1 in asymptomatic simple cysts demonstrated at post-mortem or at incidental hepatic imaging,[33] however, the ratio rises to 9:1 in symptomatic or complicated simple cysts.[34] Huge cysts affect almost exclusively women over the age of 50 years.[33]

Clinical presentation

It is rare for simple cysts to give rise to symptoms but increase in the size of such cysts produces abdominal pain, distension or discomfort. Anorexia and early satiety are not uncommon. Acute onset of pain may signal the development of intracystic haemorrhage,[34] rupture or infection. Cholestasis may result from biliary compression[34,35] and portal hypertension.[35]

A safe diagnosis can be made on the basis of abdominal ultrasonography which demonstrates a circular anechoic area with a well-defined boundary with the liver. No wall is evident and posterior acoustic enhancement arises because of the accentuation of the ultrasound waves beyond the cyst. Examination of the kidneys is useful to exclude the presence of polycystic disease. Further diagnostic investigation is rarely required, although where intervention is contemplated, computed tomography will exclude the presence of other cysts. Cysts appear as well-rounded water-dense lesions without septae (Fig. 2.3). Intravenous contrast enhancement will confirm the avascularity of these lesions. Scintigraphy and angiography are not required to make a diagnosis. Where complications such as haemorrhage occur, the simple cyst may appear relatively thick walled and may contain cystic debris. In such instances, serological tests should be undertaken to exclude parasitic infection. It should be borne in mind that calcification is absent in simple cysts but may be present with hydatid cysts.

Figure 2.3 *CT scan demonstrating a large benign cyst occupying the entire right lobe of the liver. At least two further cysts are seen in the caudate and left lobes of the liver. Note the normal left kidney. This patient underwent successful laparoscopic deroofing of the cyst.*

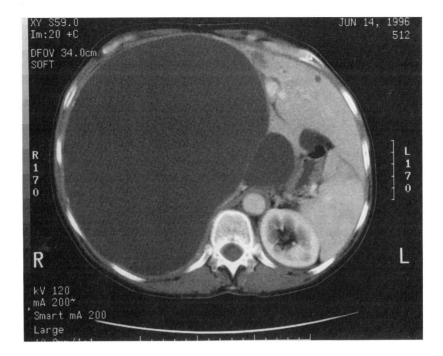

Management

There has been much recent debate regarding the management of simple liver cysts. Asymptomatic simple cysts require no treatment. Percutaneous aspiration risks introducing infection and does not provide definitive therapy.[36] For symptomatic or complicated simple cysts, partial excision or deroofing has, in the past, been the established conventional treatment. Total cystectomy is not required and is hazardous because, unlike hydatid disease, there is no plane of dissection between the cyst and the liver. In recent years, laparoscopic deroofing or fenestration of such solitary cysts has been advocated.[37,38] Few substantial series of patients have been reported, although good short-term outcome was reported in a series of four patients by Morino *et al*.[39] A longer-term follow-up in our own patient population suggests that a laparoscopic approach may not allow a sufficiently radical fenestration to prevent a recurrence in the longer term. Even at open surgery, deroofing of large centrally placed cysts may not prevent reconstitution of the cyst with recurrence of symptoms. In such patients, we would now advocate more radical resection which does not generally involve substantial sacrifice of functioning hepatic parenchyma.

Polycystic liver disease (PCLD)

Adult polycystic kidney disease (Fig. 2.4) is frequently associated with multiple liver cysts which are macroscopically and microscopically similar to simple cysts of the liver. However, in this condition, the liver cysts are multiple when present and may extensively replace both lobes of the liver. In addition to the macroscopic cysts, there are usually numerous microscopic cysts and clusters of multiple bile ductules, designated as Von Meyenburgh complexes. The condition is an autosomal dominant disorder and carries a much more sinister prognosis because of the risk of chronic renal failure. The development of liver cysts is constantly preceded by the development of renal cysts and the prevalence of macroscopic liver cysts associated with adult polycystic kidney disease increases with the age of patient.[40]

Clinical presentation

In most patients with adult polycystic kidney disease, the liver cysts are clinically silent, although these may, in a few patients, give rise to abdominal pain, distension and discomfort. There are rarely signs to suggest cholestasis, liver failure or portal hypertension and liver function tests are usually normal. Both ultrasonography and computed tomography will demonstrate multiple fluid-filled cysts with well-defined margins in the liver and the kidneys. Liver cysts increase in size slowly and complications are uncommon. Rupture and bacterial infection may arise and is said to be more common with immunosuppression.[41]

Management

Asymptomatic cysts require no treatment. Percutaneous aspiration and installation of sclerosant rarely produce satisfactory relief of symptoms. Surgical drainage or fenestration afford only temporary relief. Any form of surgery is often associated with transient but massive ascites.[42] Some have suggested that laparoscopic deroofing may provide good short-term relief of symptoms,[39] but long-term follow-up data are lacking. There is, however, recent evidence to suggest that a more aggressive open surgical approach involving resection of the liver may provide longer lasting relief of symptoms[43,44] but it should be appreciated that hepatic resection is difficult in such patients. Careful selection of patients is required, since the symptoms of abdominal pain may have both renal and hepatic components. Nonetheless, extensive resection with associated deroofing of hepatic cysts may allow the abdomen to better accommodate the enlarged residual liver (Fig. 2.4).

Summary

The key to successful management of patients with benign solid or cystic lesions of the liver is in accurate diagnosis and thorough knowledge of the natural history. Inappropriate investigation may give rise to morbidity and compromise definitive management. Modern liver resection can now be undertaken with minimal morbidity and mortality because of increasing centralisation of expertise and improved operative techniques. Nonetheless, a better understanding of the prognosis of unresected haemangioma, focal nodular hyperplasia and liver cell adenoma has made it possible to consider a more conservative approach. There seems

Figure 2.4.
(a) *Contrast-enhanced CT scan demonstrating the presence of multiple cysts within the liver and kidneys. Note the predominance of large cysts within the right lobe of the liver.*

(a)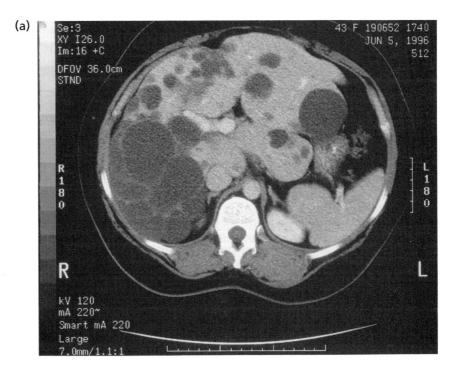

(b) *CT scan taken one month following right hepatectomy and deroofing of the residual cysts in the same patient.*

(b)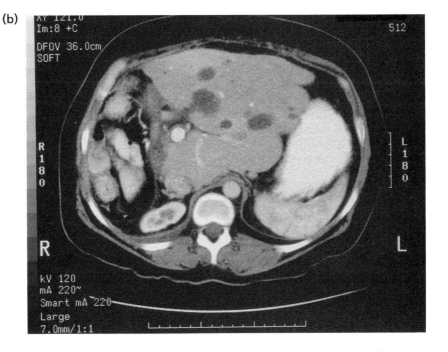

little doubt, however, that patients with symptomatic lesions or lesions which have the potential for further growth should undergo surgical treatment. Careful consideration must be given to the risk of hepatic resection against the possible morbidity or possible mortality from observation.

References

1. Edmondson HA. Benign epithelial tumours and tumorlike lesions of the liver. In: Okuda K, Peters RL (eds) Hepatocellular carcinoma. New York, John Wiley, 1976, pp. 309–30.
2. Ishak KG, Rabin L. Benign tumors of the liver. Med Clin North Am 1975; 59: 995–1013.
3. Henson SW, Gray HK, Dockerty MB. Benign tumors of the liver. Surg Gynec Obstet 1956; 103: 23–30.
4. Adams YG, Huves AG, Fortner JG. Giant hemangiomas of the liver. Ann Surg 1970; 172: 239–45.
5. Schwartz SI, Husser WG. Cavernous hemangioma of the liver: a single institution report of 16 resections. Ann Surg 1987; 205: 456–65.
6. Sewell JH, Weis K. Spontaneous rupture of hemangioma of the liver. Arch Surg 1961; 83: 105–9.
7. Trastek VF, van Heerden JA, Sheedy PF et al. Cavernous hemangiomas of the liver: resect or observe? Am J Surg 1983; 145: 49–53.
8. Farges O, Daradkeh S, Bismuth H. Cavernous hemangiomas of the liver: are there any indications for resection? World J Surg 1995; 19: 19–24.
9. Johnson CM, Sheedy PF, Stanson AW et al. Computed tomography and angiography of cavernous hemangiomas of the liver. Radiology 1985; 138: 115–21.
10. Börsch G, Uhlenbrock D, Beyer H et al. Magnetic resonance imaging in evaluating focal liver lesions. South Med J 1987; 80: 1125–8.
11. Nichols FC, van Heerden JA, Weiland LH. Benign liver tumors. Surg Clin North Am 1989; 69: 297–314.
12. Nagorney DM. Benign hepatic tumors: focal nodular hyperplasia and hepatocellular adenoma. World J Surg 1995; 19: 13–18.
13. Craig JR, Peters RL, Edmondson HA. Tumors of the liver and intrahepatic bile ducts. Atlas of tumor pathology 1989, Second Series, Fascicle 26. Washington DC: Armed Forces Institute of Pathology.
14. Rooks JB, Ory HW, Ishak KG et al. Epidemiology of hepatocellular adenoma: the role of oral contraceptive use. J Am Med Assoc 1979; 242: 644–8.
15. Kerlin P, Davis GL, McGill DB et al. Hepatic adenoma and focal nodular hyperplasia: clinical, pathologic and radiologic features. Gastroenterology 1983; 84: 994–1002.
16. Fechner RE. Benign hepatic lesions and orally administered contraceptives. Hum Path 1977; 8: 255–68.
17. Leese T, Farges O, Bismuth H. Liver cell adenomas: a 12 year surgical experience in a specialist hepatobiliary unit. Ann Surg 1988; 208: 558–64.
18. Mariani AF, Livingston AS, Pereiras Jr RV et al. Progressive enlargement of a hepatic cell adenoma. Gastroenterology 1979; 77: 1319.
19. Welch TJ, Sheedy PJ, Johnson CM et al. Focal nodular hyperplasia and hepatic adenoma: comparison of angiography, CT, US, and scintigraphy. Radiology 1985; 156: 593–5.
20. Belghiti J, Paterson D, Panis Y et al. Resection of presumed benign liver tumours. Br J Surg 1993; 80: 380–3.
21. Allaire GS, Rabin L, Ishak KG. Bile duct adenoma: a study of 152 cases. Am J Surg Path 1988; 12: 708–15.
22. Foster JH, Berman M. Solid liver tumors. Philadelphia: WB Saunders, 1977.
23. Grases PJ, Matos-Billaobos M, Arcia-Romero F, Lecuna-Torres V. Mesenchymal hamartoma of the liver. Gastroenterology 1979; 76: 1466–9.
24. Edmundson HA. Tumours of the liver and intrahepatic bile ducts. Atlas of tumor pathology 1958, Section VII, Fascicle 25, Washington DC: Armed Forces Institute of Pathology.
25. Rubin RH, Swartz MN, Malt R. Hepatic abscess: changes in clinical, bacteriological and therapeutic aspects. Am J Med 1974; 57: 601–10.
26. Pitt HA, Zuidema GD. Factors influencing mortality in the treatment of pyogenic hepatic

abscess. Surg Gynecol Obstet 1975; 140: 228–34.

27. Farges O, Leese T, Bismuth H. Pyogenic liver abscess: an improvement in prognosis. Br J Surg 1988; 75: 862–5.

28. Rintoul R, O'Riordain MG, Laurenson IF, Crosbie JL, Allan PL, Garden OJ. The changing management of pyogenic liver abscess. Br J Surg 1996; 83: 1215–18.

29. Greenstein AJ, Barth J, Dicker A *et al*. Amebic liver abscess: a study of 11 cases compared with a series of 38 patients with pyogenic liver abscess. A J Gastroenterol 1985; 80: 472–5.

30. Morris DL. Management of hydatid disease. Br J Hosp Med 1981; 25: 586–91.

31. Lewis JWJ, Koss N, Kerstein MD. A review of echinococcal disease. Ann Surg 1975; 181: 390–4.

32. Pitt HA, Korzelius J, Tompkins RK. Management of hepatic echinococcus in Southern California. A J Surg 1986; 152: 110–16.

33. Larson KA. Benign lesions affecting the bile ducts on a post-mortem cholangiogram. Acta Pathol Microbiol Immunol Scand 1961; 51: 47–62.

34. Moreaux J, Bloch P. Les kystes biliaires solitaires du foie. Arch Fr Mal App Dig 1971; 60: 203–24.

35. Johnstone AJ, Turnbull LW, Allan PL, Garden OJ. Cholangitis and Budd–Chiari syndrome as complications of simple cystic liver disease – a case report. HPB Surg 1993; 6: 223–8.

36. Saini S, Mueller PR, Ferucci JT Jr, Simeone JF, Wittenberg J, Butch RJ. Percutaneous aspiration of hepatic cysts does not provide definitive therapy. Am J Roentgenol 1983; 141: 559–60.

37. Paterson-Brown S, Garden OJ. Laser assisted laparoscopic excision of liver cyst. Br J Surg 1991; 78: 1047.

38. Tate JJ, Lau WY, Li AK. Transhepatic fenestration of liver cyst: a further application of laparoscopic surgery. Aust NZ J Surg 1994; 64: 264–5.

39. Morino M, De Giuri M, Festa Valentino, Garrone C. Laparoscopic management of symptomatic non-paracytic cysts of the liver. Ann Surg 1994; 214: 157–64.

40. Milutinovic J, Failkow PJ, Rudd TG, Agodoa LY, Phillips LA, Bryant JI. Liver cysts in patients with autosomal dominant polycystic kidney disease. Am J Med 1980; 68: 741–4.

41. Bourgeois M, Kinneart P, Vereerstraeten P, Shoutens A, Toussaint C. Infection of hepatic cysts following kidney transplantation in polycystic disease. World J Surg 1983; 7: 629–31.

42. Farges O, Bismuth H. Fenestration in the management of polycystic liver disease. World J Surg 1995; 19: 25–30.

43. Henne-Bruns D, Klomp H-J, Kremer B. Nonparasitic liver cysts and polycystic liver disease: results of surgical treatment. Hepatogastroenterology 1993; 40: 105.

44. Que F, Nagorney DM, Gross JB, Jr, Torres VE. Liver resection and cyst fenestration in the treatment of severe polycystic liver disease. Gastroenterology 1995; 108: 487–94.

3 Primary tumours of the liver

Olivier Farges
Jacques Belghiti

Hepatocellular carcinoma

Hepatocellular carcinoma (HCC) accounts for 90% of all primary liver malignancy and usually occurs on a background of chronic liver disease and in particular viral cirrhosis. HCC is therefore a major cause of death in high endemic areas of hepatitis B virus (HBV) or hepatitis C virus (HCV) infection. HCC is classically diagnosed at a late stage, and responds poorly to treatment. However, there has been considerable progress in the diagnosis and treatment of HCC over the past 10 years. HCC may now be identified at an early stage, in particular through the screening of high risk patients. Control of HCC nodules may be successfully achieved by surgical resection, transarterial chemoembolisation or percutaneous ethanol injection. The precise role of each treatment is currently being evaluated and will depend on the morphological features of the tumour and the functional status of the non-tumorous liver. These treatments, however, share a high incidence of tumour recurrence due to the persistence of the underlying cirrhosis that represents a preneoplasic condition. Liver transplantation appears as a logical alternative treatment but has its own limitations including the use of immunosuppressive agents that favour tumour recurrence (transplantation should only be indicated in patients with limited liver involvement and no extrahepatic spread), the limited availability of grafts, and its cost. The most exciting areas of progress are the control of HBV or HCV, the prevention of carcinogenesis in patients with chronic liver disease, and the development of adjuvant or neoadjuvant therapies.

Incidence

HCC is one of the most common malignant tumours in the world with an estimated number of new cases in excess of 1 million per year. The epidemiology of this disease is characterised by a striking geographic variation. It is a major cause of death in Eastern Asia, especially Taiwan (100 per 10^5 inhabitants), China (32 per 10^5 inhabitants), Japan (16 per 10^5 inhabitants), Singapore and Korea, as well as in sub-Saharan Africa, particularly Zimbabwe, Ethiopia and Mozambique (98 per 10^5 inhabitants) where it accounts for up to 50% of all malignancies. In Europe and North America, HCC occurs in 2–11 per 10^5 inhabitants and accounts for 1–2.5% of all malignancies. These geographical variations in incidence are closely related to the presence of environmental factors the most important of which are viral cirrhosis and aflatoxin B_1 exposure.

Aetiology

Liver cirrhosis and hepatitis B or C viruses

Liver cirrhosis is the predominant risk factor for the development of HCC with 80–90% of all HCC arising in cirrhotic livers. The precise nature of the relation between cirrhosis and HCC is still unclear. One mechanism may relate to the hepatocyte regeneration and increased cell proliferation associated with cirrhosis acting to promote carcinogenesis through DNA damage by environmental mutagens. This, in turn, may be favoured by a lower activity of enzymes involved in DNA repairing.[1] There is, however, no strict parallel geographical distribution of cirrhosis and HCC and the risk of HCC varies depending on the aetiology, epidemiology and natural history of cirrhosis.

HBV and HCV related cirrhosis

HBV and HCV are probably independent risk factors for hepatocarcinogenesis. This is in particular reflected by the very high rate of serological markers of HBV and/or HCV infection among HCC patients in high endemic areas (Table 3.1) and by the possible development of HCC in non-cirrhotic HBV or HCV-positive patients.[2,3]

Table 3.1 *Relative frequencies of serological markers of viral infection in HCC patients*

Country	Anti-HCV +ve HBsAg ±ve (%)	Anti-HCV −ve HBsAg +ve (%)	Anti-HCV +ve and/or HBsAg +ve (%)
Europe			
Italy, Spain, France	60–70	10–25	80–95
Germany, Switzerland	25–35	15–25	50
USA	15–40	10–30	20–70
Asia			
Taiwan, Hong Kong	10–40	50–80	80–95
Japan	50–75	15–35	70–95
South Africa	20–30	35–50	60–70

+ve: positive; −ve: negative; ±ve: positive or negative
Adapted from Caselmann WH, Alt M. J Hepatol 1996; 24 (Suppl. 2): 61–6.

In the case of HBV infection, there is evidence that HBV-DNA sequences integrate the genome of malignant hepatocytes and can be detected in the liver tissues of patients with HCC despite the absence of classical HBV serological markers.[4] HBV may be directly carcinogenic since, once integrated in the hepatocyte genome, it expresses polypeptides that transactivate cellular promoters. Furthermore, HBV may induce chronic hepatitis through its mutagenic effect by cycles of cell death and regeneration. This oncogenic potential of HBV has been confirmed by experiments using transgenic mice.[5]

The carcinogenic potential of HCV is less clear, in particular because this is an RNA virus that lacks a reverse transcriptase enzyme. Although HCV may be found in tumour cells at the molecular level, no genomic integration into the host chromosomal DNA has been documented. However, it has recently been shown that the 5′ half of the sequence encoding the HCV non-structural protein NS3 has oncogenic activity.[6] HCV could also promote hepatocarcinogenesis through chronic active hepatitis since high hepatocellular proliferation is associated with an increased risk of developing an HCC.

Although most HCC were thought initially to be HBV related, the importance of the HCV has become evident over the past 20 years. Through a better understanding of the mode of transmission of HBV infection and the development of effective vaccination plans, there has been a reduction in the proportion of HBV carriers and of HBV-related HCC. At the same time, HCV has been identified as the principal cause of non-A, non-B hepatitis and the high prevalence of HCV-infection recognised (HCV-carrier rate of 1% world-wide including Europe as compared to an HBV-carrier rate of 0.1% in Europe). It has been apparent that a high proportion of HCV-positive patients progress to cirrhosis (20–30% over a 20 year follow-up); and a comparable[7,8] or greater (up to 2.7 times[9]) carcinologic potential of HCV compared to HBV has been observed. Hence, over 60–75% of HCC patients in Japan, Italy, Spain and France are HCV positive and this trend is anticipated to become even more obvious in the near future. In other countries, the expansion of HCV infection probably accounts for the 1.7-fold increase in the age-adjusted incidence rate of HCC observed in Japan over the past 10 years. The average time interval between a contaminating blood transfusion and the occurrence of an HCC averages 30 years.[10]

Non-viral related cirrhosis

Genetic haemochromatosis is also associated with a high risk of HCC. The relative risk for the development of HCC in haemochromatosis with cirrhosis is greater than 200[11] and rises with increasing age. Among patients with cirrhosis, the cumulative incidence of HCC at 10 years is 30% but increases to 46% in patients greater than 55 years of age or who are HBsAg positive.[12] The cancer develops in highly iron-overloaded patients whether they ·have been de-ironed or not. As for viral diseases, HCC may also develop within fibrotic livers before cirrhosis develops.

Alcohol is also a classical risk factor for HCC. Its role should, however, probably be re-assessed in view of the high incidence of HCV or HBV infection in patients presumed to have an 'alcoholic' cirrhosis. The incidence of HCC in patients with autoimmune cirrhosis, biliary cirrhosis and Wilson disease are classically lower than in patients with other causes of cirrhosis. It is possible that these differences in the incidence of HCC are merely related to the gender, age, duration of exposure to the causative agent and variable natural history of each cirrhosis. The lower prevalence of HCC in biliary cirrhosis could be accounted for by the greater proportion of females than men or to the low regenerating activity of these livers. The greater proportion of HCC in viral cirrhosis and genetic haemochromatosis could be related to the longer duration of exposure to viruses in high endemic areas (where transmission occurs early in life) or to iron overload, respectively.

Risk and prevention of HCC in cirrhotic patients

The incidence of HCC in patients with cirrhosis has been calculated to be 1% per year in Europe,[13] 3% per year in Italy,[14,15] 6% per year in France[16] and 5.3–7% per year in Japan.[7,17] These variations can be accounted for by the proportion of posthepatic cirrhosis (7–14% per year) or non-viral related cirrhosis (2–4% per year)[8] in the studied populations, the mode and time of transmission of HBV or HCV (neonatal, early or late adulthood) and, yet poorly studied genetic factors. Age over 60 years, high proliferating activity of the liver and/or persistently high transaminase levels and presence of liver cell dysplasia further increase this risk.[15] In patients with chronic active hepatitis at a precirrhotic stage, the incidence of HCC is lower but figures as high as 0.5–1% have been reported. This risk seems much greater in those patients with raised α-fetoprotein (AFP) levels.

HCC is therefore a major health problem in countries, where rates of infection with HBV and HCV in the general population are high. It may for example be anticipated that the annual incidence of new HCC in Japan is 27 000 (300 000 cirrhosis × 7% + 1 200 000 chronic active hepatitis × 0.5%).

A major area of research is therefore centred on the prevention of the development of HCC in patients with chronic, viral-related, liver diseases. Recent studies have suggested that interferon (IFN) therapy in HCV-positive patients could prevent or delay the onset of HCC.[18,19] Further studies will be required to confirm or, as in the case of HBV infection, refute[20] this observation. Other drugs are also being evaluated.[21]

Aflatoxin B₁ exposure

Aflatoxin is ingested in food as a result of contamination of imperfectly stored staple crops by *Aspergillus flavus*. It is thought to induce HCC through mutation of the tumour suppressor gene P53. Although areas of high aflatoxin ingestion also have a high incidence of HBV, there is evidence both in sub-Saharan areas[22] and in China[23,24] that aflatoxin is an independent risk factor or at least that HBV and aflatoxin act as cocarcinogens.

Contraceptives and androgens
There is evidence that contraceptives and androgens are associated with the development of HCC. These risk factors however are minor when compared to cirrhosis, viral infection or aflatoxin exposure but may account for some of the HCC which develops within non-cirrhotic livers. The presumed sequence of events is that these hormones favour the development of adenoma which, in turn, may undergo malignant transformation. Although this evolution is well demonstrated, the risk of malignant transformation of an adenoma is not precisely known but is probably less than 10%.

Age and sex
In general, HCC is seen infrequently in early adulthood but the risk increases with increasing age. Peak age of onset is lower in high incidence areas being the 30s in South Africa, the 40s in Southeast Asia, the late 50s in Japan and older than 60 years in Western Europe and the United States. This is probably related to the earlier exposure to environmental factors and in particular to the mode of transmission of the HBV or HCV viruses. Men have a three to eight times greater risk of developing HCC than women.

Pathology of HCC

HCC is a malignant neoplasm composed of cells with hepatocellular differentiation. Small HCCs are defined as measuring less than 2 cm in diameter. HCC may macroscopically be stratified into a unifocal expansive type, presenting as a soft solid mass, an infiltrating type, frequently less differentiated with ill-defined margins, and a multifocal or diffuse type with multiple, minute, indistinct nodules present throughout the liver. Tumour nodules of the expansive type (as opposed to the infiltrative type) may be surrounded by a distinct fibrous capsule that results either from the compression of the non-tumorous liver as the HCC grows or from the synthesis by tumour cells of procollagen. This capsule has received considerable interest in the 1980s because it has been thought of as a barrier to the extension of the tumour in the adjacent parenchyma, and several studies have confirmed the better prognosis associated with the presence of this feature (see below). In addition, this capsule is associated with a cleavage plan allowing surgical enucleation to be performed. However, this capsule has a variable thickness, may or may not be complete, and may be infiltrated by tumour cells.

Microscopically, HCC exhibits very variable degrees of differentiation. Very well differentiated HCC can resemble normal hepatocytes and the trabecular structure may reproduce a near normal lobar architecture so that histological diagnosis by biopsy may occasionally be very difficult. Apart from this trabecular type, HCCs have also been divided into the pseudoglandular, compact, scirrhous (fibrolamellar variant), pleiomorphic, or clear cell types. The fibrolamellar variant has distinct epidemiological, histopathological and prognostic characteristics and will be studied separately in this chapter.

It is important to understand the mode of HCC expansion when assessing the rationale for, and efficacy of, the various treatment modalities. Extracapsular microscopic invasion by tumour cells is influenced by the size of the tumour and is present in a third of the tumours smaller than 2 cm in diameter as compared to two thirds of those with a larger diameter. As a result, multiple tumours are in fact present in 34% of patients with HCC less than 2 cm, 41% of those with tumours of 2–3 cm and 61% of those with tumours of 3–5 cm.[25] This low prevalence of microscopic tumour invasion from HCC nodules of less than 2 cm in diameter is the rationale for restricting the term small HCC to tumours of this size only.

HCC also have a great tendency to spread locally and to invade blood vessels, particularly the portal vein. Portal vein invasion is a frequent event estimated from autopsy series to range between 32 and 70%. This mode of extension may be observed even in small tumours (20% of minute HCC are also associated with vascular invasion) and tumour portal vein thrombosis may actually precede the radiological diagnosis of the primary tumour. The tumour thrombus has its own arterial supply, either from the vasa vasorum of the portal vein or from the site of the original venous invasion. Once HCC invades the portal vein, tumour thrombi grow rapidly in both directions and in particular towards the main portal vein without necessarily actually invading the portal vein wall. The consequences of this mode of extension are twofold. First, tumour fragments are spread throughout the liver as the thrombus crosses segmental branches. Secondly, once the tumour thrombus has extended into the main portal vein, there is a high risk for complete portal vein thrombosis and increased portal hypertension with its ensuing risk of fatal rupture of oesophageal varices, or liver decompensation including ascites, jaundice and encephalopathy. Invasion of hepatic veins is possible, although less frequent (4–23% in autopsy series). The thrombus eventually extends into the suprahepatic vena cava or the right atrium.

HCC may also more rarely (1–8%) invade the biliary tract and give rise to jaundice or haemobilia. Mechanisms of HCC-induced biliary obstruction include: (1) intraductal tumour extension; (2) obstruction by a fragment of necrotic tumour debris arising from a neoplasm that directly invades the bile duct or from necrosis of a tumour mass adjacent to a major bile duct; (3) haemorrhage of the tumour resulting in haemobilia and (4) metastatic lymph node compression of major bile ducts in the porta hepatis. Jaundice may alternatively be a late manifestation resulting from massive liver involvement by the tumour and/or liver decompensation.

When present, metastases are most frequently found in the lung, other locations being less frequent and by decreasing order of frequency the adrenal glands, the bones, the meninga, the pancreas, the brain and the kidney.

The most widely used pathological staging system for HCC is the pTNM staging system that is based on histopathological criteria that include the size, number and lobar distribution of the primary tumour, the presence of vascular invasion, lymph node involvement and distant metastasis (Table 3.2).

Dysplastic nodules represent the preneoplasic condition of HCC. They are defined as a nodular region of at least 1 mm in diameter with dysplasia but without definite histological criteria of malignancy. They are further divided into low-grade (with mild atypia) and high-grade (moderate atypia) nodules.[26] These nodules often have a soft texture, bulge above the cut surface and may either be more bile stained or paler than the surrounding liver. Necrosis and haemorrhage are not seen. As their size increases, the greater the likelihood that these nodules are in fact malignant and benign lesions are seldom larger than 2 cm. These nodules are usually supplied by portal tracts but as they enlarge, new vessels composed of non-triadal arteries develop. Differentiation between low-grade dysplastic nodules and regenerative nodules on the one hand and between high-grade dysplastic nodules and well differentiated HCC on the other hand is very difficult. Molecular genetic techniques will certainly be helpful in the future. Criteria suggesting malignancy are increased nuclear to cytoplasm ratio, irregular nuclear contour, invasion of stroma or portal tracts and at a later stage, increase

Table 3.2 *pTNM staging system for hepatocellular carcinoma*

Stage	Tumour	Lymph node	Metastasis
I	T1	N0	M0
II	T2	N0	M0
III	T1/2	N1	M0
	T3	N0/1	M0
IVa	T4	N0/1	M0
IVb	T1–4	N0/1	M1

Primary tumour. Tx: cannot be assessed; T0: no evidence of primary tumour; T1: solitary tumour ⩽ 2 cm, no vascular invasion; T2: solitary tumour ⩽ 2 cm, with vascular invasion or multiple tumours, one lobe, ⩽ 2 cm, no vascular invasion or solitary tumours > 2 cm, without vascular invasion; T3: solitary tumour > 2 cm, with vascular invasion or multiple tumours, one lobe, ⩽ 2 cm, with vascular invasion or multiple tumours, one lobe, > 2 cm, with/without vascular invasion; T4: multiple tumours, more than one lobe or any tumour(s) invading major branch of portal or hepatic veins.
Lymph nodes. Nx: cannot be assessed; N0: no regional lymph node metastases; N1: regional lymph node metastases.
Metastasis. Mx: cannot be assessed; M0: no distant metastases; M1: distant metastases.

in mitotic figures, enlargement of plates and reduction in reticulin figures.

Diagnosis of HCC

Clinical presentation

The magnitude of the clinical findings depend both on the stage of the tumour and on the functional status of the non-tumoural liver. In countries with screening programmes, a large proportion of HCCs are clinically asymptomatic and are only responsible for minor biochemical alterations. In contrast, in areas of the world without such screening programmes, HCC is diagnosed at a more advanced stage and the mode of presentation depends on whether liver cirrhosis is present or absent.

In patients with an underlying cirrhosis, the most frequently recorded clinical symptoms are those of liver decompensation (such as ascites, jaundice, encephalopathy, variceal bleeding), asthenia, anorexia or weight loss or abdominal fullness and pain. As a rule, when a patient with known cirrhosis either experiences worsening of his liver function tests, an acute complication or complains of upper abdominal discomfort, pain, or fever it should arouse suspicion of HCC. In non-cirrhotic patients, HCC tends to be discovered at a later stage. These patients may present relatively well and a liver mass is a frequent mode of revelation.

Other classical modes of presentation are the acute onset of abdominal pain resulting from the haemorrhagic rupture of a superficial HCC in the peritoneal cavity or as intermittent fever. Both modes of presentation are more frequent in South Africa (8% each) than in Asia (2–3% in Japan). Clinical symptoms resulting from biliary invasion of haemobilia are present in 2% of the patients. Metastasis is the presenting symptom in 2–5% of the patients. Possible paraneoplasic syndromes associated with HCC include polyglobulia (in less than 10% of the patients), hypercalcemia and hypoglycaemia.

Liver function tests and tumour markers

Liver function test impairment is usually non-specific and tends to reflect either the underlying liver pathology (cirrhosis or chronic active hepatitis) or the presence of a space-occupying lesion (resulting in an increase in alkaline phosphatase or gamma glutamyl transpeptidase).

Serum AFP, an α_1-globulin tumour marker introduced in 1963, is the most widely recognised serum marker of HCC but lacks sensitivity and specificity. AFP is normal in 40–50% of patients with a small HCC.[27] On the contrary, 30% of patients with chronic active hepatitis but without an HCC have increased AFP.[28] This is usually correlated with the degree of histological activity and raised levels of transaminase. In fact, it is only when the serum level exceeds $500 \, \text{ng ml}^{-1}$ that AFP can be considered as an indicator of an HCC with a 95% confidence. AFP may in addition be increased during the course of other malignancies such as testicular, gastric or pancreatic malignancies. With sophisticated biochemical techniques, it is now possible to distinguish several different AFP species and confirm or exclude HCC-derived AFP from the difference in the sugar moiety.[29]

Des-gamma-carboxyprothrombin is another serological marker of HCC which does not overlap with AFP. Sensitivities of 70% and specificity of 100% have been reported but are highly dependent on the size of the tumour and is only superior in patients with tumours larger than 5 cm.

Morphological studies

The aims of imaging in the context of HCC are: (1) to screen high-risk patients (those with cirrhosis or chronic active hepatitis); (2) to identify small lesions (only these may be anticipated to be accessible to treatments with some long-term benefit); (3) to differentiate HCC from other space-occupying lesions and (4) to help choose between the various treatments available. The number of lesions, their size and extent, the presence of daughter nodules or of vascular invasion along with extrahepatic spread and the presence of an underlying liver disease are critical in choosing the most appropriate treatment. These aims may, to some extent, be achieved by ultrasonography (US), computed tomography (CT), magnetic resonance imaging (MRI), angiography or a combination of these.

Ultrasound is the first line investigation because of its low cost, high availability and high sensitivity (greater than 90%) in identifying a focal liver mass. Tumours as small as 0.5–1 cm may be detectable and this technique is very accurate in identifying vascular or biliary invasion as well as indirect evidence of cirrhosis such as segmental atrophy, splenomegaly, ascites or collateral veins. Tumour thrombosis, as opposed to vascular thrombosis is associated with enlargement of the vascular lumen and an arterial signal may be detected by duplex doppler. This portal vein involvement is an important clue to the diagnosis of HCC as other malignancies infiltrate veins in less than 8% of cases. US cannot differentiate HCC from other tumours and a heterogeneous background pattern of cirrhosis may occasionally be difficult to differentiate from a diffuse infiltrative HCC. Typically, HCC are echoic or heterogeneous with a mosaic appearance and a hypoechoic border corresponding to the capsule. They may also be hypoechoic and homogeneous but this feature is less specific.

CT, and particularly spiral CT, is very accurate in identifying HCC. Its sensitivity is comparable to and greater than that of US or MRI for tumours larger than 5 cm and smaller than 1 cm, respectively. In addition, it is useful for identifying features of underlying cirrhosis, accurately measuring liver and tumour volumes and assessing extrahepatic tumour spread. Its drawbacks are its cost and smaller sensitivity for tumours located within the left lobe. Typically, HCC are spontaneously hypodense but up to a third may be isodense and a few HCC either appear as hyperdense (within a fatty liver) or are truly hyperdense. The most specific feature is an early uptake of contrast media, observed in 88% of the cases with a spiral CT.[30] Other characteristic features of HCC are the mosaic shape pattern (with multiple nodular areas within the tumour of different densities after contrast enhancement), an enhanced pseudocapsule, vascular invasion, fatty infiltration and an arterioportal fistula. A mosaic shape, the presence of a capsule, venous involvement, intratumoral necrosis and sinusoidal dilatation are more frequently observed in large tumours.[31]

Lipiodol has added a new dimension to the diagnosis of HCC by CT due to its ability, when injected into the hepatic artery, to be selectively retained for a prolonged period of time by the tumour. The technique introduced in the mid-1980s involves injection of lipiodol into the hepatic artery, 1–4 weeks before CT. The retained lipiodol is radiodense and reveals the tumour as a high density area thus improving the sensitivity of CT. Whereas routine CT will detect 82% of HCC less than 5 cm and 56% of those less than 2 cm, lipiodol CT is reported to have a sensitivity of 96% for lesions below 5 cm and 93% for those below 2 cm.[32] However, these figures need to be re-assessed with the development of spiral CT. Nodular uptake within the liver is not specific of HCC. All liver tumours including focal nodular hyperplasia, adenoma, angioma and metastatic lesions will retain lipiodol. This examination is therefore more valuable to assess the tumoral distribution within the liver than to confirm the diagnosis of HCC. False negative results may be observed in cases of avascular, necrotic or fibrotic tumours or if not all areas of the liver have been perfused with lipiodol because of catheter malposition or vascular interruption. It should also be borne in mind that sensitivity is low in very well differentiated HCC.

Angiography has lost its status as the primary imaging modality for HCC to the more powerful cross-sectional techniques although it is still felt by some to be the most specific imaging investigation of HCC. It can, in addition, be used for lipiodol injection. HCC is typically hypervascular and lesions as small as 3 mm may be shown. Some HCC may appear avascular either spontaneously or due to necrosis, bleeding or vascular occlusion. Other features of angiography include arterioportal or arteriovenous shunting as well as portal vein involvement.

The cost of MRI is approximately three times that of a CT scan and is therefore only used as a second or third line imaging technique. MRI tends to be more accurate than the other imaging techniques in differentiating HCC from other space-occupying lesions. As for CT, the characteristics of HCC are the mosaic shape structure and the presence of a capsule. The former is best identified on T2 sequences (50%) and the latter on T1 sequences (80%). HCC classically are hypointense on T1 weighted images and hyperintense on T2 weighted images. This differentiation may be further enhanced by hepatocyte delivered agents.

It has, however, been recognised, based on the pathological analysis of the explanted liver of liver transplant recipients that all these radiological procedures lack accuracy in detecting multiple small tumours. Overall, US, CT scanning and angiography fail to demonstrate multiple tumours in up to 50–80% of the patients.[33] This is particularly important when it comes to assessing the efficacy and results of the various treatment options.

Table 3.3 *Typical radiological features of HCC, macroregenerative nodules and borderline nodules*

		Macroregenerative	Borderline	HCC
US	– nodule	Hypoechoic	Hypoechoic	Hyperechoic
	– capsule	Absent	Absent	Hypoechoic border
	– doppler	No signal	No signal	Arterial signal
CT	– without inj.	Iso- or hyperdense	Isodense	Hypodense
	– with contrast	Isodense	Isodense	Rapid enhancement
MRI	– T1	Hypointense	Hyperintense	Variable
	– T2	Hypointense	Hypointense	Iso- or hyperintense
Angiography		Not seen	Not seen	Hypervascular

The differential diagnosis of HCC includes non-neoplasic conditions (fatty infiltration, abscesses, haematoma, complicated hydatid cyst), benign tumours (cavernous haemangioma, focal nodular hyperplasia, hepatic adenoma, nodular regenerative hyperplasia, cystadenoma) and malignant tumours (cholangiocarcinoma, angiosarcoma, metastases). However, a rising problem related to the ability of these imaging techniques to identify very small focal lesions is the differentiation of HCC from macroregenerative nodules or borderline nodules within a cirrhotic liver (Table 3.3).

Macroregenerative nodules may not be visible or only appear as a nodular modification of the outer surface of the liver. On US they are most frequently homogeneous and hypoechoic but may also appear as hyperechoic. These nodules frequently have a rich iron content which accounts for their hypodensity on CT without contrast enhancement and their hypointensity on MRI. The latter technique is currently the most reliable in differentiating regenerating nodules from HCC. Nodules larger than 2 cm are seldom macroregenerative or borderline nodules and the blood supply is predominantly portal in macroregenerative or borderline nodules and arterial in HCC.

Requirement for histological study

The approach to the diagnosis of a liver mass is dependent on whether an underlying cirrhosis is present or absent. In patients with cirrhosis, it has long been thought that a radiographically identifiable nodule was HCC unless otherwise proven. The rationale for this was that the incidence of liver metastasis from colorectal adenocarcinoma (the most frequent primary disease found in non-cirrhotic patients with liver metastasis) was low in cirrhotic patients whereas the incidence of HCC was extremely high. In addition, biopsy of the tumour is not without risk of bleeding or seeding of tumour cells along the track of the needle in the abdominal wall or the peritoneal cavity. This carcinologic risk is related to the number of needle passes and is reported to occur in up to 0.1% of cases. It is a serious concern in patients in whom a curative resection may be anticipated. However, in differentiating between regenerating or borderline nodules and HCC, the advantages and risk of liver biopsy should be assessed in each individual depending on the confidence of the diagnostic work-up and the treatment that is planned.

In patients without evidence of chronic active hepatitis or cirrhosis, with negative serological markers of HBV or HCV infection, and with normal AFP levels, the diagnosis of HCC cannot simply rely on morphological explorations. In these patients, the probability that this mass is a metastasis or a benign liver tumour is greater than the probability that it is an HCC and liver biopsy may be useful.

A histological diagnosis may be obtained either by fine needle aspiration cytology (FNAC) or by needle biopsy under US or CT guidance. The diagnostic sensitivity of FNAC ranges between 69 and 96%. The main reasons for false negative results are faulty guidance and sampling errors, necrotic tumours and well differentiated tumours. FNAC is inaccurate in differentiating HCC from adenoma or from borderline nodules. Needles less than 1 mm in diameter are associated with a mortality of 1 in 20 000 and this risk increases with increasing diameter of the needle.

Natural history of HCC

The prognosis of HCC is generally very poor due to delayed diagnosis, lack of effective treatments in symptomatic patients and frequent presence of an underlying cirrhosis that carries its own risk of complications. Based on multivariate analysis of untreated patients (or of patients thought to have received ineffective treatments), several mathematical prognosis models have been computed[34–36] to more precisely predict outcome in individual patients. None of these systems have identified factors which can be easily applied in clinical practice. Based on these models, the median survival from the time of diagnosis ranges between 1 month and 1 year (Table 3.4).

HCC has been shown by US to have a fairly long doubling time (102–195 days), although it may vary considerably between and within patients.[37–40] It has similarly been estimated that it takes 1.9 months to 3.3 years for an HCC to reach a size of 2 cm from the time of tumour onset. The reason for this variable tumour growth is unclear. Tumour doubling time does not appear to be correlated with the size of the tumour at the time of diagnosis, nor with the severity of cirrhosis. However, there are obvious ethnic variations and doubling time is, for example, particularly short in African patients.

Longer-term survival of patients receiving no specific treatment could be good provided the HCC was diagnosed at an early stage. It was in particular reported that the survival of Japanese patients with HCC less than 3 cm in diameter was 90.7% at 1 year, 55% at 2 years and 12.8% at 3 years.[38] This survival was even better in patients with well compensated

Table 3.4 *Mathematical prognosis models used to predict the survival of unresected HCC*

Reference	Model	Value of prognosis index	Survival			
			Median	1 year	2 years	5 years
Okada 1992 (Japan)[34]	(a)	<0.8	9.8 mo	41%	12%	
		0.8 ≤ - <2.0	3.8 mo	13%	0%	
		≥2.0	1.9 mo	0%	0%	
Calvet 1990 (Spain)[35]	(b)	<0.025	12.8 mo	52%	25%	
		0.025 ≤ - <0.085	3.9 mo	20%	10%	
		>0.085	1 mo	2%	0%	
Akashi 1991 (Japan)[36]	(c)	<1.0		80%		35%
		>1.0		6.3%		0%
Akashi 1991 (Japan)[36]	(d)	<1.0		88%		46%
		>1.0		35%		0%

(a) PI = 1.8109 × (0 for a performance status of 0–1 and 1 for a performance status of 2–3) + 0.9322 × (0 when tumour thrombus was absent in the main portal trunk and 1 when it was present) + 0.6996 × (0 for age <60 years and 1 for age ≥60 years).

Analysis was performed on patients with unresectable HCC, most of whom had advanced tumours and receiving various forms of systemic chemotherapy (thought not to have affected survival).

(b) PI = Exp [(0.03 × age) + (0.8281 × ascites) + (0.0137 × BUN) − (0.0538 × serum sodium) + (0.0019 × GGT) + (0.0734 × bilirubin) + (0.33 × tumour size) + (0.4965 × toxic syndrome) + (0.55 × metastasis)].

Analysis was performed on cirrhotic patients, only 10% of whom were treated with either surgery or alcoholisation.

(c) PI = Exp [1.549 × (gross appearance of HCC − 1.344) + 0.778 × (encapsulation − 1.622) + 0.818 × (clinical stage − 1.800) + 1.760 (therapy − 1.344)]

where: gross appearance is quoted 1 if nodular and 2 if massive or diffuse; encapsulation is quoted 1 if present and 2 if absent; therapy is quoted 1 if treatment was TAE and 2 if it was arterial anticancer chemotherapy. Clinical stage was quoted as follows:

Clinical stage	Ascites	Bili (mg dl^{-1})	Albumin (g l^{-1})	ICGR15 (%)	PT (%)
1	absent	≤2.0	35 ≤	≤15	80 ≤
2	responsive	2.0< ≤3.0	30 ≤ <35	15< ≤40	50 ≤ <80
3	intractable	3.0<	<3.0	40<	<50

Analysis was performed on 90 cirrhotic patients with unresectable HCC undergoing intrarterial chemotherapy with or without embolisation

(d) PI = Exp [1.210 × (extension rate − 1.576) + 1.179 × (encapsulation − 1.475) + 0.0001277 × (AFP − 1420.792) − 0.039 × (prothrombin time − 72.237) − 0.214 × (sodium − 138.427)]

Analysis was performed on the same group of patients as in (c) excluding those not receiving TAE.

cirrhosis, being 94% at 1 year, 82% at 2 years and 66% at 3 years in Child grade A patients as opposed to 76%, 35% and 0%, respectively, in Child B or C patients.[40]

These two observations have important clinical implications. First, they can be used for determining the ideal schedule of screening programmes (see below). Secondly, they underline the necessity of a control group when assessing the value of a particular treatment.

Screening for HCC

Because of the frustrations of late diagnosis and poor therapeutic results at a symptomatic stage of the disease, screening programmes were launched in high incidence areas in the 1970s. Initially, these mass screening programmes based on serum AFP measurements proved to be a complete failure in South Africa and of limited value in China. This was related to the relative lack of sensitivity of AFP in small HCC.

With improved imaging techniques and by focusing the screening on patients with cirrhosis or chronic active hepatitis, such programmes have become popular, especially in Japan where more than 1% of the screened patients were discovered to have an HCC.[41] When screening is based on US and is repeated at short time intervals (as it is the case in Japan), these HCCs are detected at an early stage,[17,42,43] 50% of the tumours being less than 2 cm and most of them (up to 80%) being unifocal. There is consequently some evidence that periodic medical screening of patients with cirrhosis is associated with an improved survival from the time of diagnosis of the HCC.[10]

In Europe on the contrary, the proportion of small tumours identified by screening programmes is less (approximately 30%) and few of these tumours prove resectable (Table 3.5). This may be related to the fact that screening programmes in Europe have usually been less repetitive than in Asia (being performed every 6 months or more in the former as compared to every 3 months in the latter). HCC in Asia and Europe may

Table 3.5 *Results of screening programmes for the detection of HCC in Japan, Italy and France*

Author (year)	Country and reference	No. of patients screened	Risk factor	Screening interval	Annual incidence	% of small HCC
Oka (1990)	Japan[17]	140	Cirrhosis	3 mo	5–11%[a]	62% ⩽ 20 cm
Tanaka (1990)	Japan[43]	179	Cirrhosis	3 mo	6%	50% ⩽ 2 cm
		481	CAH	6 mo	0.6%	
Colombo (1991)	Italy[14]	447	Cirrhosis	12 mo	3%	28% isolated and <3 cm
Pateron (1994)	France[16]	118	Cirrhosis	6 mo	5.8%	21% isolated and <3 cm

CAH, chronic active hepatitis.
[a] incidence at 5 years was 35%.

also have different doubling time. Up to 50% of patients presenting with an HCC in Northern Europe have previously undiagnosed cirrhosis and therefore escape screening programmes. With this limitation in mind, the high risk patients who should most benefit from screening are patients with posthepatic cirrhosis (regardless of virus) above 45 years of age and patients with cirrhosis related to other causes (in particular haemochromatosis) above 55 years. Attempts have been made to further identify a subgroup of cirrhotic patients at particular high risk of developing an HCC. One model[44] is based on the calculation of a score according to the following formula:

$$S = (6 \times age) + (4 \times sex) + (3 \times EV) + (3 \times PT) + (3 \times AFP) + (3 \times anti\text{-}HVB \text{ antibodies})$$

A score <11 and a score >11 are associated with a cumulated incidence of HCC at 3 years of 0 and 24%, respectively. This risk may be further refined by taking into account the presence or absence of liver cell dysplasia at liver biopsy, which, when present in patients with a high risk score, is associated with a cumulative incidence of HCC of 72% at 3 years. The prognosis value of an even slightly increased AFP level in cirrhotic patients has been confirmed by other studies[45] and are in keeping with the previously mentioned influence of superimposed chronic active hepatitis activity on the risk of developing an HCC.

Whether screening programmes are justified is, however, still controversial. The ultimate parameters that should be taken into account when evaluating these programmes are: (1) the overall increase in life duration resulting from treatment at an earlier stage; (2) the costs of these treatments as compared to only conservative management, had these patients been diagnosed at a later stage; and (3) the additional cost resulting from these screening programmes. Such parameters can only be assessed on a national basis and be adapted to the policy of each National Health Service and the ethnic growth characteristics of the tumour.

Treatment

A number of treatments are available for patients with an HCC. These include: (1) surgical resection through either partial or total liver resection (i.e. liver transplantation); (2) less-invasive procedures aiming at physically destroying the tumour such as ethanol injection, cryotherapy or microwave coagulation[46] and (3) systemic or regional chemotherapy or radiotherapy.

Patient eligibility for treatment depends on tumour characteristics and on liver status. The clinical status may be staged using either the Child Pugh classification or the clinical staging system proposed by the Liver Cancer Study Group of Japan (see Table 3.4). The efficacy of each treatment should be weighed against the possible long-term spontaneous survival of patients with small HCC and well compensated cirrhosis.

Liver resection of HCC

Liver resection has long been considered as the only potentially curative treatment of HCC, which was confirmed by a National Institutes of Health Consensus Conference held in 1986. Tumour spread on the one hand and coexistence of an underlying liver cirrhosis on the other hand are, however, important limitations to liver resection so that less than 10–30% of HCC patients are in fact potential candidates for resection. Indeed, whereas a carcinologic resection would often require that a large resection be indicated, the presence of an underlying cirrhosis prevents such a large resection being performed.

Liver cirrhosis is an important risk factor for postoperative complications in patients undergoing liver resection due to the poor functional reserve of the liver and/or to the impaired and delayed ability of the liver to regenerate.[47,48] The overall incidence of in-hospital death following liver resection for HCC in the most recent studies ranges between 0 and 20% with an average of 12%.[49–51] Hospital mortality lies between 0 and 5.8% in patients without cirrhosis but between 7 and 25% in patients with liver cirrhosis. The predominant cause of death in these cirrhotic patients is from liver failure which is best assessed on a modification of Child's classification.[52] Any resection is contraindicated in patients who are grade C at the time of surgery and only limited resection is possible in patients who are grade B. However, even in grade A cirrhotic patients with apparently normal liver function, the risk of liver surgery is increased and several models have been developed to assess the extent of a safe resection as a function of bromosulphalein or indocyanine green clearance, glucose tolerance, redox tolerance index, volume of the remnant liver[53] or a combination of these.

Although there is growing evidence that some selected cirrhotic patients can undergo major resections,[54] the tendency is to try to remove as little liver as possible. This may best be achieved through enucleation of the HCC, which may prove easy to perform in superficially located encapsulated tumours. Such non-anatomical resections often prove to be non-carcinologic due to the mode of tumour extension. Tumour cells may seed more distally in the liver segments or proximally where they can be carried into an adjacent portal venous branch (Fig. 3.1). In this way, it is possible to account for step-by-step intrahepatic dissemination, ranging from satellite metastases in the immediate vicinity of a large mass or in adjacent segments and ultimately a complete liver lobe or bilateral spread. These principles are the basis of segmental or subsegmental liver resections guided by intraoperative US. Alternatively, a dye may be injected at the time of surgery in portal radicles under US control to more accurately define their limits.

The development of new surgical techniques and the emergence of a generation of specialised surgeons have contributed to reduce the risk of liver resection such that the experience of the surgeons[55] and/or the time period of hepatectomy[56] significantly influence outcome, and that any comparison with historical controls is inappropriate. Improved results may be related to better patient selection, reduced intraoperative

Figure 3.1
Propagation of HCC throughout the liver as a consequence of tumour thrombosis in the portal vein.

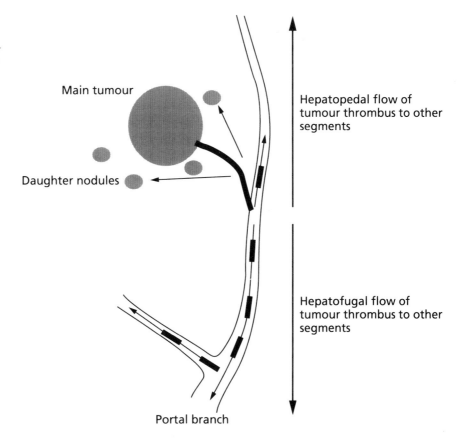

Main tumour

Daughter nodules

Portal branch

Hepatopedal flow of tumour thrombus to other segments

Hepatofugal flow of tumour thrombus to other segments

transfusion,[52,56] and better postoperative management of cirrhotic patients.[57]

The largest report of resected patients comes from the Liver Cancer Study Group in Japan that has reported 1-, 3- and 5-year survival rates of 82%, 62% and 44%, respectively in 3205 patients undergoing curative resection between 1982 and 1989.[58] Comparable results have been reported by other groups world-wide (Table 3.6). Survival rates as high as 60% at 5 years may be achieved in patients with tumours of 2 cm in diameter or less and even up to 78% in patients aged less than 65 years, Child grade A, well-nourished with well-encapsulated tumours less than 2 cm.[59] However, less than 10% of patients fit these selection criteria.

There is no prospective study comparing resection with no treatment. However, most retrospective matched controlled studies have shown that survival following resection was significantly greater than that of a population of untreated patients matched for prognosis variables (Table 3.7). This was particularly so for single HCC, less than 5 cm in patients with Child grade A cirrhosis.[60] This has nevertheless been challenged by uncontrolled studies showing that in early detected HCC (by screening programmes), survival following resection was not different from that of untreated patients[61] at least over a short-term follow-up.

Table 3.6 *Results after curative surgical resection of HCC in the most recent studies*

Reference /source	Study period	No. of patients	Cirrhosis	ϕ <5 cm	In hospital mortality	1-yr	2-yr	3-yr	5-yr
						(in-hosp death excluded)			
Franco 1990 France/Italy	1983–1988	72	100%	59.7%	6.9%	67.5%	55%	51%	—
		54	Child A		3.7%	80.2%	76.5%	56.7%	—
		18	Child B/C		16.7%	55.6%	12.2%	12.2%	—
Nagasue 1993 Japan[52]	1980–1990	229	76.6%	75%	10.5%	79.8%	—	51.3%	26.4%
Ikeda 1993 Japan[70]	1983–1990	83	91.6%	—	0%	95.0%	77.7%	69.1%	65.3%
Sugioka 1993 Japan[73]	1973–1990	137	62%	53%	11.3%	—	—	58%	49%
Castells 1993 Spain[134]	1987–1991	33	100%	100%	9.0%	81%	73%	44%	—
Izumi 1994 Japan[65]	1976–1990	104	80.7%		7.1%	87.8%	74.5%	65.4%	58.8%
Chen 1994 Taiwan[69]	1977–1991	205	49.8%	30.2%	4.4%	55.8%	40.4%	35.6%	28.2%
Kawasaki 1995 Japan[50]	1990–1993	112	67.9%	83%	1.8%	92.4%	85.0%	78.9%	—
Mazziotti 1995 Italy	1983–1994	174	100%	61%	6.3%	82.4%	—	64.2%	41.4%
Lai 1995 Hong Kong[56]	1972–1987	149	69%	13%	21.5%	48%	—	21%	14%
	1987–1991	128	78%	29%	14.8%	68%	—	44%	35%
	1991–1994	66	74%	32%	6%				
Takenaka 1996 Japan[49]	1985–1993	280	52%	—	2%	88%	—	70%	50%
Authors' experience	1986–1995	226	84%	45%	8.4%	82%	69%	59%	39%

Recurrence following resection of HCC

Tumour recurrence is the major cause of death following resection of HCC both in cirrhotic[52] and non-cirrhotic livers.[62] Recurrence is a very common event and prognosis following recurrence is usually dismal with a median survival of 1 year. The frequency of tumour recurrence is estimated to range between 20 and 64% within the first year, between 57 and 81% at 3 years and between 75 and 100% at 5 years.[56,62–70] Recurrence within the liver is multifocal in 45–64% of the patients and is associated with distant metastasis in 12–26%, especially in the lungs

Table 3.7 *Results of studies comparing the efficacy of resection, percutaneous ethanol injection (PEI) and transarterial embolization (TAE) (number in parentheses refer to the number of patients treated in each group)*

Study	Selection of patients	End-point	Resection	PEI	TAE	Control	P<
Unicentric retrospective[61]	Asymptomatic HCC	1-year survival	92% (12)			96% (25)	n.s.
		2-year survival	39% (12)			50% (25)	n.s.
Unicentric retrospective[62a]	Unselected	2-year survival	73% (28)			18% (28)	0.003
	single HCC ≤ 5 cm	2-year survival	90% (19)			22% (19)	0.0005
Multicentric retrospective[136b]	Child A, single HCC < 5 cm	3-yr survival	79% (82)	71% (105)		26% (73)	
	Child B, single HCC < 5 cm	3-yr survival	26% (38)	30% (50)		13% (43)	
Unicentric retrospective[134c]	Single HCC ≤ 4 cm	4-yr survival	44% (33)	34% (30)			n.s.
Multicentric retrospective[51d]	Okuda stage I	3-yr survival	43% (30)		54% (42)	11% (33)	
	single HCC < 5 cm	3-yr survival	65% (9)		50% (4)	0% (5)	
Unicentric retrospective[92e]	Child A	2-yr survival	61% (46)		65% (10)		n.s.
	Child B	2-yr survival	55% (20)		56% (19)		n.s.
Unicentric retrospective[135f]	Unselected	3-year survival	74% (67)		50% (20)		0.05
		5-year survival	54% (67)		17% (20)		
Unicentric retrospective[124g]	Unselected	1-yr survival			59% (30)	0% (30)	0.001
		2-yr survival			30% (30)	0% (30)	
Unicentric retrospective[119h]	Okuda stage 1 or 2	1-yr survival			65% (50)	42% (50)	0.01
	Child A or B	2-yr survival			38% (50)	20% (50)	0.01
Multicentric prospective[129i]	Child A, all HCC	1-yr survival			62% (50)	43% (46)	n.s.
		2-yr survival			38% (50)	26% (46)	
Multicentric prospective[128j]	Unresectable HCC	1-year survival			24% (21)	31% (21)	n.s.
Unicentric prospective[127k]	Unresectable HCC	1-yr survival			42% (21)	13% (21)	0.01
		2-year survival			25.3% (21)	12.8% (21)	

[a] Control group consisted of untreated patients matched for prognosis factors seen over the same period of time.

[b] The control group consisted of patients seen during the same period of time but who refused any treatment, had contraindications to surgery while PEI was not available. Resection and PEI were not significantly different from one another but both were significantly superior to the control group.

[c] Treatment consisted of repeated courses of PEI. Resection was associated with improved survival only in patients with tumours larger than 3 cm.

[d] The control group in this study includes patients fulfilling all the criteria to undergo TOCE.

[e] Treatment consisted of repeated courses of TAE. TAE group had a higher rate of TNM stage III or IV tumours.

[f] Most patients received a single course of TAE. TAE patients were selected on the basis that they could also have undergone a surgical treatment.

[g] Treatment consisted of repeated courses of TAE. Comparison was made with a group of patients seen during the same period of time and matched for cause of cirrhosis, age, Okuda's staging, Child's Pugh class, serum bilirubin and AFP levels, size of the main tumour mass, and cancerous thrombosis of the right or left branch of the portal vein.

[h] Treatment consisted of a single course of TAE. Comparison was made with the expected survival had these patients been not treated using a mathematical prognosis model from data on a historical series of untreated patients.

[i] Treatment consisted of repeated courses of TAE.

[j] Treatment consisted of repeated courses of TAE.

[k] Treatment consisted of repeated courses of TAE. Control consisted of patients receiving systemic chemotherapy alone. Difference was not significant during the first 8 months but was significant thereafter.

and the bones, and more rarely in the adrenal gland.[71–74] Extrahepatic recurrence without simultaneous intrahepatic recurrence is infrequent in cirrhotic livers.

The predominant cause of tumour recurrence is probably metachronous carcinogenesis since the precursor condition (cirrhosis) persists after surgery. Alternative possibilities include seeding of tumour cells as a result of surgical manipulation and pre- or intraoperative incomplete diagnosis. Indeed, 20–60% of small HCC are multifocal and as stated above, it is very difficult even with preoperative lipiodol injection and intraoperative ultrasound to comprehensively assess this diffusion. Some have advocated repeating systematically morphological investigations 1 month after surgery prior to considering surgical resection as curative.

Variables that have been found to be significantly associated with a greater incidence of recurrence are the presence and severity of an underlying cirrhosis,[52,75] alcohol abuse,[66] the presence of more than one nodule,[55,74,70] a tumour of more than 5 cm,[55,74] the lack of a capsule,[52] an aneuploid DNA content,[66] a moderately or poorly differentiated HCC,[76] the presence of daughter nodules,[50,52,74] venous invasion,[50,52,66] an infiltrating rather than an expansive tumour, an insufficient cancer-free margin[52] and intraoperative blood transfusion.[77] The relative weight of each of these parameters is difficult to assess because most overlap (it is, for example, generally accepted that the incidence of portal vein invasion and intrahepatic metastasis correlate with the tumour size). Using multivariate analysis, presence of tumour thrombus in the portal vein, invasion of the resection margin, intraoperative transfusion and/or tumour size[65,73,77,78] were independent prognostic factors with portal invasion carrying the worst influence. This has led to the proposition[65] of a modified TNM classification (Table 3.8) that better correlates with outcome than the classical TNM stratification. Other parameters such as

Table 3.8 *Modified TNM staging system for hepatocellular carcinoma*

Stage	Tumour	Lymph node	Metastasis
I	T1	N0	M0
II	T2	N0	M0
III	T3	N0	M0
	Any T	N1	M0
IV	Any T	Any N	M1

Primary tumour. T1: solitary tumour without vascular invasion; T2: solitary or multiple tumours with vascular invasion; T3: solitary or multiple tumours with invasion of major branch of portal or hepatic veins.
Lymph nodes. N0: no regional lymph node metastases; N1: regional lymph node metastases.
Metastasis. M0: no distant metastases; M1: distant metastases including remote lymph node metastasis.

an age greater than 50 or 70 years,[52,50] males[52,74] and high preoperative serum AFP levels[52] also tend to be associated with a greater incidence of recurrence.

The importance of a resection margin free of tumour has been stressed in some clinical studies but remains controversial.[79,80,83] The rationale for a wide resection margin is the presence of microsatellites and histological venous permeation whereas capsular invasion or direct liver invasion pose little threat to an incomplete resection.[80] The latter two features are confined to within 2 mm from the main tumour nodule. On the other hand, the furthest distance microsatellites have been measured is 11–34 mm for HCC <5 cm and 24–97 mm for HCC ⩾5 cm. Histologic venous permeation was noted between 9 and 28 mm for HCC <5 cm and 17 and 80 mm for HCC ⩾5 cm. A surgical resection margin of 1 cm would appear not to achieve safe clearance in most patients. Nonetheless a compromised surgical margin with exposure of the tumour capsule is not always incompatible with long-term survival.

Recent studies assessing the risk of recurrence have focused on the outcome of small resected HCC[81–83] in a less heterogeneous population to determine whether this is related to multifocal tumorigenesis rather than incomplete tumour resection. In these patients, a low serum albumin level or Child B grade, high ALT concentrations, a high proliferating activity in the non-tumorous liver and the presence of active inflammation were associated with an increased risk of recurrence whereas wedge resection of tumour, presence of a fibrous capsule, histological grade and the number of nodules or vascular invasion had no or little influence. Disease-free survivals following resection of single or multiple (2–3) HCC smaller than 2 cm are not significantly different (38% vs. 23% at 3 years).[83,84] Impaired immune function and active inflammation may increase the risk of tumour recurrence, an observation in keeping with the influence of a high proliferating activity index of *de novo* malignancy within a cirrhotic liver (see above).

Treatment of recurrence following resection of HCC

Although recurrence following resection of HCC has traditionally been associated with a very poor outcome, there is growing evidence that some patients will benefit from a more aggressive approach and that some form of treatment should be considered, provided recurrence is limited to the liver. It is, therefore, important to monitor resected patients by measurement of serum AFP levels and US. Serum AFP levels may be normal at the time of recurrence despite being raised at the time the first HCC was diagnosed.[85]

The choice of treatment should be governed by the extent of the tumour and by the functional status of the liver. Repeat liver resection is technically possible and has proved to be safe in experienced hands[50,72,86–89] although the resectability rate is less than 30% due to extrahepatic spread of tumour or to worsening liver function. In patients with non-cirrhotic livers, resectability rates for recurrent tumours are greater.[62]

Repeat hepatectomy for recurrent HCC appears to be associated with a long-term outcome comparable to that of first hepatectomy and improves the overall survival of patients undergoing a first resection for HCC.[72,85,87,88] Survival beyond 5 years has been described after repeat hepatectomy.[68,85,89] There is evidence that regional therapy also improves survival once recurrence has occurred.[90,91] Median survival following resection or embolisation for recurrent HCC ranges between 18 and 36 months.[50,68,71,72]

Prevention of recurrence after liver resection

Neoadjuvant therapy In an attempt to reduce the risk of recurrence, preoperative chemoembolisation has been advocated. The rationale for this neoadjuvant treatment is to induce tumour necrosis and hence favour the efficacy of resection. Results are controversial but most studies have shown no influence on disease-free survival.[52,62,66,92] In addition, preoperative embolisation may, in this setting, be associated with the development of hypervascular adhesions, gallbladder infarction or difficulty in identifying the tumour intraoperatively, all of which may complicate surgery. In addition, the development of partial tumour necrosis (as opposed to complete or no necrosis) may theoretically favour the dislodgement of tumour residual cells into the bloodstream at the time of surgery thereby favouring the development of distant metastasis. Although there are no controlled data available, preoperative embolisation may be of value in controlling bleeding of a ruptured resectable HCC (see below), or in reducing the size of a large HCC, allowing a more limited liver resection to be performed[62] or even converting an irresectable tumour into a resectable one.[93]

Adjuvant therapy Postoperative adjuvant therapy is currently the subject of a number of trials that have however only recently been launched and there is currently no consensus agreement on if and how it should be administered. Postoperative chemotherapy may kill any shed tumour cells potentially released by surgical manipulation and may destroy small, intrahepatic metastases that may not have been detected during surgery. Postoperative systemic chemotherapy has not, however, been widely employed due to its toxicity, its possible adverse effect on liver regeneration and its lack of efficacy as a primary treatment of HCC. One study failed to demonstrate an influence on patient or disease-free survival when 5-fluorouracil (5-FU) derivatives were administered orally from the first month after the operation when compared to patients receiving no adjuvant therapy[94] whereas, in a further study, this treatment was associated with increased patient and disease-free survival in clinical stage I patients with stage II HCC.[95]

There is, however, growing evidence that regional chemotherapy is more effective since unlike systemic chemotherapy, it is better tolerated and may be more appropriate since intrahepatic recurrence predominates. An uncontrolled study has shown that, in patients at high risk of tumour recurrence (surgical margins less than 1 cm, intrahepatic metastasis, tumour invasion into the second branch or more proximal sites of portal vein, and lack of fibrous capsule around the tumour), arterial 5-FU chemotherapy started 2–6 weeks after operation and repeated every 3 months for 1 year was associated with improved patient survival.[96] In a prospective randomised controlled trial, patients who had undergone curative resection but were at high risk of recurrence due to vascular invasion and/or intrahepatic metastasis received a single intra-arterial bolus infusion of lipiodol containing doxorubicin and mitomycin C within 3 months of resection. This regimen improved disease-free survival (32% vs. 11% in patients receiving no adjuvant therapy at 3 years, $P = 0.02$) but failed to reduce recurrences in the long-term or to improve patients survival.[97] On the other hand, in patients who had undergone curative resection, lipiodolisation with epirubicin performed once or twice a year was associated with improved disease-free survival when compared to patients receiving no adjuvant therapy (86% vs. 15% at 3 years, $P = 0.001$) and the actuarial 4 year survival rate was 100%.[94] However, a recent controlled trial of systemic and intra-arterial chemotherapy in unselected patients with HCC failed to demonstrate any benefit of adjuvant chemotherapy and was actually associated with reduced disease-free survival and a greater incidence of extrahepatic metastases (Lai, 1996, submitted for publication). Further studies are obviously needed to define the group of patients (if any) who may most benefit from these treatments.

Finally, there is recent but yet unconfirmed evidence that chemoprevention of hepatocarcinogenesis through the administration of polyprenoic acid reduces the incidence of secondary tumours.[98]

Liver transplantation

Liver transplantation is obviously the most attractive therapeutic option for HCC because it removes both detectable and undetectable tumour nodules together with all the preneoplastic lesions that are present in the cirrhotic liver. In addition, it simultaneously treats the underlying cirrhosis and prevents the development of postoperative or distant complications associated with portal hypertension and liver failure.

Liver transplantation was initially performed in patients in whom partial liver resection could not be contemplated due to the high number and/or large size of the tumours. Early studies, however, reported very high recurrence rates and disappointing long-term survival of 18–35% at 5 years[99,100] when compared to the 65–75% 5-year survival rates in patients undergoing liver transplantation for non-tumoral chronic liver disease. The high incidence of recurrence is probably related to the use of immunosuppressive agents that lack specificity, preventing both rejection of the graft and the immune response against microbial or tumoral antigens. Evidence for this comes from the observation that the tumour doubling time of liver transplant patients with recurrent HCC under cyclosporin–steroid based therapy is 26 days as compared to the average 6 months (range 1–19 months) reported in the literature in nontransplanted patients. Because of these poor results, the proportion of patients transplanted for malignancy has fallen world-wide from 25% to 12%.

On the other hand, it should also be noted that the outcome in patients transplanted with an HCC incidentally discovered by pathological examination of the explanted liver is extremely favourable. In these patients, the incidence of tumour recurrence is small and survival is comparable to patients transplanted without malignancy. In Pittsburgh, the 5-year survival of 16 such patients who underwent transplantation for chance-discovered HCC was 90%. These observations therefore led several groups to perform liver transplantation in patients with limited tumour involvement as an alternative to partial liver resection.

Based on these retrospective studies,[101,102] certain clinicopathological features have been identified which may influence survival following transplantation (Table 3.9). It is clear that distant and nodal tumour spread is a contraindication to liver transplantation with few patients surviving a year. Because it is almost impossible to assess lymphatic spread preoperatively, in cirrhotic patients who tend to have enlarged lymph nodes, some centres plan a back-up for non-cancer patients. Multiple and large nodules as well as the presence of vascular invasion have a significant deleterious impact on outcome. These observations are best illustrated by the difference in the 5-year survival rates of patients with TNM stage I (75%), II (68%), III (52%) and IV (11%) HCC.[103] It is therefore considered that the best results of transplantation may be achieved in patients with less than three nodules and with tumours less than 3 cm in diameter and without vascular involvement. Using these strict selection criteria, up to 80% survival at 4 years has been reported.[104] In this setting, liver transplantation is more likely to be curative than liver resection[105] and this is particularly true when assessing tumour-free rather than patient survival.[102] However, as stated in a recent Consensus Conference on the indications of liver transplantation:[106] 'liver transplantation in patients with primary liver cancer must be thoroughly evaluated and must be compared with other

Table 3.9 *Results of studies comparing partial and total liver resection in patients with HCC (number in parentheses refer to the number of patients treated in each group)*

Reference	Study	Selection of patients	End point	Resection	OLT	*P*
Iwatsuki 1991[101]	Retrospective	Overall	5-yr survival	32.9% (76)	35.6% (105)	n.s.
		HCC with cirrhosis	5-yr survival	0% (17)	40.7% (71)	0.00001
		HCC without cirrhosis	5-yr survival	43.7% (59)	26.0% (34)	
Bismuth 1993[102]	Retrospective	Overall	3-year survival	52% (60)	49% (60)	n.s.
		size < 3 cm	3-year survival	39% (25)	60% (28)	n.s.
		< 3 nodules < 3 cm	3-year survival	41% (60)	83% (60)	0.05
Tan 1995[105]	Retrospective	Tumour diam < 8 cm	2-years DF survival	41%	73%	0.1

DF: disease free.

methods such as excision, alcoholization and chemoembolization'. The results of retrospective matched-controlled studies and current prospective controlled trials are awaited with interest. Improved outcome following liver transplantation might be expected through improved pretransplant evaluation, more specific immunosuppressive regimens, by limiting manipulation of the tumour at the time of surgery so as to prevent tumour seeding, and by defining antitumoral protocols aimed at controlling tumour growth both prior to and following transplant. As for liver resection, pre- intra- or postoperative chemotherapy and radiotherapy is currently the subject of several studies.[107,108] Comparison with historical controls indicates that an aggressive regimen of postoperative chemotherapy improves survival through a reduction in tumour recurrence.[109] Of interest in this particular setting is the fact that cyclosporin, when used as the main immunosuppressant may block the activity of the drug resistance gene p-glycoprotein (see below) and hence potentiate chemotherapy.

There are, however, several limitations to this further development of liver transplantation besides cost. Liver transplantation is not easily available or not available at all in high endemic areas. Furthermore, in countries where a liver transplant programme does exist, waiting lists are becoming so long due to a relative scarcity of donor organs that a patient initially felt to be a good transplant candidate may no longer be so at the time transplantation is actually performed.

Systemic and regional chemotherapy of HCC

Systemic chemotherapy has very limited value as a primary treatment modality for HCC and only a small number of patients will obtain meaningful palliation. Its ineffectiveness may be due to the expression of a multidrug-resistance gene known as p-glycoprotein that acts as an efflux pump therefore preventing intracellular accumulation of some agents such as doxorubicin. Other confounding factors include the frequent multiclonality of the tumour nodules, and the relatively slow mean tumour volume doubling time which is characteristic for chemoresistant tumours. The best responses have been obtained with intravenous 5-FU or doxorubicin in combination with other drugs. However, even with the best combination, the response rate is less than 20%, the median survival is under 6 months and fewer than 25% of the patients are alive at one year. In randomised controlled trials, systemic chemotherapy has not only failed to prolong patient survival but has also been associated with significant morbidity.[110] Recombinant interferon has also been used as an antitumour agent. Although initial experience was disappointing, two recent controlled trials have shown that high dose interferon was associated with improved survival when compared to no treatment or adriamycin.[111,112]

The poor results with intravenous chemotherapy have prompted trials of hepatic arterial infusion in an attempt to achieve higher local levels of agents with lower systemic toxicity. Liver tumours derive their blood supply principally from the hepatic artery, rather than from the portal vein. Direct infusion of the drug into the hepatic artery may therefore be anticipated to increase the concentration of the drug and the time during which it is in contact with the tumour. For these reasons, drugs with short half-lives are particularly appropriate for this route of administration. However, drugs currently available have either a short half-life but minimal activity on the tumour (such as 5-FU) or better activity but a long half-life (such as anthracyclines). It is currently believed that hepatic artery infusion chemotherapy is more effective than intravenous chemotherapy but does not, however, demonstrate a definitive survival advantage.[113,114] This may be due to the fact that the periphery of the HCC may still receive some of its blood supply from the portal vein.

Transarterial embolisation (TAE) of HCC

Interruption of the arterial blood supply has been undertaken from the early 1970s for hypervascular tumours (such as HCC or neuroendocrine liver metastasis) and has been associated with symptomatic palliation but no substantial impact on survival. To improve the efficacy of locoregional chemotherapy, hepatic artery infusion therapy has been combined with the embolisation of the tumour arterial supply by the injection of iodised oil.

Iodised oil (Lipiodol) is cleared from the normal hepatic parenchyma within 7 days but is retained in malignant tumours several weeks to over a year. This accumulation is not associated with significant adverse effects or with any apparent antitumour effect. This property may, however, be used for targeting cytotoxic drugs by increasing their concentration in the tumour cells. Such drugs have included 5-fluoro-deoxyuridine, emulsified hydrosoluble agents (such as doxorubicin, mitomycin C, epirubicin or cisplatin) and ^{131}Iodine. There is now clear evidence that lipiodol results in a 10 times greater concentration of the drug within the tumour as compared to the adjacent tissue. The response rates following chemo-lipiodolisation have consistently been better than those achieved by systemic or intra-arterial chemotherapy.[117] Similarly, lipiodol-based chemotherapy followed by transcatheter arterial embolisation produces superior results to those obtained by embolisation alone.[115,116] Not surprisingly, there is a good correlation between the efficacy of this treatment and the intensity with which the tumours have been labelled by lipiodol.[117] Lipio-chemo-embolisation is therefore the current locoregional treatment of choice of HCC.

A variety of protocols have been advocated which differ in the method of embolisation (polyvinyl alcohol, gelfoam particles, gelfoam powder or autologous blood clot) and chemotherapy used (cisplatin or doxorubicin, the former seeming more effective than the latter[118]) and the frequency with which embolisations are performed. Encapsulated tumour may become completely necrotic after TAE but a more frequent finding is the presence of necrosis in the central area and persistence of cancer cells in the peripheral area and in the capsular and subcapsular regions due to persisting portal venous supply.

A typical postembolisation syndrome consisting of fever, abdominal pain and nausea occurs in 88% of the patients[119] but, in most patients, these symptoms are self limiting and last for less than 1 week. These symptoms are either related to the necrosis of the tumour or to an effect of this treatment on the non-tumoral adjacent parenchyma. More severe complications are rare and include, by decreasing order of frequency, cholecystitis or gallbladder infarction, upper gastrointestinal bleeding, gastric or duodenal wall necrosis, acute pancreatitis, hepatic abscess formation or rupture of the tumour.[120] These latter complications have become less frequent with the use of supraselective embolisation and are thought to be related to inadequate superselectivity, regurgitation of embolus, anatomical variations, injury of vessel intima or pseudoaneurysm formation. Antibiotics do not prevent the development of the postembolisation syndrome but anti-H_2 receptor blockade should be routinely used and an ultrasound and a serum amylase should be performed in patients who experience delayed or worsening symptoms. Long-term side effects of repeated TAE include the progressive development of distal arterial injuries (comparable to that described after locoregional chemotherapy of liver metastasis) which favour the development of hepatic artery thrombosis. It has been suggested that TAE can be associated with an increase in the incidence of pulmonary metastasis,[124] as a result of the release of tumour cells, and may therefore adversely affect survival. This is especially so with solitary tumours greater than 10 cm in diameter, multiple tumours with the main tumour measuring 5 cm or more, diffuse HCC, intrahepatic portal vein thrombosis, arterioportal or arteriovenous shunt, and in the presence of incomplete tumour necrosis after TAE.[121]

Contraindications to TAE include portal vein thrombosis (as a simultaneous arterial embolisation may lead to liver necrosis), liver decompensation and impaired kidney function. This treatment is suitable, therefore, for probably less than 50% of symptomatic HCC. The mortality associated with this procedure usually ranges between 0 and 2%.[119,120,129] It should, however, be noted that the risk increases rapidly with deteriorating liver function, being 2.8%, 8% and 37% in Child's grade A, B and C, respectively.[122] After recovery from the postembolisation syndrome, most patients maintain at least the same performance status as before treatment and usually recover liver function within the first month of follow-up.[123]

Case-control studies have shown that TAE is associated with a decrease in tumour size (in 50–80% of patients) and AFP levels as well as an improvement in patient survival.[122,124,125] This response after a single TAE is, however, not long lasting and the probability of maintaining response 2 years after TAE has been estimated to be around 10%.[119] In addition, disease reactivation is frequently associated with deteriorating health, worsening liver function or extrahepatic spread so that further TAE is compromised. TAE can be repeated to prolong its beneficial effect, but repeated TAE is associated with an increased risk of hepatic artery thrombosis. At least two courses of TAE are normally delivered at 1 or 2 months interval and subsequent TAE can be undertaken according to the clinical condition and to the objective parameters of tumour growth. A controlled study has also shown that TAE combined with percutaneous injection of ethanol resulted in a better survival than TAE alone in patients with unresectable tumours greater than 3 cm.[126]

However, randomised trials have failed to demonstrate that the inhibition of tumour growth has been associated with a significant effect on long-term patient survival.[127–129] It should be noted that patients enrolled in these studies were unselected and that survival was better in the TAE than in the control group during, at least, the first 2 years after onset of treatment. Furthermore, TAE provides effective symptomatic relief of pain in the majority of patients.[122]

Independent variables of good prognosis after TAE are an age less than 60 years, a Child–Pugh grade A and/or a preserved performance status, a total serum bilirubin less than $1 \, mg \, dl^{-1}$, tumour diameter less than 5 cm, low AFP concentrations, a lack of cancerous portal vein thrombosis and good lipiodol labelling.[116,119,122,125] In addition, reduction in tumour size or AFP levels following a first course of TAE is a good independent predictor of favourable prognosis.[116]

Percutaneous ethanol injection (PEI) of HCC

Absolute ethanol can be used to induce a coagulative necrosis of HCC. This necrosis is followed by the formation of fibrotic and granulomatous tissue and thrombosis of small vessels.

Under local anaesthesia a 22-gauge Chiba needle is introduced into the tumour periphery under US guidance and 2–6 ml of ethanol are slowly injected. The needle should preferentially not enter the tumour directly but through the hepatic parenchyma so as to prevent intraperitoneal bleeding or seeding of tumour cells.

Side effects occur in less than a third of patients and include pain and fever. Complications are rare and result from the passage of ethanol into the bile ducts (resulting in cholangitis) or the portal radicles (resulting in thrombosis). The mortality rate associated with this procedure is minimal and it can usually be performed on an outpatient basis twice a week. Consensus is currently lacking on the ideal method of PEI but promoters of the method stress that PEI should be repeated. Lesions smaller than 2 cm are treated in three to six sessions, whereas lesions of 3.5–5 cm may require 12–15 sessions.[130] Thereafter, PEI is repeated if there is evidence of recurrence upon follow-up. The presence of ascites is a relative contraindication because it will prevent adhesions between the liver and the abdominal wall and hence favour intraperitoneal bleeding. Lesions located in the upper part of segment 7 or 8, may be difficult to identify and/or to puncture without entering the pleural cavity. It may be difficult to achieve a transparenchymal route in pedunculated tumours of the left lobe or of segment 6. Finally, although large HCC (up to 10 cm) may be successfully treated by PEI,[131] it has become clear that the smaller the tumour, the greater the probability of achieving a complete response.[132,133] Hence, the rate of complete tumour necrosis may range between 60 and 100% (depending on the size of the tumour and the frequency of the injections). Recurrence rates are 28.3% within 1 year, 54% within 2 years and 63% within 3 years. The survival of PEI-treated Child grade A patients with HCC less than 5 cm range between 68 and 79% at 3 years and between 47 and 51% at 5 years.

These figures are close to those reported after surgical resection. Retrospective matched controlled studies have suggested that the outcome of these two treatments is comparable in single HCC less than 5 cm in diameter. Liver resection is associated with a greater early risk than PEI but results in a greater radicality (as evidenced by a lower recurrence rate) except in patients with single HCC less than 3 cm in which both procedures are associated with comparable survival rates.[134] Since the safety and costs of PEI and resection differ appreciably, a randomised clinical trial comparing the efficacy of these two treatments in Child grade A patients appears worthwhile especially in high endemic areas.

Comparison of treatments

Although few controlled studies are currently available, there is substantial evidence from retrospective studies using a matched control population that liver resection, percutaneous ethanol injection and TAE improve survival at least in selected patients (Table 3.7).

Accurate comparison between these treatments will only be possible through controlled trials but from available retrospective studies,[51,60,119,124,127–129,134–136] a number of conclusions can be drawn. Surgery and PEI probably achieve comparable results in patients with single HCC less than 2–3 cm provided they can be easily accessed percutaneously. Surgery achieves a better chance of cure for single tumours larger than 3 cm. The risk of surgery is greater than that of PEI in Child B patients and TAE is best indicated in patients with large and/or multiple HCC.

Other palliative treatments

Radiation therapy of HCC

External beam radiation therapy has been of limited value in treating HCC since the tumour is relatively radioresistant whereas the normal liver parenchyma is very radiosensitive. Maximum tolerance of the normal liver to irradiation is generally accepted to be between 2500 and 3000 cGy (a cirrhotic liver is probably even more susceptible). Above these values, the risk of radiation hepatitis increases rapidly and is associated with a mortality rate close to 50%. In addition, it is difficult to protect the surrounding organs such as the colon, duodenum and kidney.

Greater interest has therefore been placed on targeted therapy with either intravenously administered radiolabelled ([131]iodine or [90]yttrium) xenogeneic monoclonal antibodies directed against tumour markers (such as AFP or ferritin) or intra-arterially administered [131]iodine-radiolabelled lipiodol. Intravenous administration of radiolabelled monoclonal antibodies suffers from several limitations, in particular the relatively low radiation dose achieved within the tumour (calculated to be in the order of 1000–1200 cGy), the bone marrow toxicity due to the intravenous route of administration of the compound and the progressive immunisation of the patient against the xenogeneic antibodies. Nevertheless, this method appears more effective than external irradiation and is associated with similar response rates to systemic chemotherapy. The injection of radioisotopes directly into the hepatic artery offers the advantage of increased delivery of isotope within the tumour and decreased systemic toxicity. Mean cumulative radiation dose in the tumour has been shown to be 6240 cGy as compared to 555 cGy in the normal liver and 290 cGy in the lungs.[137] The limitations of this method are that the tumour has to be hypervascular but devoid of arteriovenous shunts and to be of small size due to the relative low energy of [131]iodine. Overall, an objective tumour response is observed in 40% of the patients.[137] In patients with HCC less than 5 cm, a reduction in size of the tumour is obtained in 75% of the patients and complete necrosis may even be obtained for smaller lesions.[138] This technique can be used in patients with portal vein thrombosis and may result in the disappearance of the thrombus. In this setting, a recent controlled trial has shown that intra-arterial injection of [131]iodine-iodised oil was associated with a 6 months survival rate of 48% as compared to 0% in a control group receiving only medical support.[139]

Antiandrogen treatment

Both antiandrogen and antioestrogenic treatments have been used as a palliative treatment of HCC. The rationale for antiandrogen treatment is based on the following observations: (1) the incidence of HCC is higher in men than in women and some studies have also reported an influence of sex on the incidence of recurrence following resection; (2) sex steroid hormones and their receptors are closely involved in hepatocyte regeneration and carcinogenesis; (3) there is experimental evidence that antiandrogen treatments reduce the size and number of HCC. However, results with antiandrogen have been disappointing.

There has been more interest over the past 5 years regarding the use of oestrogenic treatment with tamoxifen. Preliminary uncontrolled studies have yielded encouraging results. Results of controlled studies are controversial with three studies[140–142] demonstrating a 4 to 5-fold improvement in patient survival in patients unsuitable for surgery or alcoholisation although two further studies have shown no benefit.[143,144] Other trials are in progress assessing tamoxifen alone or in combination with antiandrogens. Tamoxifen is cheap, well tolerated and easy to administer although its mechanism of action is not yet clearly defined. It could act through an antioestrogenic effect (although the relevance of the oestrogen receptors in hepatocarcinogenesis is controversial) or through alternative pathways linked to the ability of tamoxifen to also bind to calmodulin or triphenylethylene derivates.

Treatment of complicated HCC

Treatment of HCC with portal vein invasion

Portal vein invasion usually occurs as a relatively late complication of large or diffuse HCC and is associated with a dismal prognosis with a median survival time after its discovery of 4 months. Patients with this mode of extension have therefore traditionally been considered unsuitable for treatment. There are, however, a few patients in whom the HCC from which the thrombus originates is not so advanced. In these patients the risk is not related to the primary tumour but more to the possible extension of the thrombus into the main portal vein resulting in death from acute portal hypertension. Although a classical contraindication to TAE, more recent experience has shown that in some cases, TAE can be performed and is effective. Provided that the tumour is limited to one or two hepatic segments and there is good hepatic function (Child's class A), TAE can be safely performed, may result in partial or even complete remission of the thrombus[122] and is associated with a 3-year survival rate of 24%.[145] Targeted radiotherapy has also been performed (see above). Regression of tumour thrombus has similarly been (although rarely) reported after US-guided injection of chemotherapy or alcohol within the thrombus.

Treatment of ruptured HCC

Spontaneous rupture of HCC occurs in 10–15% of patients and accounts for up to 10% of deaths. This complication is observed particularly in patients with large superficial or protruding tumours.

Ruptured HCC should be suspected in patients with a known HCC or cirrhosis presenting with acute epigastric pain as well as in Asian or African men who develop an acute abdomen or signs of a haemoperitoneum. The majority of patients are not known to have hepatic malignancy before their index admission for bleeding. Bleeding from ruptured HCC is not always exsanguinating, nor necessarily progressive. Minor rupture manifests as abdominal pain or haemorrhagic ascites and hypovolaemic shock is only present in 60% of the patients. However, biological or clinical evidence of liver decompensation is frequent.

Without any treatment, rupture of an HCC is almost always lethal due to persistent bleeding even in patients with normal coagulation. The primary aim of treatment is to stop the bleeding as ascites and/or impaired coagulation usually prevent spontaneous haemostasis. Emergency resection may appear to be the ideal treatment and may indeed be performed if the tumour is small and pedunculated. However, if a formal hepatectomy is required, this should be avoided as the length of time required, the associated blood loss and resection of functional tissue may precipitate or worsen liver decompensation. Patients particularly at risk include those who already have severe cirrhosis or have experienced systemic consequences of their bleeding such as poor liver perfusion, kidney failure, acidosis or hypothermia. In addition, experience with emergency liver resection has shown that clear margins are rarely achieved. In-hospital mortality rates as high as 75% have been reported in patients undergoing one-stage lobectomy.[146]

An alternative is therefore first to achieve haemostasis and delay resection until the patient has recovered from the episode of haemorrhage, and an accurate appraisal of the limits of the tumour and of the functional liver reserve has been made. Several methods of emergency haemostasis have been advocated. Local control through suture plication, packing or argon beam coagulation are usually ineffective. Hepatic artery ligation, although logical because the HCC mainly derives its blood supply from the hepatic artery is frequently effective in controlling bleeding. However, this technique is associated with a high risk because the cirrhotic liver has a reduced portal inflow and hence is more dependent on the arterial supply. In addition, hepatic artery ligation may be ineffective if there is a collateral vascularisation. TAE is therefore currently the treatment of choice, because it has the advantage over hepatic artery ligation of being more selective, but requires the availability of an experienced radiologist. The need for a second stage hepatectomy is dependent on the morphological characteristics of the tumour and on the severity of liver disease. Although rupture of an HCC is probably associated with peritoneal seeding of tumour cells, this should not be regarded as a contraindication to subsequent radical treatment. Data available from the literature indicate that the 1-year survival of patients undergoing second-stage hepatectomy is 40%[147] and long-term survival has been reported.

Fibrolamellar carcinoma

Fibrolamellar carcinoma (FLC) has several pathological and clinical features distinct from that of HCC. It is most frequently observed in the Western hemisphere, where it accounts for 7–20% of primary liver malignancies, and is much less common in Asia. These tumours occur at a younger age than HCC (between 20 and 30 years) and there is no apparent relationship with gender. Most importantly, FLC rarely occurs on a background of chronic liver disease and the prevalence of HBV infection is less than 10%. The most common presenting symptoms are a palpable mass, abdominal pain, weight loss, malaise and anorexia. AFP levels are raised in less than 5% of the patients. FLC usually presents as a large (mean 10–15 cm) solitary hypervascular liver mass. The most characteristic features include the presence of calcification in 40–60% of the patients and a central hypodense region due to central necrosis or fibrosis. Histology demonstrates deeply eosinophilic, polygonal neo-plastic cells surrounded by a dense layered fibrous stroma.

Although the natural history of FLC is ill-defined, these tumours are usually considered as having a relatively better prognosis than HCC. Prolonged survival has been reported even in patients with advanced tumour stage and metastatic spread. The 5-year survival following resection ranges between 40 and 65%. However, it is still unclear whether the histology alone, the absence of underlying chronic liver disease or the greater resectability rate account for the better prognosis of FLC.

Epithelioid haemangio-endothelioma

Epithelioid haemangioendothelioma (EHE) is a rare tumour that develops from the endothelial cells lining the sinusoids and progresses along the sinusoids, hepatic venules and portal vein branches. The neoplastic cells have an epithelioid or a dendritic shape but their vascular origin is identified by antibodies against factor VIII-related antigen or other endothelial markers. The stroma of this tumour has a myxoid appearance that may become fibrotic. Calcification is identified on abdominal radiograph or CT scans in 10–30% of the patients.

The tumour usually develops in young adults but no risk factors have been identified. It does not generally arise on a background of chronic liver disease although an association with cirrhosis or nodular regenerative hyperplasia is reported.[148] The tumour usually has a multifocal distribution in the liver and 20% of the patients have lung (or more rarely bone) metastasis at the time of diagnosis.

MRI is the most reliable radiological investigation[149] but is not specific and a biopsy is mandatory to confirm the diagnosis. It is, however, important to be aware that EHE can occasionally be very difficult to differentiate from other tumours (such as cholangiocarcinoma or angiosarcoma) due to the epithelioid shape of the tumour cells and the dense fibrotic stroma.

The natural history is highly variable and prolonged survival of more than 10 years has been reported without any treatment. However, 20% of patients are dead within 2 years of diagnosis and 20% survive more than 5 years.[150] Although the potentially lengthy clinical course following diagnosis favours resection, partial hepatectomy is rarely feasible due to the usually multifocal involvement of the liver. Total liver resection (i.e. liver transplantation) has been performed in a limited number of patients some of whom had metastasis at the time of transplantation. The actuarial survival after transplantation is 82% at 2 years and 43% at 5 years with most of the deaths being due to tumour recurrence[99] although metastatic tumour regression has been described after transplantation.[151] There is no evidence that liver transplantation improves the prognosis of these patients. The current shortage of liver grafts and the prolonged waiting time, may dictate that liver transplantation only be indicated in very selected patients. Chemotherapy, chemoembolisation or radiotherapy do not appear to be effective.

Angiosarcoma

Angiosarcoma are the most frequent sarcoma of the liver but remain rare tumours. Their prevalence in autopsy series ranges between 0.002% and 0.01% and they account for 0.5–1.8% of primary liver malignancies. The tumour develops from endothelial cells lining the hepatic sinusoids, and grows along sinusoids, hepatic venules and portal vein branches. Disruption of hepatic plates may result in the development of cavities filled with tumour debris or clotted blood which favour the invasion of hepatic and portal veins. These tumours have ill-defined borders and typically involve the entire liver.

There is a clear association of angiosarcoma with prior exposure of the patient to thorium dioxide (Thorotrast, a contrast medium used in radiology during the first half of the 20th century), arsenicals or vinyl chloride (used in the manufacture of plastics). An association with androgenic anabolic steroids, oestrogens, oral contraceptives, phenelzine and culpric acid has also been reported. Overall, up to 50% of angiosarcoma are associated with previous exposure to a chemical carcinogenic agent. These risk factors may account for the male predominance (sex ratio of 3/1) and the age at the time of diagnosis (50–70 years). It has also been suggested that angiosarcoma may represent progression of an haemangioendothelioma into the malignant condition. Evidence to support this evolution is the possible occurrence of angiosarcoma in children and the coexistence, within the same tumour, of features of angiosarcoma and of cavernous haemangioma.[152] Liver cirrhosis is not a risk factor for angiosarcoma.

Angiosarcoma are rapidly growing tumours and, because they are frequently discovered at a late stage, median survival is 6 months.[153] Deaths may result from liver failure or from intraperitoneal bleeding due to rupture of the tumour. Bleeding is favoured by the hypervascularisation of the tumour by thrombocytopenia as part of a consumption coagulopathy or by liver failure. Prolonged survival beyond 7 years has, however, been reported.[153,154] It is, therefore, reasonable to attempt resection (whenever possible) and to administer adjuvant chemotherapy. Liver transplantation has not been associated with survival beyond 3 years due to tumour recurrence, and is therefore not indicated in patients with angiosarcoma. Radiation therapy may have some value in this particular tumour.

Malignant lymphoma

The liver is frequently involved by lymphoma (5–10% for Hodgkin's disease, 15–40% for non-Hodgkin's lymphoma) but primary lymphoma of the liver is rare (10 cases had been published by 1986). They develop predominantly in men (90%) and present either as multiple nodules or, in 50% of the patients, as a solitary large mass.[155]

Because primary lymphoma of the liver is not necessarily a disseminated disease from its inception, resection should be considered, when possible, in addition to chemotherapy.

References

1. Collier JD, Guo K, Burt AD, Bassendine MF, Major GN. Deficient repair of DNA lesion O6-methylguanine in cirrhosis. Lancet 1993; 341: 207–8.

2. De Mitri MS, Poussin K, Baccarini P et al. HCV-associated liver cancer without cirrhosis. Lancet 1995; 345: 413–15.

3. El-Refaie A, Savage K, Bhattacharya S et al. HCV-associated hepatocellular carcinoma without cirrhosis. J Hepatol 1996; 24: 277–85.

4. Paterlini P, Gerken G, Nakajima E et al. Polymerase chain reaction to detect hepatitis B virus DNA and RNA sequences in primary liver cancers from patients negative for hepatitis B surface antigen. N Engl J Med 1990; 323: 80–5.

5. Kim CM, Koike K, Saito L, Miyamura T, Jay G. HBx gene of hepatitis B virus induced liver cancer in transgenic mice. Nature 1991; 351: 317–20.

6. Sakamuro D, Furukawa T, Takegami T. Hepatitis C virus nonstructural protein NS3 transforms NIH 3T3 cells. J Virol 1995; 69: 3893–6.

7. Tsukuma H, Hiyama T, Tanaka S et al. Risk factors for hepatocellular carcinoma among patients with chronic liver disease. N Engl J Med 1993; 328: 1797–801.

8. Kato Y, Nakata K, Omagari K et al. Risk of hepatocellular carcinoma in patients with cirrhosis in Japan. Analysis of infectious hepatitis viruses. Cancer 1994; 74: 2234–8.

9. Takano S, Yokosuka O, Imazeki F, Tagawa M, Omata M. Incidence of hepatocellular carcinoma in chronic hepatitis B and C: a prospective study of 251 patients. Hepatology 1995; 21: 650–5.

10. Shiratori Y, Shiina S, Imamura M et al. Characteristic difference of hepatocellular carcinoma between hepatitis B- and C- viral infection in Japan. Hepatology 1995; 22: 1027–33.

11. Niederau C, Fisher R, Sonnenberg A, Stremmel W, Trampisch HJ, Strohmeyer G. Survival and cause of death in cirrhotic patients with primary hemochromatosis. N Engl J Med 1985; 31: 1256–83.

12. Fargion S, Fracanzani AL, Piperno A et al. Prognostic factors for hepatocellular carcinoma in genetic hemochromatosis. Hepatology 1994; 20: 1426–34.

13. Fattovich G, Giustina G, Schalm SW et al. Occurrence of hepatocellular carcinoma and decompensation in Western European patients with cirrhosis type B. Hepatology 1995; 21: 77–82.

14. Colombo M, de Franchis R, Del Ninno E et al. Hepatocellular carcinoma in Italian patients with cirrhosis. N Engl J Med 1991; 325: 675–80.

15. Borzio M, Bruno S, Roncalli M et al. Liver cell dysplasia is a major risk factor for hepatocellular carcinoma in cirrhosis: a prospective study. Gastroenterology 1995; 108: 812–17.

16. Pateron D, Ganne N, Trinchet JC et al. Prospective study of screening for hepatocellular carcinoma in Caucasian patients with cirrhosis. J Hepatol 1994; 20: 65–71.

17. Oka H, Kurioka N, Kim K et al. Prospective study of early detection of hepatocellular carcinoma in patients with cirrhosis. Hepatology 1990; 12: 680–7.

18. Nishiguchi S, Kuroki T, Nakatani S et al. Randomised trial of effects of interferon-α on incidence of hepatocellular carcinoma in chronic active hepatitis C with cirrhosis. Lancet 1995; 346: 1051–5.

19. Mazzella G, Accogli E, Sottili S et al. Alpha interferon treatment may prevent hepatocellular carcinoma in HCV-related liver cirrhosis. J Hepatol 1996; 24: 141–7.

20. Lok ASF. Does interferon therapy for chronic hepatitis B reduce the risks of developing cirrhosis and hepatocellular carcinoma. Hepatology 1995; 22: 1336–7.

21. Oka H, Yamamoto S, Kuroki T et al. Prospective study of chemoprevention of hepatocellular carcinoma with Sho-saiko-to (TJ)ç). Cancer 1995; 76: 743–9.

22. Peers FJ, Bosch FX, Kaldor JM, Linsell CA, Pluijmen M. Aflatoxin exposure, hepatitis B virus and liver cancer in Swaziland. Int J Cancer 1987; 39: 545–53.

23. Ross RK, Yuan JM, Yu MC et al. Urinary aflatoxin biomarkers and risk of hepatocellular carcinoma. Lancet 1992; 339: 943–6.

24. Chen CJ, Wang LY, Lu SN et al. Elevated aflatoxin exposure and increased risk of

hepatocellular carcinoma. Hepatology 1996; 24: 38–42.

25. Ohto M, Kondo F, Ebara M. Pathology, diagnosis and treatment of small liver cancer. In: Tobe T, Kaneda H, Okudaira M et al. (eds) Primary liver cancer in Japan. Tokyo: Springer, 1992.

26. International working party. Terminology of nodular hepatocellular lesions. Hepatology 1995; 22: 983–93.

27. Chen DS, Sung JL, Sheu JC et al. Serum alpha-fetoprotein in the early stage of human hepatocellular carcinoma. Gastroenterology 1984; 86: 1404–9.

28. Bloomer JR, Waldmann TA, McIntyre KR, Klatskin G. Alpha-fetoprotein in non-neoplastic hepatic disorders. JAMA 1975; 233: 38–41.

29. Sato Y, Nakata K, Kato Y et al. Early recognition of hepatocellular carcinoma based on altered profiles of alpha-fetoprotein. N Engl J Med 1993; 328: 1802–6.

30. Ueda K, Kitagawa K, Kadoya M, Matsui O, Takashima T, Yamahana T. Detection of hypervascular hepatocellular carcinoma by using spiral volumetric CT: comparison of US and MR imaging. Abdom Imaging 1995; 20: 547–53.

31. Stevens WR, Johnson CD, Stephens DH, Batts KP. CT findings in hepatocellular carcinoma: correlation of tumor characteristics with causative factors, tumor size, and histological tumor grade. Radiology 1994; 191: 531–7.

32. Choi BI, Park JH, Kim BH, Kim SH, Han MC, Kim CW. Small hepatocellular carcinoma: detection with sonography, computed tomography (CT), angiography and lipiodol CT. Br J Surg 1989; 62: 897–903.

33. Rizzi PM, Kane PA, Ryder SD et al. Accuracy of radiology in detection of hepatocellular carcinoma before liver transplantation. Gastroenterology 1994; 107: 1425–9.

34. Okada S, Okazaki N, Nose H, Yoshimori M, Aoki K. Prognostic factors in patients with hepatocellular carcinoma receiving systemic chemotherapy. Hepatology 1992; 16: 112–17.

35. Calvet X, Bruix J, Gines P, Bru C, Sole M, Vilana R, Rodes J. Prognostic factors of hepatocellular carcinoma in the West: a multivariate analysis in 206 patients. Hepatology 1990; 12: 753–60.

36. Akashi Y, Koreeda C, Enomoto S et al. Prognosis of unresectable hepatocellular carcinoma: an evaluation based on multivariate analysis of 90 cases. Hepatology 1991; 14: 262–8.

37. Sheu JC, Sung JL, Chen DS et al. Growth rate of asymptomatic hepatocellular carcinoma and its clinical implications. Gastroenterology 1985; 89: 259–66.

38. Ebara M, Ohto M, Shinagawa et al. Natural history of minute hepatocellular carcinoma smaller than 3 cm complicating cirrhosis. Gastroenterology 1986; 90: 289–98.

39. Okazaki N, Yoshino M, Yoshida T et al. Evaluation of the prognosis for small hepatocellular carcinoma based on tumor volume doubling time. Cancer 1989; 63: 2207–10.

40. Barbara L, Benzi G, Gaiani S et al. Natural history of small untreated hepatocellular carcinoma in cirrhosis: a multivariate analysis of prognostic factors of tumor growth rate and patient survival. Hepatology 1992; 16: 132–7.

41. Itaya H, Fukuda M, Mima S. Studies on early detection of hepatocellular carcinoma. HCC cases detected by ultrasound mass survey with subsequent therapeutic results. In: Hepatocellular carcinoma in Asia. Kobe, Japan: International center for Medical Research, 1985; 183–95.

42. Kobayashi K, Sugimoto T, Makino H et al. Screening methods for early detection of hepatocellular carcinoma. Hepatology 1985; 5: 1100–5.

43. Tanaka S, Kitamura T, Nakanishi K et al. Effectiveness of periodic checkup by ultrasonography for the early diagnosis of hepatocellular carcinoma. Cancer 1990; 66: 2210–14.

44. Ganne-Carrié N, Chastang C, Chapel F et al. Predictive score for the development of hepatocellular carcinoma and additional value of liver large cell dysplasia in Western patients with cirrhosis. Hepatology 1996; 23: 1112–18.

45. Oka H, Tamori A, Kuroki T, Kobayashi K, Yamamoto S. Prospective study of α-fetoprotein in cirrhotic patients monitored for development of hepatocellular carcinoma. Hepatology 1994; 19: 61–6.

46. Sato M, Watanabe Y, Ueda S et al. Microwave coagulation therapy for hepatocellular carcinoma. Gastroenterology 1996; 110: 1507–14.

47. Lin TY, Lee CS, Chen CC, Liau KY, Lin WSJ. Regeneration of human liver after hepatic

lobectomy studied by repeated liver scanning and repeated needle biopsy. Ann Surg 1979; 190: 48.

48. Nagasue N, Yakaya H, Kohno H. Human liver regeneration after major hepatic resection. A study of normal liver and livers with chronic hepatitis and cirrhosis. Ann Surg 1987; 206: 30.

49. Takenaka K, Kawahara N, Yamamoto K *et al.* Results of 280 liver resections for hepatocellular carcinoma. Arch Surg 1996; 131: 71–6.

50. Kawasaki S, Makuuchi M, Miyagawa S *et al.* Results of hepatic resection for hepatocellular carcinoma. World J Surg 1995; 19: 31–4.

51. Bronowicki JP, Boudjema K, Chone L *et al.* Comparison of resection, liver transplantation and transcatheter oily chemoembolization in the treatment of hepatocellular carcinoma. J Hepatol 1996; 24: 293–300.

52. Nagasue N, Kohno H, Chang YC *et al.* Liver resection for hepatocellular carcinoma. Results of 229 consecutive patients during 11 years. Ann Surg 1993; 217: 375–84.

53. Yamanaka N, Okamoto E, Kuwata K, Tanaka N. A multiple regression equation for prediction of posthepatectomy liver failure. Ann Surg 1984; 200: 658–63.

54. Fan ST, Lai ECS, Lo CM, Ng IOL, Wong J. Hospital mortality of major hepatectomy for hepatocellular carcinoma associated with cirrhosis. Arch Surg 1995; 130: 198–203.

55. Pite J, Houssin D, Kracht M. Resection of hepatocellular carcinoma. A multicenter study of 153 patients. Gastroenterol Clin Biol 1993; 17: 200–6.

56. Lai ECS, Fan ST, Lo CM, Chu KM, Wong J. Hepatic resection to hepatocellular carcinoma: an audit of 343 patients. Ann Surg 1995; 221: 291–8.

57. Fan ST, Lo CM, Lai ECS, Chu KM, Liu CL, Wong J. Perioperative nutritional support in patients undergoing hepatectomy for hepatocellular carcinoma. N Engl J Med 1994; 331: 1547–52.

58. The Liver Cancer Study Group in Japan. Predictive factors for long term prognosis after partial hepatectomy for patients with hepatocellular carcinoma in Japan. Cancer 1994; 74: 2772–80.

59. Yamanaka N, Okamoto E. Conditions favoring long-term survival after hepatectomy for hepatocellular carcinomas. Cancer Chemother Pharmacol 1989; 23: S83–86.

60. Bruix J, Cirera I, Calvet X *et al.* Surgical resection and survival in Western patients with hepatocellular carcinoma. J Hepatol 1992; 15: 350–5.

61. Cottone M, Virdone R, Fusco G *et al.* Asymptomatic hepatocellular carcinoma in Child's A cirrhosis. Gastroenterology 1989; 96: 1566–71.

62. Bismuth H, Chiche L, Castaing D. Surgical treatment of hepatocellular carcinomas in noncirrhotic liver: experience with 68 liver resections. World J Surg 1995; 19: 35–41.

63. Nagasue N, Uchida M, Makina Y *et al.* Incidence and factors associated with intrahepatic recurrence following resection of hepatocellular carcinoma. Gastroenterology 1993; 105: 488–94.

64. Ouchi K, Matsubara S, Fukuhara K, Tominaga T, Matsuno S. Recurrence of hepatocellular carcinoma in the liver remnant after hepatic resection. Am J Surg 1993; 166: 270–3.

65. Izumi R, Shimizu K, Li T *et al.* Prognostic factors of hepatocellular carcinoma in patients undergoing hepatic resection. Gastroenterology 1994; 106: 720–7.

66. Okada S, Shimada K, Yamamoto J *et al.* Predictive factors for postoperative recurrence of hepatocellular carcinoma. Gastroenterology 1994; 106: 1618–24.

67. Belghiti J, Panis Y, Farges O *et al.* Intrahepatic recurrence after resection of hepatocellular carcinoma complicating cirrhosis. Ann Surg 1991; 214: 114–17.

68. Lui WY, Chau GY, Loong CC *et al.* Hepatic segmentectomy for curative resection of primary hepatocellular carcinoma. Arch Surg 1995; 130: 1090–7.

69. Chen MF, Hwang TL, Jeng LB, Wang CS, Jan YY, Chen SC. Postoperative recurrence of hepatocellular carcinoma. Two hundred and five consecutive patients who underwent hepatic resection in 15 years. Arch Surg 1994; 129: 738–42.

70. Ikeda K, Saitoh S, Tsubota A *et al.* Risk factors for tumor recurrence and prognosis after curative resection of hepatocellular carcinoma. Cancer 1993; 71: 19–25.

71. Takayasu K, Wakao F, Moriyama N *et al.* Postresection recurrence of hepatocellular

carcinoma treated by arterial embolization: analysis of prognostic factors. Hepatology 1992; 16: 906–11.

72. Lee PH, Lin WJ, Tsang YM *et al.* Clinical management of recurrent hepatocellular carcinoma. Ann Surg 1995; 222: 670–6.

73. Sugioka A, Tsuzuki T, Kanai T. Postresection prognosis of patients with hepatocellular carcinoma. Surgery 1993; 113: 612–18.

74. Jwo SC, Chiu JH, Chau GY, Loong CC, Lui WY. Risk factors linked to tumor recurrence of human hepatocellular carcinoma after hepatic resection. Hepatology 1992; 16: 1367–71.

75. Nagashima I, Hamada C, Naruse K *et al.* Surgical resection for small hepatocellular carcinoma. Surgery 1996; 119: 40–5.

76. Sasaki Y, Imaoka S, Ishiguro S *et al.* Clinical features of small hepatocellular carcinomas as assessed by histological grades. Surgery 1996; 119: 252–60.

77. Yamamoto J, Kosuge T, Takayama T *et al.* Perioperative blood transfusion promotes recurrence of hepatocellular carcinoma after hepatectomy. Surgery 1994; 115: 303–9.

78. Lai ECS, Ng IOL, Ng MMT *et al.* Long-term results of resection for large hepatocellular carcinoma: a multivariate analysis of clinicopathological features. Hepatology 1990; 11: 815–18.

79. Yoshida Y, Kanematsu T, Matsumata T, Takenaka K, Sugimachi K. Surgical margin and recurrence after resection of hepatocellular carcinoma in patients with cirrhosis. Further evaluation of limited hepatic resection. Ann Surg 1989; 209: 297–301.

80. Lai ECS, You KT, Ng IOL, Shek TWH. The pathological basis of resection margin for hepatocellular carcinoma. World J Surg 1993; 17: 786–91.

81. Adachi E, Maeda T, Matsumata T *et al.* Risk factors for intrahepatic recurrence in human small hepatocellular carcinoma. Gastroenterology 1995; 108: 768–75.

82. Chiu JH, Wu LH, Kao HL *et al.* Can determination of the proliferative capacity of the nontumor portion predict the risk of tumor recurrence in the liver remnant after resection of human hepatocellular carcinoma. Hepatology 1993; 18: 96–102.

83. Nakajima Y, Shimamura T, Kamiyama T *et al.* Evaluation of surgical resection for small

hepatocellular carcinoma. Am J Surg 1996; 171: 360–3.

84. Takenaka K, Adachi E, Nishizaki T *et al.* Possible multicentric occurrence of hepatocellular carcinoma: a clinicopathological study. Hepatology 1994; 19: 889–94.

85. Suenaga M, Sugiura H, Kobuka Y, Uehara S, Kurumiya T. Repeated hepatic resection for recurrent hepatocellular carcinoma in eighteen cases. Surgery 1994; 115: 452–7.

86. Lange JF, Leese T, Castaing D, Bismuth H. Repeat hepatectomy for recurrent malignant tumors of the liver. Surg Gynecol Obstet 1989; 169: 119–26.

87. Shimada M, Matsumata T, Taketomi A, Yamamoto K, Itasaka H, Sugimachi K. Repeat hepatectomy for recurrent hepatocellular carcinoma. Surgery 1994; 115: 703–6.

88. Nagasue N, Kohno H, Hayashi T *et al.* Repeat hepatectomy for recurrent hepatocellular carcinoma. Br J Surg 1996; 83: 127–31.

89. Matsuda Y, Ito T, Oguchi Y, Nakajima K, Izukara T. Rationale of surgical management for recurrent hepatocellular carcinoma. Ann Surg 1993; 217: 28–34.

90. Sasaki Y, Imaoka S, Fujita M *et al.* Regional therapy in the management of intrahepatic recurrence after surgery for hepatoma. Ann Surg 1987; 206: 40–7.

91. Furuta T, Kanematsu T, Matsumata T *et al.* Lipiodolization prolongs survival rates in postoperative patients with a recurrent hepatocellular carcinoma. Hepatogastroenterology 1990; 37: 494–7.

92. Shirabe K, Kanematsu T, Matsumata T, Adachi E, Akazawa K. Sugimachi K. Factors linked to early recurrence of small hepatocellular carcinoma after hepatectomy: univariate and multivariate analysis. Hepatology 1991; 14: 802–5.

93. Yu YQ, Xu DB, Zhou XD, Lu JZ, Tang ZY, Mack P. Experience with liver resection after hepatic arterial chemoembolization for hepatocellular carcinoma. Cancer 1993; 71: 62–5.

94. Takenaka K, Yoshida K, Nishizaki T *et al.* Postoperative prophylactic lipiodolization reduces the intrahepatic recurrence of hepatocellular carcinoma. Am J Surg 1995; 169: 400–5.

95. Yamamoto M, Arii S, Sugahara K, Tobe T. Adjuvant oral chemotherapy to prevent

recurrence after curative resection for hepatocellular carcinoma. Br J Surg 1996; 83: 336–40.

96. Nonami T, Isshiki K, Katoh H *et al*. The potential role of postoperative hepatic artery chemotherapy in patients with high-risk hepatomas. Ann Surg 1991; 213: 222–6.
97. Izumi R, Shimizu K, Iyobe T *et al*. Postoperative adjuvant hepatic arterial infusion of lipiodol containing anticancer drugs in patients with hepatocellular carcinoma. Hepatology 1994; 20: 295–301.
98. Muto Y, Moriwaki H, Ninomiya M *et al*. Prevention of second primary tumors by an acyclic retinoid, polyprenoic acid, in patients with hepatocellular carcinoma. N Engl J Med 1996; 334: 1561–7.
99. Penn I. Hepatic transplantation for primary and metastatic cancers of the liver. Surgery 1991; 110: 726–35.
100. Yokoyama I, Sheahan DG, Carr B *et al*. Clinicopathological factors affecting patient survival and tumor recurrence after orthotopic liver transplantation for hepatocellular carcinoma. Transplant Proc 1991; 23: 2194–6.
101. Iwatsuki S, Starzl TE, Sheahan DG *et al*. Hepatic resection versus transplantation for hepatocellular carcinoma. Ann Surg 1991; 214: 221–9.
102. Bismuth H, Chiche L, Adam R, Castaing D, Diamond T, Dennison A. Liver resection versus transplantation for hepatocellular carcinoma in cirrhotic patients. Ann Surg 1993; 218: 145–51.
103. Selby R, Kadry Z, Carr B, Tzakis A, Madariaga JR, Iwatsuki S. Liver transplantation for hepatocellular carcinoma. World J Surg 1995; 19: 53–8.
104. Mazzaferro V, Regalia E, Doci R *et al*. Liver transplantation for the treatment of small hepatocellular carcinomas in patients with cirrhosis. N Engl J Med 1996; 334: 693–9.
105. Tan KC, Rela M, Ryder SD *et al*. Experience of liver transplantation and hepatic resection for hepatocellular carcinoma of less than 8 cm in patients with cirrhosis. Br J Surg 1995; 82: 253–6.
106. Consensus Conference on indications of liver transplantation. In: Bismuth H (ed) Hepatology 1994; 20: 66S.
107. Stone MJ, Klintmalm GB, Polter D *et al*. Neoadjuvant chemotherapy and liver transplantation for hepatocellular carcinoma: a pilot study in 20 patients. Gastroenterology 1993; 104: 196–202.
108. Cherqui D, Piedbois P, Pierga JY *et al*. Multimodal adjuvant treatment and liver transplantation for advanced hepatocellular carcinoma. A pilot study. Cancer 1994; 73: 2721–6.
109. Olthoff KM, Rosove MH, Shackleton CR *et al*. Adjuvant chemotherapy improves survival after liver transplantation for hepatocellular carcinoma. Ann Surg 1995; 221: 734–43.
110. Lai C, Wu P, Chan G *et al*. Doxorubicin versus no antitumour therapy in inoperable hepatocellular carcinoma. A prospective randomized trial. Cancer 1988; 62: 479–83.
111. Lai CL, Mu PC, Lok ASF. Recombinant alpha-2-interferon is superior to doxorubicin for inoperable hepatocellular carcinoma: a prospective randomised trial. Br J Cancer 1989; 60: 928–33.
112. Lai CL, Lau JYN, Wu PC *et al*. Recombinant interferon-alpha in inoperable hepatocellular carcinoma: a randomized controlled trial. Hepatology 1993; 17: 389–94.
113. Nerenstone SR, Ihde DC, Friedman MA. Clinical trials in primary hepatocellular carcinoma: current status and future directions. Cancer Treat Rev 1988; 15: 1–31.
114. Ramming KP. The effectiveness of hepatic artery infusion in treatment of primary hepatobiliary tumors. Semin Oncol 1983; 10: 199–205.
115. Takayasu K, Shima Y, Muramatsu Y *et al*. Hepatocellular carcinoma: treatment with intraarterial iodized oil with and without chemotherapeutic agents. Radiology 1987; 162: 345–51.
116. Mondazzi L, Bottelli R, Brambilla G *et al*. Transarterial oily chemoembolization for the treatment of hepatocellular carcinoma: a multivariate analysis of prognostic factors. Hepatology 1994; 19: 1115–23.
117. Kanematsu T, Furuta T, Takenaka K *et al*. A 5-year experience of lipiodolization: selective regional chemotherapy for 200 patients with hepatocellular carcinoma. Hepatology 1989; 10: 98–102.
118. Kasugai H, Kojima J, Tatsuta M *et al*. Treatment of hepatocellular carcinoma by transcatheter arterial embolization combined with intraarterial infusion of a mixture of cisplatin

and ethiodized oil. Gastroenterology 1989; 97: 965–71.

119. Bruix J, Castells A, Montanya X et al. Phase II study of transarterial embolization in European patients with hepatocellular carcinoma: need for controlled trials. Hepatology 1994; 20: 643–50.

120. Jeng KS, Ching HJ. The role of surgery in the management of unusual complications of transcatheter arterial embolization for hepatocellular carcinoma. World J Surg 1988; 12: 362–8.

121. Liou TC, Shih SC, Kao CR, Chou SY, Lin SC, Wang HY. Pulmonary metastasis of hepatocellular carcinoma associated with transarterial chemoembolization. J Hepatol 1995; 23: 563–8.

122. Bismuth H, Morino M, Sherlock D, Castaing D, Miglietta C, Cauquil P, Roche A. Primary treatment of hepatocellular carcinoma by arterial chemoembolization. Am J Surg 1992; 163: 387–94.

123. Miyoshi S, Minami Y, Kawata S et al. Changes in hepatic functional reserve after transcatheter embolization of hepatocellular carcinoma. Assessment by maximal removal of indocyanine green. J Hepatol 1988; 6: 332–6.

124. Vetter D, Wenger JJ, Bergier JM, Doffoel M, Bockel R. Transcatheter oily chemoembolization in the management of advanced hepatocellular carcinoma in cirrhosis: results of a Western comparative study in 60 patients. Hepatology 1991; 13: 427–33.

125. Stefanini GF, Amorati P, Biselli M et al. Efficacy of transarterial targeted treatments on survival of patients with hepatocellular carcinoma. Cancer 1995; 75: 2427–34.

126. Tanaka K, Nakamura S, Numata K et al. Hepatocellular carcinoma: treatment with percutaneous ethanol injection and transcatheter arterial embolization. Radiology 1992; 185: 457–60.

127. Lin DY, Liaw YF, Lee TY, Lai CM. Hepatic arterial embolization in patients with unresectable hepatocellular carcinoma – a randomized controlled trial. Gastroenterology 1988; 94: 453–6.

128. Pelletier G, Roche A, Ink O et al. A randomized trial of hepatic arterial chemoembolization in patients with unresectable hepatocellular carcinoma. J Hepatol 1990; 11: 181–4.

129. Groupe d'Etude et de Traitement du Carcinome Hépatocellulaire. A comparison of lipiodol chemoembolization and conservative treatment for unresectable hepatocellular carcinoma. N Engl J Med 1995; 332: 1256–61.

130. Livraghi T, Bolondi L, Lazzaroni S et al. Percutaneous ethanol injection in the treatment of hepatocellular carcinoma in cirrhosis. Cancer 1992; 69: 925–9.

131. Shiina S, Tagawa K, Unuma T et al. Percutaneous ethanol injection therapy of hepatocellular carcinoma. Analysis of 77 patients. Am J Roentgenol 1990; 155: 1221.

132. Vilana R, Bruix J, Bru C, Ayuso C, Sole M, Rodes J. Tumor size determines the efficacy of percutaneous ethanol injection for the treatment of small hepatocellular carcinoma. Hepatology 1992; 16: 353–7.

133. Ohnishi K, Nomura F, Ito S, Fujiwara K. Prognosis of small hepatocellular carcinoma (less than 3 cm) after percutaneous acetic acid injection: study of 91 cases. Hepatology 1996; 23: 994–1002.

134. Castells A, Bruix J, Bru C et al. Treatment of small hepatocellular carcinoma in cirrhotic patients: a cohort study comparing surgical resection and percutaneous ethanol injection. Hepatology 1993; 18: 1121–6.

135. Kanematsu T, Matsumata T, Shirabe K et al. A comparative study of hepatic resection and transcatheter arterial embolization for the treatment of primary hepatocellular carcinoma. Cancer 1993; 71: 2181–6.

136. Livraghi T, Bolondi L, Buscarini L et al. No treatment, resection and ethanol injection in hepatocellular carcinoma: a retrospective analysis of survival in 391 patients with cirrhosis. J Hepatol 1995; 22: 522–6.

137. Raoul JI, Bretagne JF, Caucanas JP et al. Internal radiation therapy for hepatocellular carcinoma. Results of a French multicenter phase II trial of transarterial injection of iodine 131-labeled lipiodol. Cancer 1992; 69: 346–52.

138. Yoo HS, Park CH, Lee JT et al. Small hepatocellular carcinoma: high dose internal radiation therapy with superselective intra-arterial injection of I-131-labeled lipiodol. Cancer Chemother Pharmacol 1993; 33: S128–33.

139. Raoul JL, Guyader D, Bretagne JF et al. Randomized controlled trial for hepatocellular carcinoma with portal vein thrombosis:

intraarterial iodine-131-iodized oil versus medical support. J Nucl Med 1994; 35: 1782–7.

140. Farinati F, Salvagnini M, de Maria N et al. Unresectable hepatocellular carcinoma: a prospective controlled trial with tamoxifen. J Hepatol 1990; 11: 297–301.

141. Cerezo FJ, Tomas A, Donosco L et al. Controlled trial of tamoxifen in patients with advanced hepatocellular carcinoma. J Hepatol 1994; 20: 702–6.

142. Manesis EK, Giannoulis G, Zoumboulis P, Vafiadou I, Hadziyannis SJ. Treatment of hepatocellular carcinoma with combined suppression and inhibition of sex hormones: a randomized, controlled trial. Hepatology 1995; 21: 1535–42.

143. Coll S, Sola R, Vila MC et al. Treatment with tamoxifen in patients with advanced hepatocellular carcinoma. Results of a randomized placebo controlled trial (abstract). Hepatology 1995; 22 (suppl): 404A.

144. Castells A, Bruix J, Bru C et al. Treatment of hepatocellular carcinoma with tamoxifen: a double-blind placebo-controlled trial in 120 patients. Gastroenterology 1995; 109: 917–22.

145. Chung JW, Park JH, Han JK, Choi BI, Han MC. Hepatocellular carcinoma and portal vein invasion: results of treatment with transcatheter oily chemoembolization. Am J Roentgenol 1995; 165: 315–21.

146. Lai ECS, Wu KM, Choi TK, Fan ST, Wong J. Spontaneous ruptured hepatocellular carcinoma. An appraisal of surgical treatment. Ann Surg 1989; 210: 24–8.

147. Zhu LX, Wang GS, Fan ST. Spontaneous rupture of hepatocellular carcinoma. Br J Surg 1996; 83: 602–7.

148. Ishak KG, Sesterhenn IA, Goodman ZD et al. Epithelioid hemangioendothelioma of the liver: a clinicopathologic and follow-up study of 32 cases. Hum Pathol 1984; 15: 839–52.

149. Beers BV, Roche A, Mathieu D et al. Epithelioid hemangioendothelioma of the liver: MR and CT findings. J Comput Assist Tomogr 1992; 16: 420–4.

150. Radin DR, Craig JR, Colletti PM, Ralls PW, Halls JM. Hepatic epithelioid hemangioendothelioma. Radiology 1988; 169: 145–8.

151. Marino IR, Todo S, Tzakis AG et al. Treatment of hepatic epithelioid hemangioendothelioma with liver transplantation. Cancer 1988; 62: 2079–84.

152. Tohme C, Drouot E, Piard F et al. Cavernous hemangioma of the liver associated with angiosarcoma: malignant transformation? Gastroenterol Clin Biol 1991; 15: 83–6.

153. Locker GY, Oroshow JH, Zwelling LA, Chabner BA. The clinical features of hepatic angiosarcoma: a report of four cases and a review of the English literature. Medicine 1979; 58: 48–64.

154. Paliard P, Valette PJ, Berger F, Contassot JC, Partenski C. Peliosis hepatis of late onset in a patient exposed to vinyl chloride and treated for hepatic angiosarcoma. Gastroenterol Clin Biol 1991; 15: 445–8.

155. Ryoo JW, Manaligod JR, Walker MJ. Primary lymphoma of the liver. J Clin Gastroenterol 1986; 8: 308–11.

4 Hepatic metastases

Thomas J. Hugh
Graeme J. Poston

Introduction

The liver is a common site of metastatic spread of tumours, especially those originating in the gastrointestinal tract. In autopsy studies of patients who die of malignant disease, hepatic metastases are found in up to 36% of cases. The six commonest primary sites responsible for liver metastases are colon and rectum, bronchus, pancreas, breast, stomach and 'primary of unknown origin'.[1] The prognosis of untreated hepatic metastases is generally very poor, especially when derived from oeso-phageal, stomach, pancreas, colorectal, or breast primary tumours. If left untreated, the majority of patients will succumb to their disease within 12 months of diagnosis.[2,3] Recent increases in the number of patients developing certain tumours, such as colonic and oesophagogastric adenocarcinoma[4,5] have coincided with improvements in imaging tech-niques that allow better detection of metastatic disease. In conjunction with this, the introduction of screening programmes for a variety of other tumours, including breast carcinoma, has meant that metastatic disease is being detected at an earlier stage and hence increasing the dilemma as to whether aggressive treatment is appropriate.

This chapter starts by examining the aetiology and modes of presenta-tion of hepatic metastases, and goes on to describe the relevant investi-gations and management options of this condition, with a particular emphasis on surgical resection. This is followed by a discussion on the various cytoreductive treatments as well as several newer options for dealing with advanced disease which have been investigated in the experimental or clinical setting.

Aetiology and patho-physiology of hepatic metastases

Almost half of all patients who die of cancer of the stomach, pancreas or breast are found to have liver metastases at autopsy; with endometrial tumours, metastatic spread to the liver occurs in approximately 40% of cases. Liver metastases may be present in as many as 35% of patients with colorectal cancer at the time of operation and another 8–30% will subsequently be found to have liver metastases.[6] The 5-year survival following an apparently curative resection of a colorectal primary tumour is only 50% and the liver is the most frequent site of relapse.[7]

The predilection for metastases to develop in the liver is partly related to the fact that the liver receives the portal drainage of the gastrointestinal tract from where tumour cells can embolise via the mesenteric veins.[8] However, less than 0.1% of circulating tumour cells survive the mechanical trauma and host defence mechanisms encountered during their passage through the vascular and lymphatic vessels and those that do develop into a metastasis are a selected subpopulation.[9] This subpopulation is more homogeneous compared to the primary tumour since they are a clonal expansion of a few highly metastatic cells which have arrested in the capillary beds of the liver.[10] The process of invasion and metastasis of a malignant cell involves a series of linked, sequential steps necessitating detachment from the primary tumour, invasion of the extracellular matrix and subsequent reattachment and independent growth in the new environment.[11] The complex tumour cell interactions that occur with the lining endothelial and lymphatic cells are, in part, what determines their final organ distribution.[12] Also, tumour cells 'recognise' tissue-specific motility factors which direct their movement and invasion properties.[13] The complete explanation as to why a cancer cell leaves the circulation at a specific organ is not known but is thought to involve a homing receptor on the cancer cell and an addressin on the endothelial cell.[14] The fact that tumours from outside the gastrointestinal tract also commonly spread to the liver suggests that organ preference for metastases is not purely anatomical and the 'seed and soil' hypothesis, first proposed by Paget in 1889, is still tenable.[15]

In several experimental tumour models of liver metastasis it has been shown that metastatic cells first come into contact with, and implant in the portal endothelium, within a limited portion of the sinusoid.[16] From here, tumour cells may break off into a portal radical and re-seed close to the initial lesion or may spread by periportal lymphatic pathways. Such satellite formation close to a large liver metastasis is common with secondary tumours of the liver.[3] Also, approximately 10% of patients with colorectal cancer who are candidates for liver resection are found to have spread to extrahepatic lymph nodes, highlighting the importance of this mode of spread which, if found, excludes the possibility of cure.[17]

The right lobe of the liver is involved with metastases more frequently than the left lobe although the reasons for this remain unclear as there is no gross difference of either arterial or portal venous blood received by each lobe.[18] It may be that this reflects the fact that the right lobe is usually larger than the left lobe but may also be a consequence of portal vein 'streaming' resulting in tumour emboli preferentially entering the right portal vein branches. Approximately one third of patients with colorectal liver metastases will have disease limited to one lobe[19] whereas multiple deposits throughout the liver are more commonly seen in patients with breast, oesophageal, gastric and pancreatic cancer and are indicative of a more widespread metastatic process.[20]

Although there are no lymphatic channels draining directly to the liver from the gastrointestinal tract, a metastatic deposit may arise by sequential lymphatic spread from draining lymph nodes. Tumour cells that invade lymphatics may also spread haematogenously via veno-lymphatic communications or directly via the thoracic duct.[21] Certainly, liver metastases develop in the absence of lymph node involvement, and presumably this occurs via the haematogenous route. Some large metastases do not demonstrate spread to local periportal lymph nodes even in the presence of extensive disease within the liver.[22]

Macroscopically, liver metastases are usually more lightly coloured and firmer to palpation than the surrounding normal liver tissue. They enlarge by concentric growth with extension in all directions and surface lesions may show central umbilication, probably as a result of infarction when the tumour outgrows its blood supply. A liver metastasis may attain an enormous size, sometimes occupying much of the liver and may occasionally spread to adjacent structures, such as the diaphragm, by penetrating the usually unyielding Glisson's capsule.[3]

Presentation of hepatic metastases

Liver metastases detected at the time of presentation of primary disease are termed synchronous metastases, those detected after presentation are termed metachronous. The aim of a thorough preoperative work-up and routine follow-up after resection of a primary tumour is to identify metastases as early as possible in order to select patients who might benefit from further surgery, adjuvant or palliative chemotherapy and exclude those for whom such treatment might not be helpful.

Small lesions within the liver are usually asymptomatic and are difficult to detect with conventional imaging techniques. Patients with advanced disease usually present with a combination of upper abdominal discomfort, weight loss and general malaise. Pain may be due to unremitting rapid growth of large metastases and is occasionally referred to the right shoulder. Central necrosis and infarction of a metastasis may also cause pain and pyrexia but these are usually only transient symptoms. Hepatomegaly is indicative of advanced disease and may occasionally be accompanied by fulminant hepatic failure if the metastases are rapidly growing. Evidence of advanced liver failure such as jaundice, ascites and occasionally portal hypertension, are late signs and are indicative of an extremely poor prognosis.[3]

In patients with carcinoid, the first presentation may be with the carcinoid syndrome, characterised by diarrhoea, flushing and wheezing due to excessive secretion of serotonin and tachykinin peptides from the hepatic metastases.

Investigation of hepatic metastases

Blood tests may or may not be abnormal in patients with liver metastases. Serum levels of alkaline phosphatase, aspartate aminotransaminase, γ-glutamyl transferase, carcinoembryonic antigen (CEA), and occasionally, alphafetoprotein may be elevated in the presence of liver metastases[23] but may also be affected in benign disease or metastatic disease without liver involvement. The biochemical tests combining the highest sensitivity (42–47%) with the highest specificity (95–97%) for detecting liver metastases are the serum alkaline phosphatase and serum γ-glutamyl transferase. Simultaneous and significantly elevated serum alkaline phosphatase, lactate dehydrogenase (LDH) and γ-glutamyl transferase levels are thought to be highly predictive of liver metastases,[23] although these blood tests are rarely used alone as absolute criteria of liver involvement. Serum CEA levels are frequently used to follow-up patients with colorectal primary tumours and in approximately 90% of patients with hepatic metastases CEA levels will also be elevated.[24] Other tumour markers (CA19-9, CA15-3 and CA-125) may also be elevated in the presence of liver metastases (dependent on the primary site) but are not specific enough to be used for screening.

Preoperative organ imaging and, more recently intraoperative imaging, are routinely used to detect liver metastases. The greatest difficulties in imaging the liver are being able to distinguish metastases from incidental benign focal liver lesions and being able to detect small metastases less than 2 cm in diameter.

Percutaneous ultrasound

This is the most widely used imaging technique as it is relatively inexpensive and non-invasive. Real-time evaluation in any plane makes it possible to determine the relation of metastatic lesions to biliary and vascular structures.[25] However, it is operator dependent and therefore not as reproducible as computed tomography (CT) or magnetic resonance image (MRI) scanning. Difficulties in interpreting percutaneous ultrasound images may occur as a result of obesity, intestinal gas overlying the liver, or a liver situated high under the costal margin, all of which interfere with the echo signal and occasionally mean that a satisfactory scan cannot be achieved using this modality.

Liver metastases from the gastrointestinal and urogenital tracts are generally hyperechoic on ultrasound although they may be echo-free when there is extensive necrosis within the tumour.[26] Incidental haemangiomata are similarly hyperechoic and may be difficult to differentiate from metastatic tumours on ultrasound.[25] Those hepatic metastases arising from breast, lung, melanoma and lymphoma are usually echopoor whereas metastasis arising from mucin-secreting tumours may occasionally appear cystic.

Preoperative percutaneous ultrasound is a highly sensitive (94%) technique for detecting metastatic lesions >2 cm in diameter but often fails to identify smaller lesions which may reduce the sensitivity of this test to only 56%.[27]

CT scanning

Conventional unenhanced and intravenous contrast-enhanced CT scanning may be used to detect liver metastases although, increasingly, bolus dynamic CT, delayed-scan CT, EOE-13 CT (ethiodised oil emulsion-13 enhanced CT), and dynamic CT scanning during arterial portography (CTAP) have superseded these investigations because of improved sensitivity and better image definition.

Bolus dynamic CT is achieved with rapid cycle, late generation scanners and is associated with detection rates of 87–93% although this figure drops to 68% for nodules <1 cm in diameter.[26] Delayed-scan CT exploits the fact that metastatic deposits excrete iodine slowly and may be detected 4–5 h after intravenous injection of contrast. Attenuation of hepatic parenchyma is increased and vascular structures are visualised which may be an advantage in determining the presence of clear margins adjacent to major structures.[24] This technique is equivalent to bolus dynamic scanning in terms of sensitivity and specificity although it has the disadvantage of requiring higher doses of contrast material.

CTAP involves selective catheterisation of the superior mesenteric artery (SMA) followed by bolus contrast injection and CT scanning of the liver during the portal phase. The necessity to perform angiography in order to deliver the contrast agent has restricted its use, although CTAP is particularly helpful for detecting lesions <5 mm in diameter and may allow precise localisation of the tumour within the hepatic segments.[26] In a prospective evaluation of the accuracy of preoperative imaging in patients undergoing liver resection for colorectal metastases, Yamaguchi et al.[28] have shown that CTAP was significantly better than ultrasound, contrast CT or hepatic angiography in detecting metastases <10 mm in diameter.

In a comparison of the different CT scan modalities in 109 patients with various hepatic tumours, Karl et al.[29] demonstrated that CTAP was significantly more sensitive than either delayed or conventional CT in assessing the distribution of intrahepatic disease. Delayed CT was no more sensitive than conventional CT at detecting either hepatic or extrahepatic disease. Besides being invasive, the other major limitation of CTAP is the number of false-positive findings caused by defects of perfusion from flow artefacts.[30]

Typical liver metastases are hypodense on CT scanning but may be surrounded by a hyperdense ring due to contrast uptake in the compressed surrounding parenchyma. Unenhanced CT scanning may detect hepatic metastases but some are only seen after contrast enhancement. Bolus CT scanning usually allows clear demarcation from adjacent normal liver and the intrahepatic biliary and vascular structures. Occasionally a metastasis may appear dense due to haemorrhage or calcification and if there is extensive central necrosis they may also appear cystic. Most liver metastases are hypovascular and therefore may be distinguished from hypervascular lesions such as hepatocellular carcinomas, adenomas, and focal nodular hyperplasia.

Magnetic resonance imaging (MRI)

The exact role of MRI in the detection of liver metastases has yet to be established. Several different contrast agents are used but superpara-

Figure 4.1 *T1-weighted MRI scan showing a large, solitary liver metastasis.*

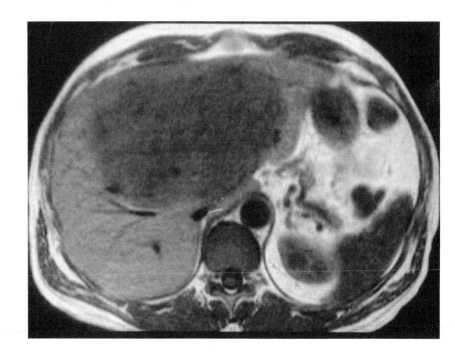

magnetic iron oxide particles, which are preferentially taken up by the reticuloendothelial system, appear to improve the sensitivity of MRI for liver metastases, especially in high-field-strength imaging.[31] MRI scans of liver metastases are characterised by a prolonged relaxation time in T1 and T2. On T1-weighted images (Fig. 4.1), metastatic lesions appear hypointense, sometimes associated with a 'doughnut' appearance whereas T2-weighted images tend to be hyperintense compared to the surrounding normal liver parenchyma.[26,32]

Comparisons of preoperative imaging techniques

Several studies have compared the sensitivity of the various imaging techniques for detecting hepatic metastases.[31,33,34] Chezmar *et al.*[33] showed that MRI scan and bolus dynamic or delayed CT scan were equally sensitive in detecting hepatic metastases, although CT scan was still superior at detecting extrahepatic disease. Ward *et al.*[34] compared several preoperative imaging techniques in 19 patients undergoing resection for colorectal liver metastases and found comparable sensitivities between EOE CT scan (83%), MRI (84%), CTAP (78%), and delayed CT scan (82%). CTAP had the highest false positive rate (63%) whereas T1-weighted MRI had the lowest false positive rate (11%). All are limited in the ability to reliably detect lesions <10 mm and it is these occult metastases which have the most significant impact on long-term survival.[35]

Intraoperative ultrasound

Several studies have confirmed that intraoperative ultrasound is highly sensitive and specific for detecting liver metastases compared with preoperative ultrasound, CT scan, or palpation at laparotomy.[31,36]

Previously undetected lesions may be seen and, prior to resection of known lesions, it is possible to clearly delineate anatomical landmarks in relation to the tumour. Intraoperative ultrasound may also be useful for identifying lesions deep within the liver, particularly those <10 mm in diameter,[37] and these findings may tip the balance against a curative resection. Anatomical variations which may make the resection more difficult, such as accessory hepatic veins or common origins of the portal pedicles, may also be identified.[37]

Additional liver metastases may be found in as many as 33% of patients with lesions detected by preoperative imaging[38] and in those with negative preoperative scans a further 5% will be found to have occult disease.[39]

Laparoscopic ultrasonography

Staging laparoscopy with laparoscopic ultrasonography has recently been reported using specially designed probes inserted through standard laparoscopic ports. This work was pioneered by Japanese workers in the 1960s and recent technical advances in probe design have yielded commercially available systems.[40] Accurate preoperative hepatic staging may be provided by laparoscopic ultrasonography with the added bonus that peritoneal involvement may also be assessed. Needle biopsy of hepatic lesions is possible during the laparoscopy although it is not recommended because of the potential for metastatic seeding of the port sites.[41]

Early experience with this technique suggests it may provide additional staging information which may alter management[40] although further experience is needed to determine whether the additional benefits justify the technical demands and expense of this technique.

Hepatic perfusion index

Hepatic flow scintigraphy and Duplex colour ultrasound scanning allow measurement of the Hepatic Perfusion Index (HPI), which has been used to detect liver metastases; the HPI is altered in patients with metastases as a result of a relatively increased hepatic arterial flow and decreased portal venous flow.[42,43] Duplex doppler ultrasound is a more reliable means of measuring the HPI (doppler perfusion index or DPI) than dynamic scintigraphy and is particularly attractive because it is non-invasive.[43] Leen *et al.*[44] have shown that patients with colorectal cancer who have an elevated DPI are more likely to develop hepatic metastases than those with a normal DPI. In their hands, the sensitivity, accuracy, and negative predictive rate of DPI for detecting colorectal liver metastases is 100%, 86% and 100% respectively. These results are generally better than achieved by either standard CT, transabdominal US, or palpation at laparotomy[44] and appear to be superior to Dukes staging in predicting survival from colorectal cancer.[45] However, measurement of the DPI is highly operator dependent and not easy to reproduce.[46] The effectiveness of DPI in detecting liver metastases needs to be confirmed in further clinical trials.

Staging

The extent of liver involvement by metastatic tumour is an important determinant of long-term survival[47] and hence accurate staging of liver metastases may provide a guide to the likelihood of success following surgical intervention. Also, staging systems allow meaningful comparisons of treatments for liver metastases by classifying patients into matched groups. Several staging systems for liver metastases from colorectal carcinomas have been proposed and the prognostic significance of each system has been evaluated although unfortunately, no single system is universally accepted.

A staging system, modified from the International Union Against Cancer (UICC) and The American Joint Committee on Cancer (AJCC) recommendations for primary hepatobiliary tumours, has recently been proposed (Table 4.1).[48] In this system tumour size, tumour distribution, number of metastatic lesions, and the extent of extrahepatic disease are incorporated. In an analysis of 204 patients who underwent potentially curative hepatic resection for metastatic colorectal cancer in Pittsburgh, Gayowski et al.[48] confirmed that stage I and II cases (unilobar solitary tumours of any size, or unilobar multiple tumours of 2 cm or smaller without nodal disease or direct invasion) had an overall 5-year survival of 61% while those with stage III, IVa and IVb (unilobar disease with multiple lesions greater than 2 cm, bilobar involvement, and nodal involvement or extrahepatic disease, respectively) had overall 5-year survivals of 28%, 20% and 0%, respectively. Despite the fact that stage III and IV disease was generally associated with a poor outcome, a small

Table 4.1 *Staging system for hepatic metastases*

Stage I	mT1	N0	M0
Stage II	mT2	N0	M0
Stage III	mT3	N0	M0
Stage IVa	mT4	N0	M0
Stage IVb	Any mT	N1	M0, M1
		N0, N1	M1

mT1, Solitary $\leqslant 2$ cm; mT2, solitary > 2 cm, unilobar; multiple, $\leqslant 2$ cm, unilobar; mT3, multiple > 2 cm, unilobar; mT4, solitary or multiple, bilobar, invasion of major branch of portal or hepatic veins or bile ducts: N1, abdominal lymph node; M1, extrahepatic metastases or direct invasion to adjacent organs.

Reproduced with permission from Gayowski et al. Surgery 1994; 116: 703–11.

percentage of patients with stage IV disease were still alive and disease-free five years after resection, suggesting that patients should not always be rejected for surgery on the basis of stage of liver metastases alone.[48]

Natural history of untreated liver metastases

The two most important factors known to influence the survival of patients with untreated liver metastases are the extent of hepatic involvement at the time of diagnosis and the histological grade of the primary tumour. Other factors that indicate a poor outlook in untreated patients are the presence of abnormal liver function tests, spread of tumour to extrahepatic sites, and primary tumours that are not resected.[49] Thus, in untreated patients, tumour burden is the major determinant of outcome and patients with solitary metastases usually live longer than those with multiple, bilobar disease.[50] However, prolonged follow-up of untreated patients, even with solitary hepatic metastases, has confirmed that survival beyond five years is rare. This is in contrast to results from most series of hepatic resection for colorectal metastases where 5-year survival rates are approximately 25–35% and where 10 and even 20-year survivors following resection have been documented[51] (Fig. 4.2).

The natural history of liver metastases in untreated patients has been studied and tumour doubling times for these metastases have been shown to be between 50–95 days.[52] By assuming that a tumour requires approximately 30 tumour volume doublings to reach 1 cm in diameter it has been estimated that the subclinical phase of a liver metastasis (i.e. from metastatic implantation to clinical appearance) may be 2.5–5 years.[52] This suggests that survival rates may be improved if liver metastases are detected much earlier.

Figure 4.2 *The survival rates of patients treated by resection compared with survival rates of patients who had biopsy-proven solitary (n = 39) and multiple unilobar (n = 31) metastases that were not resected.*

Reproduced with permission from Adson MA. World J Surg 1987; 11: 511–20.

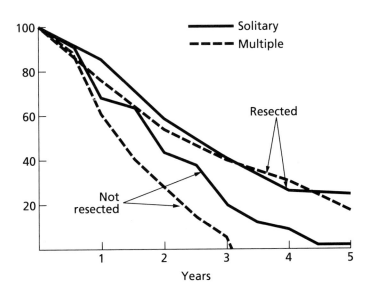

Overt liver metastases sometimes appear years after apparently successful resection of the primary tumour. This long delay in the development of clinically detectable metastases suggests that in such patients host defence mechanisms have induced tumour dormancy following initial treatment.[3]

Resection of hepatic metastases

In 1963 Woodington and Waugh[53] published their experience of resection of colorectal metastases at the Mayo Clinic and demonstrated that a 20% 5-year survival was possible for selected patients, and these results were confirmed by an early experience of liver resection for metastases from a variety of gastrointestinal primary tumours.[54] In 1976 Wilson and Adson[55] reported a further series of liver resections for colorectal metastases from the Mayo Clinic with follow-up data extending to 23 years. They documented a 5-year survival of 28% and recommended aggressive surgical treatment of apparent solitary lesions.

Most of the data concerning resection of liver metastases come from patients with colorectal cancer as isolated liver metastases occur more frequently than in other cancers. However, only 7–10% of all patients with colorectal liver metastases will ultimately benefit from resection. Despite this apparently small proportion of the total number of patients with colorectal cancer it has been estimated that in the United States some 5000 patients each year might be suitable for resection of liver metastases[56] and, extrapolated to the United Kingdom, this figure would be in excess of 1000 patients annually.

There is still a degree of nihilism among clinicians regarding the treatment of patients with hepatic metastases although there is now ample evidence that survival may be improved by resection of isolated hepatic metastases from renal, adrenal and carcinoid tumours, as well as those from colorectal cancer.[57]

The current success of liver resection is due to major advances in metabolic, haemodynamic, and respiratory support as well as to developments in surgical technique. The need for detailed knowledge of liver anatomy as a prerequisite for liver resection has been emphasised by Starzl et al.[58] Better understanding of liver inflow and outflow control to reduce intraoperative blood loss and the use of intraoperative ultrasound, ultrasonic dissection, argon beam coagulation, and topical haemostatic agents have all contributed to accurate segmental resection with minimal postoperative morbidity or mortality.

Resection of hepatic metastases, with acceptable blood loss and transfusion requirements, is accomplished by controlling the hilar structures, with or without the use of the Pringle manoeuvre, and extrahepatic control of the hepatic veins. Placing the patient in the Trendelenberg position and maintaining a low central venous pressure have also been shown to reduce the likelihood of bleeding during the resection.[59]

Morbidity and mortality after resection

Because the long-term survival benefit of liver resection for metastases is relatively small, the risks of surgery assume great significance. Perioperative morbidity should be low and the perioperative mortality must be less than the anticipated 5-year survival rate.

In the larger series of patients undergoing resection of colorectal liver metastases reported operative mortality rates vary from 0 to 8%. Most patients have a postoperative stay of 10–12 days and operative morbidity rates range from 10 to 39%.[6,48,50,55,56,60–64]

In a review of morbidity and mortality after hepatic resection of colorectal liver metastases, Doci et al.[64] noted that intra-abdominal sepsis was the most frequent 'major' complication and pulmonary infection or atelectasis was the most frequent 'minor' complication reported. A large residual cavity is often left after partial hepatectomy and this may fill with blood or bile and, combined with sloughing of devitalised tissue at the resection line, may lead to intra-abdominal infection.[64] Simultaneous hepatectomy and gastrointestinal resection with anastomosis during 'one-stage' procedures may lead to postoperative intra-abdominal infection. Elias et al. have examined this issue in a retrospective study of 53 patients with colorectal cancer and showed that postoperative complications could be minimised by thoroughly preparing the bowel preoperatively and by using a defunctioning colostomy to protect low anastomoses.[65]

Most postoperative complications after liver resection can be managed without re-operation and percutaneous drainage of perihepatic collections and endoscopic stenting of biliary leaks are now routine.[63]

Excessive bleeding during hepatic resection is a major complication associated with a perioperative mortality as high as 17%.[62] However, the introduction of newer technology (ultrasonic dissectors, intraoperative ultrasound, argon beam coagulator and fibrin glue) has improved control of haemorrhage although surgeons must still be familiar with the established techniques of finger fracture and hepatic vascular isolation.

Hepatic failure occasionally occurs following liver resection for metastases and is often a lethal complication.[64] The probability of postoperative hepatic failure depends on the volume and function of the residual liver and there is evidence that a preoperative estimate of a postresection liver volume of at least 35% is predictive of a good outcome.[66] In general, the larger the hepatic resection the greater the probability of postoperative complications. Therefore, hepatic metastases should ideally be removed with a satisfactory clear margin, preferably by segment orientated resections, but at the same time spare as much normal liver as possible.

Most of the larger published series of resection of liver metastases report a gradual improvement in perioperative mortality rates over time as experience and technical skill with resection have developed and, as such, there is general agreement that liver resection is most safely performed by surgeons in specialised units.[63]

Survival following resection

Hepatic resection offers the only chance of cure from certain metastases confined to the liver, although significant survival benefit is only seen if resection is performed with minimal morbidity and mortality.

The reported overall 5-year survival rates following hepatic resection of colorectal metastases range from 16 to 48%.[6,48,50,56,60–63,67–73] A few series have extensive follow-up data and are able to document actual survival figures[50,56,63,72] but most long-term figures are predicted from early survival curves. Many of these studies do not take perioperative deaths into account when calculating survival data and thus tend to distort the true survival picture.

A survival plateau is noted above five years after resection of liver metastases.[74,75] These patients subsequently have a similar life expectancy to a matched non-cancer cohort.[74] Ten-year survival rates after hepatic resection for colorectal metastases are approximately 24%[63,74] and some even report 20-year survival rates approaching 20%.[63]

There has never been a controlled trial to address the question of resection versus non-resection or conservative treatment of potentially resectable colorectal liver metastases. Therefore, these figures for survival after resection need to be compared with survival rates of untreated, historical controls. Studies of the natural history of untreated liver metastases have revealed that a minority of patients with limited disease may live for long periods without treatment and this group offers the most realistic comparison with patients undergoing liver resection.[47] Even though some of these patients have 'favourable' tumour biology, possibly allowing prolonged survival without treatment, long-term survival beyond five years is rare without liver resection.[47] This compares to overall 5-year survival rates of 25–35% reported in most series following resection of colorectal liver metastases.[60] However, overall survival figures may give an over-optimistic impression of the curative benefit of resection and a substantial percentage of patients may remain alive but with recurrent disease.[6] In a large multi-institutional study of liver resections for colorectal metastases (Table 4.2), overall 5-year survival was 32% but only 24% of patients were disease free.[76] Despite the frequency of relapse following surgery, the natural history of the disease is probably altered by hepatic resection, as evidenced by the unusual sites of colorectal cancer recurrence that occur in these patients, such as in the lungs.[75]

Factors affecting survival after resection of liver metastases

Many factors have a significant influence on survival following resection of colorectal liver metastases. This information provides a valuable

Table 4.2   *Survival following resection of colorectal liver metastases*

Reference	No. of patients	Operative morbidity (%)	Operative mortality (%)	Median survival (months)	3-yr survival (%)	5-yr survival (%)
Fortner et al. (1984)[67]	65	27	7	—	57	30
Adson et al. (1984)[50]	141	—	4	—	—	25
Ekberg et al. (1986)[68]	72	15	5.6	22	30	16[b]
Cobourn et al. (1987)[69]	41	—	0	—	—	25
Bradpiece et al. (1987)[8]	24	25	8.3	30	44[b]	—
Hughes et al. (1988)[77a]	859	—	—	—	—	33
Holm et al. (1989)[70]	35	46	0	—	31	—
Doci et al. (1991)[71]	100	39	5	28	—	30
Steele et al. (1991)[56a]	150	13	2.7	26	53	—
van Ooijen et al. (1992)[61a]	118	35	7.6	26	—	21
Rosen et al. (1992)[72]	280	—	4	34	47	25[b]
French Association of Surgery (1992)[62a]	1818	24	2.4	—	41	25[b]
Sugihara et al. (1993)[73]	109	22	4	—	57	48
Gayowski et al. (1994)[48]	204	—	0	33	43	32
Scheele et al. (1995)[63]	434	16	4.4	40	—	39
Jatzko et al. (1995)[6]	66	20	4.5	25	—	30

[a]Multi-institutional series.
[b]Includes perioperative death.

guide to patient selection for hepatic resection and may prevent unnecessary surgery in patients who will gain no survival benefit in the remaining months of their lives. Many studies have used univariate analysis of these factors to determine their prognostic significance although this may be misleading because of the influence of the multiple factors involved in liver resection. Therefore, the following paragraphs concentrate on data obtained from studies which examined the various prognostic factors by multivariate analysis.

Number and distribution of metastases

There is no significant difference in long-term outcome following resection of one, two or three metastases. The current consensus of the maximum number of metastases that can safely be resected, with a likelihood of cure, is three and some authors advise against resection if there are four or more lesions because, in their experience, long-term survival is rare.[68] However, Scheele et al.[63] describe patients with up to five randomly distributed metastases who have survived more than five years after complete resection, and argue that the limiting factor to the number of lesions that can be resected is whether it is technically possible to remove all of the tumour.[63] In a recently published series of hepatic resections from Starzl's unit in Pittsburgh, survival was adversely affected by the presence of more than three metastases although 20% of the patients in this group still survived to five years.[48] These authors, and others, suggest that the presence of multiple metastases should not be an absolute contraindication to resection.[6,48,63,67,71] Multivariate analysis of the number of metastases present has been shown to be a significant factor for long-term survival[48,60–62,68] but not all studies have found this association.[63,67,71] Most of these reports also show that the distribution of metastases to one or both lobes of the liver does not affect prognosis. It is therefore reasonable to consider resection for more than three metastases if the procedure can be done with a low risk of liver failure. This is particularly the case where a cluster of similar-sized metastases (suggestive of a common tumour embolic event) has clearly occurred in a segment or lobe, and the residual liver is disease free. It is debatable whether the presence of satellite metastases have any impact on survival.[63]

Resection margins

There is considerable debate concerning the ideal resection margin of healthy liver tissue that must be obtained around the metastasis to maximise the benefit of resection. Data from the Registry of Hepatic Metastases, a multi-institutional database of liver resections, showed that a margin > 1 cm was associated with a 45% 5-year survival, but only 23% survived five years if the margin was less. However, this factor was not found to be statistically significant as information on margin size was not available for many cases.[77] Conventional teaching advocates a margin of at least 10 mm clear of microscopic disease and this is supported by the results from several series which document a statistically significant poorer overall and disease-free 5-year survival in patients with margins less than 10 mm.[62,68] However, this teaching is challenged by others who argue that strict adherence to obtaining a margin > 10 mm may not be important.[63] A margin that may appear to be adequate during resection, may subsequently be reported as inadequate by the pathologist who may note microscopic involvement of resection margins. It may also be possible to destroy a field of liver parenchyma adjacent to the resection margin with either argon beam coagulation or wide-field cryotherapy to a depth of several millimetres. A recent pathological study of resected colorectal liver metastases documented that many metastases have a thick fibrous pseudocapsule which allow adequate clearance of tumour by shaving non-cancerous tissue.[78]

Protagonists of generous resection margins cite evidence of a higher incidence of hepatic recurrence associated with narrow margins. This may reflect the extent of liver involvement, necessitating a greater resection with tight margins to preserve residual liver function. It is our experience that when disease recurs in the liver it is more often at some site distant from the original resection line and we assume most likely to have arisen in undetected micrometastases present at the time of original liver resection. Therefore, ideally, a resection margin of at least 10 mm should be attempted, judged by intraoperative ultrasonography, but if this is not technically possible narrow margins should not be an absolute contraindication to resection.

Size of metastases

Clearly the size of a metastasis is related to its 'age' since onset of the malignant process. Larger liver metastases have usually been present for a longer time than smaller lesions. Metastases of differing sizes are probably indicative of showers of tumour emboli occurring at different times. In several large studies metastases >5 cm were associated with poorer survival than smaller metastases[60,62,79] although multivariate analysis of this factor in other studies has failed to show an influence on survival.[68] In some situations, extended (and occasionally non-anatomical) resections are required to remove very large deposits. Usually these resections are dictated by the extent and number of deposits and are indicative of a more aggressive malignant process with a poorer outcome, regardless of intervention. In the specific situation of a giant solitary metastasis, tumour biology is such that the capacity for multiple metastases may well be limited, and therefore outcome may be good after resection. On balance, the size of a metastasis is probably not a significant influence on subsequent survival after hepatectomy.

Synchronous versus metachronous disease

There is controversy over the value of resection of liver metastases found synchronously with the primary lesion. Several studies have documented poorer outcome in patients who undergo resection of synchronous metastases and, conversely, better survival in patients with disease-free intervals of one or more years after resection of their primary tumours.[60,62] This may reflect better tumour biology in lesions detected at a later date since it is likely that these deposits were present, but undetectable at the time of resection of the primary lesion. In interpreting data concerning the benefits of resection of metachronous versus synchronous metastases, consideration should be given to progress in methods of earlier detection (see above). However, several other studies have shown that when analysed by multivariate analysis, the prognosis after resection is not dependent on the time of detection of metastatic disease.[6,61,68,71,80] Therefore, if patients have potentially resectable synchronous metastases and are otherwise well, they should be considered for hepatectomy after they have been appropriately staged.

Resection in the presence of extrahepatic metastases

The presence of extrahepatic disease significantly reduces the likelihood of long-term survival[62,68] and is usually a contraindication to liver resection. Palliation of symptoms may be attained by resection of a large tumour but, in most cases, this has no beneficial effect on survival.[63] However, there are certain circumstances where long-term survival has been achieved after liver resection in the presence of extrahepatic disease. Patients with resectable pulmonary or adrenal gland metastases may survive for more than five years after a successful liver resection, although most will develop further recurrence during that time.[32] Anecdotal reports cite successful resection of solitary cerebral metastases after resection of liver metastases, but there are no verifiable 5-year survival data to support such interventions.

Occasionally a subcapsular hepatic metastasis appears to invade an adjacent structure (mostly the diaphragm). This attachment is usually fibrotic and probably represents an inflammatory response to the tumour.[81] If frozen section analysis of the area is clear of malignant disease then the outcome after resection is similar to those without extrahepatic attachment.

Hepatic pedicle lymph node involvement may be present in 20–30% of patients with hepatic metastases and almost none of these patients survive five years after hepatectomy.[60,82] Some studies suggest benefit from radical excision of nodes in the region of the hepatic pedicle[62,83] although this is not widely practised.

Type of resection

Simple 'shelling out' of metastases is associated with higher recurrence rates than formal resections which remove a margin of normal liver tissue.[60,79] In addition, non-segmental resection may compromise the vascularity of adjacent residual liver tissue and may be technically more difficult.[60,84] Consequently hepatic segmentectomy is preferable for small, localised lesions unless this increases the risk of postoperative liver failure. Multivariate analysis in several studies has shown that anatomical resections have a significant survival benefit over lesser procedures[6,63] although these findings have not been confirmed in other studies.[62,68] It is important that all tumour is removed with an adequate margin and for larger tumours this may be difficult with non-anatomical wedge excisions. Clearly, for small awkwardly located lesions (such as at the apex of segment VIII in the axilla of the right and middle hepatic veins), local resection might be preferable to formal hemi-hepatectomy, whereby a whole, healthy lobe may need to be sacrificed for a small deposit. A diligent search for other metastases should be carried out using intraoperative ultrasound before attempting to 'wedge out' an apparently superficial tumour nodule. For larger metastases or multiple deposits standard anatomical resections based on Couinaud segments should ensure adequate margins.[60,63]

If more radical procedures (right and left trisegmentectomy) are necessary to obtain adequate clearance the prognosis is poorer.[85] Extensive disease requiring an extended (one lobe plus one or two segments of the other lobe) resection to obtain clearance are obviously likely to have more disease than those with tumour confined to one anatomical lobe. However, there are 5-year survivors following extended hepatectomy[85] and therefore this criterion alone should not preclude a patient from resection.

Patient age

In a multi-institutional study by Hughes *et al.*[77] the patient's age was shown significantly to influence the outcome after resection of liver metastases although this relationship has not been observed in other studies.[6,62,63,67] It is reasonable to base the decision to offer liver resection to patients on biological rather than chronological age as it has been shown that there is no difference in perioperative mortality or morbidity between elderly and young patients following hepatectomy.[86] The major determinant of success in the elderly (>80 years of age) is the volume of residual liver (since liver adaptations following resection diminishes with age), and fitness for general anaesthesia.

Gender

It has been suggested that males have a poorer survival than females after resection of liver metastases[70] although most studies do not confirm this.[6,61,62,67,71,79] This should therefore not be a factor in the decision whether or not to offer liver resection to patients.

Operative blood loss

Major operative blood loss has been related to a poorer prognosis following partial hepatectomy for colorectal metastases.[61,72,87] Obviously this finding may be confounded by the fact that larger tumours are likely to be associated with greater blood loss during resection. Some authors have shown that perioperative transfusion requirements were not an independent prognostic factor in survival.[48] This is not a factor which can be taken into account preoperatively when selecting patients for resection.

Site of primary tumour

Several groups have noted that the site of the primary tumour was an independent predictor of survival in patients with colorectal liver metastases.[6,49,88] Rougier *et al.*[49] have demonstrated that in patients whose liver metastases are left untreated (or received palliative chemotherapy), those whose primary tumours arose in the right colon fared worse than those whose primary developed elsewhere in the colon or rectum. Younes *et al.*[88] confirmed these findings in patients who underwent resection of the liver metastases although a contradictory finding was reported by Jatzko *et al.*[6] who noted that patients with rectal tumours had a worse survival than those patients with colon tumours. Whether these results reflect later presentation of right-sided disease or higher local recurrence rates of rectal cancers is speculative.

In most series, however, the site of the primary colorectal cancer has not been shown to influence the long-term outcome following hepatectomy for liver metastases.[48,61–63,67,71,89]

Grade of primary tumour

Some authors have noted that patients with histologically high grade primary tumours have poorer survival after resection of liver metastases.[6,63] This is not surprising as the grade of the primary tumour is known to influence survival after resection of the primary tumour, independent of whether liver metastases are present. However, in other studies multivariate analysis of the grade of primary tumour has not been found to be an independent predictor of survival.[48,61,68,89] The majority of liver metastases are either moderately or poorly differentiated and were likely to have arisen from similarly differentiated primary tumours. Since we would not advocate tumour biopsy prior to hepatectomy, in order to reduce the risk of tumour spill (the liver resection is the biopsy), then such information regarding differentiation of the metastasis is not available preoperatively. Regardless, there are survivors alive, and disease free, five years after resection of poorly differentiated liver metastases.

Stage of primary tumour

Several authors have reported a statistical correlation between the stage of primary tumour and outcome after hepatectomy[6,47,60,62,63,67,71] although others have not recorded this relationship.[48,61,68,88] Tumours that have the capacity to invade and metastasise to lymphatics are clearly more aggressive than those without this potential and, conceivably may by-pass the liver, by spreading to pre-aortic lymph nodes, and beyond to the thoracic duct and systemic circulation. Although there may be a correlation between primary tumour stage and survival, the relationship is not strong enough to preclude liver resection for patients with more advanced primary tumours.

Carcinoembryonic antigen (CEA)

Several studies have shown that an elevated preoperative serum level of CEA is an independent predictor of poor survival in patients who undergo hepatectomy.[62,88]

Contraindications to liver resection

Absolute contraindications for resection of colorectal liver metastases have not been clarified, but most would agree that patients should not be offered resection if they have uncontrolled primary disease or such widespread intrahepatic involvement that the residual liver function after resection would be inadequate. Relative contraindications include situations where resection of an hepatic metastasis is not easily performed such as those involving the caudate lobe (segment I) or tumours invading the inferior vena cava. Tumour involvement of the portal vein confluence would also limit the potential curability of the resection.

Preoperative work-up Prior to undergoing resection of liver metastases, patients should undergo colonoscopy to exclude local recurrence or metachronous primary disease. Some authors use serum CEA levels as a guide to local control but this may also be elevated due to the liver metastases. Radioimmunoguided surgery may offer a more accurate guide to recurrent primary disease but this investigation is not widely used.

Liver function tests and coagulation studies should be performed and a chest X-ray and abdominal ultrasound arranged, as a minimum. Ideally patients should also undergo a CT scan of the chest and abdomen to exclude pulmonary metastases or intra-abdominal spread beyond the liver. If hepatic resection is being considered, CTAP or MRI may provide accurate localisation of metastases and reveal small lesions not detected by ultrasound or conventional CT scan.

Hepatic angiography may be helpful to identify vascular anomalies such as aberrant right or left hepatic arteries if hepatic artery cannulation is to be considered for regional chemotherapy. Magnetic resonance cholangiography is an emerging non-invasive technique that may allow detailed definition of segmental invasion by metastatic tumours.

Valuable preresection information may be obtained by staging laparoscopy which can accurately identify extrahepatic local spread or peritoneal carcinomatosis and possibly prevent an unnecessary laparotomy. If laparoscopic ultrasonography is available this may also be used. Preoperative histological proof of metastatic disease is seldom required because preoperative imaging techniques are sensitive enough to distinguish metastatic disease from most other lesions.

There appears to be no advantage in delaying hepatic resection following diagnosis (old dogma that a waiting period is necessary to evaluate tumour aggressiveness is no longer tenable) and patients should undergo surgery as soon as is feasible.

Re-resection of liver metastases

Recurrence may occur in up to 65% of patients following liver resection for metastases, the most common site being in the liver.[62] Approximately 20% of these patients have liver-only recurrence and hence may be suitable for re-resection.[90] However, most series of repeat hepatectomies for metastatic disease involve only small numbers of patients and hence firm conclusions regarding indications for repeat resection are difficult to make. Intrahepatic recurrence after resection of metastases may arise from inadequate clearance of tumour or may be due to residual micrometastatic disease elsewhere in the liver. In a large multicentre study from the French Association of Surgery, 23% of patients underwent repeat hepatectomy following resection of colorectal liver metastases. Recurrent disease occurred in the opposite side of the liver in more than a third of cases.[62] Repeat hepatectomy is often more difficult than the initial procedure because of dense adhesions and because the liver parenchyma may be more friable or fibrotic.[91] Surprisingly, reported mortality and morbidity rates after repeat liver resection of metastases are similar to those reported after initial hepatectomy.[90] Survival figures from the larger series of repeat hepatic resection of colorectal metastases are also similar to those achieved after the first procedure. As with the initial resection, the presence of extrahepatic disease or incomplete tumour clearance are associated with a poorer outcome.[90]

The majority of patients who develop recurrence following hepatic resection of colorectal metastases relapse within two years of surgery; aggressive surveillance with regular serum CEA levels, abdominal and chest CT or conventional ultrasound following resection may improve the detection of recurrent disease.[90] In patients who do develop recurrence it seems reasonable to consider these lesions in the same way as the first metastasis and offer re-resection to patients based on operative risk and probable survival.

Resection of non-colorectal hepatic metastases

Improvements in perioperative mortality of major hepatic resection have led to a more liberal application of this procedure for metastatic disease. Hepatic resections of metastases from non-colorectal primary tumours have occasionally been reported although all have involved relatively small numbers of patients.[57] Resection of non-colorectal liver metastases is not performed routinely because widespread hepatic infiltration occurs more frequently with non-colorectal liver metastases. In a recent review of the literature on hepatic resection for non-colorectal, non-neuroendocrine metastases, Schwartz suggested that resection of confined liver metastases arising from primary renal cell carcinomas, Wilms' tumours, and adrenocortical carcinomas may improve long-term survival. Five-year survival rates following partial hepatectomy for these metastases are equivalent to those achieved following resection of colorectal metastases and it seems reasonable, therefore, to offer resection to patients with resectable lesions who can tolerate surgery.[57] However, experience with metastases from other non-colorectal primary tumours would indicate that there is no survival advantage in performing liver resection although palliation of symptoms from bulky metastases may be achieved by resection in selected patients.[57]

Elias *et al.*[92] have reported a series of 21 patients who underwent hepatectomy for liver metastases from breast carcinoma. Preoperative and postoperative chemotherapy were also used for many of these patients, which makes interpretation of the survival data difficult. They reported an overall 5-year survival rate of 24% from commencement of combined therapy although only 9% of patients were alive five years after surgery. Unsuspected metastases were found at laparotomy in 22% of patients and the authors conceded that hepatectomy for metastases from breast carcinoma was mainly a cytoreductive procedure which did not prolong survival.[92]

Hepatic resection of metastases from soft-tissue sarcomas have been reported, most commonly from primary visceral leiomyosarcomas.[93] The experience of the Memorial Sloan–Kettering Cancer Center suggests that patients with retroperitoneal leiomyosarcomas are most at risk of metastasising to the liver whereas sarcomas of the extremity rarely spread in this fashion. In 14 patients who underwent hepatic resection all developed recurrent disease, which was mainly within the liver, and there were no 5-year survivors. These authors conclude that resection of hepatic metastases from primary sarcomas is only indicated if it is feasible to completely remove all tumour from the liver and, even if this is undertaken, survival beyond five years is rare.[93]

True isolated metastatic deposits from gastric or gallbladder adenocarcinoma are rare and there are few reported long-term survivors in patients who have undergone resection of metachronous hepatic metastases. However, some authors suggest that isolated metastatic deposits of gastric cancer may be resected, with a chance of cure, if the original primary tumour showed no evidence of serosal invasion, lymphatic or vascular involvement.[94]

Isolated reports of liver resection of metastases from gynaecological, pancreatic and oesophageal primary tumours would suggest there is little survival benefit from this procedure.[57] Hepatic resection of metastatic neuroendocrine tumours, such as carcinoids and VIPomas, have been performed on the basis that these tumours are slowly growing and clinical symptoms are known to correlate directly with tumour bulk. Several studies have reported excellent palliation of symptoms and even long-term survivors after this procedure.[95]

In situ destruction

Cryotherapy

Hepatic cryotherapy using insulated probes containing liquid nitrogen has been used successfully by several groups to treat liver metastases.[96–98] The aim of this treatment in unresectable hepatic metastases is to reduce tumour burden, although there have been a few reports of long-term survival following this procedure.[96] The indications for hepatic cryotherapy have not been clearly defined but broadly include patients with unresectable metastases who can tolerate general anaesthesia. The presence of extrahepatic disease is generally considered a contraindication and in patients with multiple hepatic deposits cryotherapy is usually only undertaken in patients with less than 10 metastases.[99] CEA levels have been shown to fall following cryotherapy of colorectal liver metastases and may be used as a guide to effective control of disease.[98] A laparotomy is required for direct application of the cryotherapy probes and intraoperative ultrasound guides and monitors the freezing process.[100] Several groups have reported no deaths following hepatic cryotherapy[96,100] although others have documented postoperative deaths due to uncontrollable coagulopathy and subsequent multisystem organ failure.[97] Reported complications following this procedure include hepatic bleeding, thrombocytopenia, hypothermia, myoglobinuria, pleural effusions, acute tubular necrosis, hepatic abscess and bile duct injury.[97,101]

Recurrent disease following cryotherapy of unresectable colorectal liver metastases occurs frequently and may be due to residual disease at the site of cryotherapy or due to growth of micrometastatic disease elsewhere in the liver. In our experience of cryotherapy for hepatic metastases in 53 patients, less than 20% are alive at 2-year follow-up.

Cryotherapy may be useful to treat small lesions in the contralateral lobe during resection of a large metastasis. There are reports of cryo-assisted hepatic resection of metastases which allow controlled resections with well-defined margins, thereby maximising preservation of functional parenchyma.[102] However, the follow-up of these patients is too short to determine if improved recurrence rates are achieved by this technique.

Cryotherapy and regional chemotherapy

A retrospective study of 38 patients examined the effect of combined hepatic cryotherapy and regional chemotherapy in patients with colorectal liver metastases.[103] This suggested that patients who had more than three months of hepatic artery chemotherapy (5-fluorouracil and folinic acid) following hepatic cryotherapy had a longer survival compared with those who did not receive this treatment. Phase I and II trials are currently being conducted to examine this issue further.

Other forms of cytoreductive therapy

Other cytoreductive techniques which produce controlled hepatic destruction include ethanol injection, thermotherapy and interstitial radiotherapy. The aim of these treatments is to palliate patients with unresectable liver metastases. They have the advantage of being performed percutaneously but with the disadvantage of not being able to visualise and therefore control the scale of tissue destruction by intra-operative ultrasound.

Percutaneous alcohol injection has been used to treat unresectable colorectal liver metastases but usually produces only partial responses and early recurrence of tumour is common. Although this technique has been shown to be safe for treating liver metastases, pain following the injection has been reported and because of poor response rates there is little to recommend this form of treatment.[104] Furthermore, the technique may be ineffective as the alcohol tends to spread out into the hepatic parenchyma in preference to penetrating the dense tumour stroma.

Thermotherapy of hepatic metastases using either saline-enhanced radiofrequency, low-level direct electrical current, or laser has been reported but only appears to be suitable for small lesions. This therapy suffers from the same problem as ethanol injection in not being able satisfactorily to monitor treatment-induced destruction.[105]

Radioactive implants have been used to treat gross residual disease or to sterilise known positive margins following hepatic resection of colorectal metastases, although early resection margin recurrence, as well as distant recurrence commonly occurs.[106] Selective internal radiation (SIR) of hepatic metastases involves embolising radioactive microspheres into the hepatic arterial circulation. Recently this technique has been shown, in an animal model, to have a potential role as an adjuvant treatment for patients who are at high risk of developing liver metastases.[107]

Hepatic artery ligation

Hepatic artery ligation has been advocated as a treatment of liver metastases based on the fact that metastases principally derive their blood supply from the hepatic artery.[108] However, peritoneal arterial communications and portal venous tributaries may supply the tumour after hepatic artery ligation. This technique alone is not recommended for the treatment of hepatic metastases.

Chemotherapy

The majority of patients with liver metastases are not suitable for resection and chemotherapy offers the only hope of palliation. It is not possible to cure patients with liver metastases by using chemotherapy but symptom palliation and prolonged survival has been reported for patients with disseminated disease.[109] Chemotherapy may be administered systemically or regionally via the hepatic artery or portal vein. Chemotherapy may be given as the sole form of treatment in patients with unresectable disease (palliative) or may be given prior to resection (neoadjuvant) or following resection (adjuvant). However, adjuvant chemotherapy has not been shown to improve the outcome following hepatectomy for metastases in any randomised, controlled trials. Adjuvant chemotherapy has also been used in conjunction with various cytoreductive procedures.

Systemic chemotherapy

The most widely used agent for systemic treatment of colorectal liver metastases is the antimetabolite, 5-fluorouracil (5-FU). This agent is a prodrug which is metabolised by cells to active cytotoxic species which can inhibit the key enzyme, thymidylate synthase. In patients given 5-FU alone an objective tumour response is seen in 5–18% of cases[110] although this has had little effect on survival. Folinic acid (leucovorin) may be combined with 5-FU to enhance overall cytotoxicity by promoting its transformation into FUdMP.[111] Mean response rates are approximately 30% with median survivals of approximately 12 months which is significantly better than seen in untreated patients or those treated with 5-FU alone.[110] The only other chemotherapeutic agent proven equal to 5-FU combined with folinic acid is Tomudex which has recently been licensed in the UK for the palliative treatment of colorectal cancer.[112]

Neoadjuvant therapy

Initially unresectable hepatic metastases may be made resectable by pretreating with high dose chemotherapy. Bismuth *et al.*[113] have resected tumours in 53 patients, initially evaluated as unresectable, following courses of intravenous, chronomodulated chemotherapy combining 5-FU, folinic acid, and oxaliplatinum.[113] The 3-year survival rate in these patients was 55%, which is comparable to survival rates of patients undergoing resection without prior chemotherapy.

Regional chemotherapy

Hepatic metastases exclusively derive their blood supply from the hepatic artery and regional perfusion of established liver metastases allows delivery of high doses of chemotherapeutic agents directly to the tumour while avoiding high systemic levels since much of the drug will be eliminated by the liver.[114] The two most frequently used agents for hepatic artery infusion (HAI) are 5-FU and FUDR (5-fluoro-2-deoxyuridine).[110] Intraportal chemotherapy is of no greater benefit than systemic chemotherapy and is normally reserved for adjuvant treatment of micrometastases following primary colorectal excision.

HAI is usually indicated in patients with unresectable hepatic metastases which are confined to the liver. Preoperative angiography will identify variations in arterial anatomy, especially a right hepatic artery arising from the superior mesenteric artery. A laparotomy is performed and a catheter inserted and fixed at the proximal end of the gastroduodenal artery. A cholecystectomy is usually required to avoid subsequent chemical cholecystitis. Satisfactory liver perfusion may be confirmed intraoperatively by injecting fluorescein or methylene blue through the subcutaneous port of the catheter.[110] Implantable constant-infusion devices connected to inert, siliconised catheters can be used and allow longer, more tolerable infusions than previously possible with external pump devices.

Response rates of intra-arterial chemotherapy have appeared higher than those seen with systemic chemotherapy although only one study has documented marginal survival benefit over systemic chemotherapy.[115] Allen-Mersh et al.[116] have demonstrated that hepatic artery infusion of 5FUDR also contributes to improved quality of life. HAI has been studied in combination with systemic chemotherapy for the treatment of unresectable colorectal metastases and has not been shown to be superior to HAI alone.[117] However, complications of regional chemotherapy such as biliary sclerosis, chemical hepatitis, arterial thrombosis, infections, catheter displacement, gastroduodenal inflammation and peritonitis are not uncommon. The addition of dexamethasone to the hepatic artery infusion may reduce the toxicity of regional chemotherapy and possibly increase response rates, although the mechanism of these actions are unclear.[118] Close monitoring of liver function tests is necessary when patients undergo hepatic artery infusion and abnormalities, particularly a rising bilirubin, are usually indicative of hepatocyte toxicity, requiring cessation of treatment.[119] In an attempt to improve the results of regional chemotherapy some authors have used vasoactive agents, such as angiotensin or vasopressin, to try and alter the pharmacokinetics of bolus HAI 5-FU although there is no evidence this significantly alters survival. Synchronous primary tumour resection and regional hepatic chemotherapy have been reported and shown to be well tolerated.[120]

Chemo-embolisation

This involves the selective injection into the hepatic artery of a combination of cytotoxic drugs with an occluding agent such a gelfoam or starch microspheres. The aims of this treatment are to combine two forms of local treatment, namely acute ischaemia and chemotherapy, and localise the chemotherapy in the liver. Experimental and clinical work has suggested that embolisation may promote arterial perfusion of under-perfused metastases and at the same time block the arterioles to the healthy liver, the effect being to enhance cytotoxicity.[110,121] However, there is no evidence that this form of treatment confers any significant survival benefit over regional chemotherapy alone in patients with colorectal liver metastases.

Role of transplantation
Pichlmayr et al.[122] have demonstrated that liver transplantation may have a role in the treatment of selected patients with liver metastases from neuroendocrine primary tumours. However, in the limited number of patients with a variety of non-neuroendocrine hepatic metastases who have undergone liver transplantation no survivors beyond three years have been documented. These results are in agreement with the data from the Cincinnati Transplant Tumor Registry where early recurrence following transplantation occurred in 59% of patients with liver metastases from a variety of primary tumours.[123] Most authors agree that because of the high probability of recurrence there is no role, at present, for liver transplantation in the treatment of non-neuroendocrine hepatic metastases.

Immuno-therapy
Treatments aimed at reversing the depression of host defences in the perioperative period may reduce the dissemination of disease that invariably occurs after hepatectomy and thereby improve the long-term results of surgery. Interleukin-2 (IL-2) has been used as a neoadjuvant therapy in patients with resectable colorectal liver metastases.[124] In a phase II randomised study prehepatectomy recombinant interleukin-2 increased the mean lymphocyte count in the postoperative period and was associated with an acceptable level of toxicity.[124] Theoretically, this would mean that immune-stimulated patients are less susceptible to micrometastatic dissemination at the time of surgery and in the early postoperative period. Further clinical trials are required to confirm this hypothesis.

Targeting of liver metastases with monoclonal antibodies recognising specific antigens within tumour cells has also been investigated.[125] The major difficulty associated with this technique is the poor specificity of the antibodies and carriers, such as chemotherapeutic agents or isotopes, may also be directed at cells within normal tissue. In a recent phase I study the monoclonal antibody, F19, which recognises a cell surface glycoprotein abundantly expressed in epithelial tumours, was shown to be highly selective for colorectal hepatic metastases allowing imaging of lesions as small as 1 cm in diameter.[125] If the sensitivity of this monoclonal antibody is confirmed it may serve to identify patients with previously undetected disease who would benefit from surgery and prevent patients with disseminated spread from undergoing unnecessary liver resections.

Another interesting application of immunotherapy for the treatment of liver metastases involves the use of specific immunisation with vaccines.[126] In a phase II clinical trial, Schlag et al.[126] immunised 23 patients with autologous, irradiated, metastasis-derived tumour cells following resection of their colorectal liver metastases. After a follow-up of 18 months only 61% of the immunised group developed recurrence as compared to 87% in the group treated by resection alone.[126] Prospective, randomised trials are required to further evaluate this form of treatment.

Future treatment options

Future therapeutic options for treating hepatic metastases may include the use of gastrointestinal hormone antagonists directed at receptor positive tumour cells[127] and the targeting of micrometastases using specific angiogenesis inhibitors.[128] In addition there are likely to be future clinical applications of gene therapy which have resulted from recent advances in the understanding of the genetic events underlying the progression to malignancy.[129]

References

1. Willis RA. The spread of tumours in the human body. London: Butterworths, 1973.
2. Bengtsson G, Carlsson G, Hafstrom L, Jonsson P. Natural history of patients with untreated liver metastases from colorectal cancer. Am J Surg 1981; 141: 586–9.
3. Foster JH, Lundy J. Liver metastases. Curr Probl Surg 1981; 18: 158–204.
4. Vukasin AP, Ballantyne GH, Flannery JT, Lerner E, Modlin IM. Increasing incidence of cecal and sigmoid carcinoma – Data from the Connecticut Tumor Registry. Cancer 1990; 66: 2442–9.
5. Blot WJ, Devesa SS, Fraumeni JF. Continuing climb in rates of esophageal adenocarcinoma – An update. JAMA 1993; 270: 1320.
6. Jatzko GR, Lisborg PH, Stettner HM, Klimpfinger MH. Hepatic resection for metastases from colorectal carcinoma – a survival analysis. Eur J Cancer 1995; 31A: 41–6.
7. Gordon NLM, Dawson AA, Bennett B, Innes G, Eremin O, Jones PF. Outcome in colorectal adenocarcinoma – 2 7-year studies of a population. Brit Med J 1993; 307: 707–10.
8. Fisher ER, Turnbull RB. The cytological demonstration and significance of tumor cells in the mesenteric venous blood in patients with colorectal carcinoma. Surg Gynecol Obstet 1955; 100: 102–8.
9. Fidler IJ. Metastasis: quantitative analysis of distribution and fate of tumor emboli labeled with I-5-iodo-2-deoxyuridine. J Nat Cancer Inst 1970; 45: 773–82.
10. Poste G, Fidler IJ. The pathogenesis of cancer metastasis. Nature 1980; 283: 139–46.
11. Nigam AK, Pignatelli M, Boulos PB. Current concepts in metastasis. Gut 1994; 35: 996–1000.
12. Naito S, Giavazzi R, Fidler IJ. Correlation between the in vitro interaction of tumor

cells with an organ environment and metastatic behavior in vivo. Invasion Metastasis
1987; 7: 16–29.

13. Nicolson GL, Dulski KM. Organ specificity of
metastatic tumor colonization is related to
organ-selective growth-properties of malignant cells. Int J Cancer 1986; 38: 289–94.

14. Jiang WG, Puntis MC, Hallett MB. Molecular
and cellular basis of cancer invasion and
metastasis: implications for treatment. Br J
Surg 1994; 81: 1576–90.

15. Paget S. The distribution of secondary
growths in cancer of the breast. Lancet 1889;
i: 571–3.

16. Barberaguillem E, Alonsovarona A, Vidalva-
naclocha F. Selective implantation and
growth in rats and mice of experimental liver
metastasis in acinar zone-one. Cancer Res
1989; 49: 4003–10.

17. August DA, Sugarbaker PH, Schneider PD.
Lymphatic dissemination of hepatic metastases – implications for the follow-up and
treatment of patients with colorectal cancer.
Cancer 1985; 55: 1490–4.

18. Holbrook RF, Rodriguezbigas MA, Rama-
krishnan K, Blumenson L, Petrelli NJ. Patterns of colorectal liver metastases according
to Couinauds segments. Dis Colon Rectum
1995; 38: 245–8.

19. Cady B, Stone MD. The role of surgical resection of liver metastases in colorectal carcinoma. Semin Oncol 1991; 18: 399–406.

20. Pickren JW, Tsukada Y, Lane WW. Liver
metastasis: analysis of autopsy data. In:
Weiss L, Gilbert HA (eds) Liver metastasis.
Boston: GK Hall Medical Publishers, 1982: 2–
19.

21. Fisher B, Fisher ER. The interrelationship of
hematogenous and lymphatic tumor cell dissemination. Surg Gynecol Obstet 1966; 122:
791–8.

22. Dworkin MJ, Earlam S, Fordy C, Allen-Mersh
TG. Importance of hepatic artery node involvement in patients with colorectal liver
metastases. J Clin Pathol 1995; 48: 270–2.

23. Huguier M, Lacaine F. Hepatic metastases in
gastrointestinal cancer – diagnostic value of
biochemical investigations. Arch Surg 1981;
116: 399–401.

24. Sugarbaker PH. Surgical decision-making for
large bowel cancer metastatic to the liver.
Radiology 1990; 174: 621–6.

25. Metha S, Johnson RJ, Schofield PF. Review.
Staging of Colorectal Cancer. Clin Radiol
1994; 49: 515–23.

26. Tubiana JM, Deutsch JP, Taboury J, Martin B.
Imaging of hepatic colorectal metastases:
diagnosis and resectability. In: Nordlinger B,
Jaeck D (eds) Treatment of hepatic metastases
of colorectal cancer. Paris: Springer-Verlag,
1992, pp. 55–69.

27. Sheu JC, Sung JL, Chen DS et al. Ultrasonography of small hepatic tumors using high-
resolution linear-array real-time instruments.
Radiology 1984; 150: 797–802.

28. Yamaguchi A, Ishida T, Nishimura G et al.
Detection by CT during arterial portography
of colorectal cancer metastases to liver. Dis
Colon Rectum 1991; 34: 37–40.

29. Karl RC, Morse SS, Halpert RD, Clark RA.
Preoperative evaluation of patients for liver
resection – appropriate CT imaging. Ann
Surg 1993; 217: 226–32.

30. Soyer P, Lacheheb D, Levesque M. False
positive CT portography – correlation with
pathological findings. Am J Roentgenol 1993;
160: 285–9.

31. Hagspiel KD, Neidl KFW, Eichenberger AC,
Weder W, Marincek B. Detection of liver
metastases: comparison of superparamagnetic iron oxide-enhanced and unenhanced
MR imaging at 1.5 T with dynamic CT, intraoperative US, and percutaneous US. Radiology 1995; 196: 471–8.

32. Launois B, Landen S, Heautot JF. Colorectal
metastatic liver tumours. In: Terblanche J (ed)
Hepatobiliary malignancy. Its multidisciplinary management. London: Edward Arnold,
1994, pp. 271–300.

33. Chezmar JL, Rumancik WM, Megibow AJ,
Hulnick DH, Nelson RC, Bernardino ME.
Liver and abdominal screening in patients
with cancer – CT versus MR imaging. Radiology 1988; 168: 43–7.

34. Ward BA, Miller DL, Frank JA et al. Prospective evaluation of hepatic imaging studies in
the detection of colorectal metastases – correlation with surgical findings. Surgery 1989;
105: 180–7.

35. Finlay IG, McArdle CS. Occult hepatic metastases in colorectal carcinoma. Br J Surg 1986;
73: 732–5.

36. Rafaelsen SR, Kronborg O, Larsen C, Fenger
C. Intraoperative ultrasonography in detec-

tion of hepatic metastases from colorectal cancer. Dis Colon Rectum 1995; 38: 355–60.

37. Castaing D. The role of intraoperative ultrasound in the surgical treatment of hepatic metastases of colorectal origin. In: Nordlinger B, Jaeck D (eds) Treatment of hepatic metastases of colorectal cancer. Paris: Springer-Verlag, 1992, 71–3.

38. Paul MA, Mulder LS, Cuesta MA, Sikkenk AC, Lyesen GKS, Meijer S. Impact of intraoperative ultrasonography on treatment strategy for colorectal cancer. Br J Surg 1994; 81: 1660–3.

39. Soyer P, Elias D, Zeitoun G, Roche A, Levesque M. Surgical treatment of hepatic metastases – impact of intraoperative sonography. Am J Roentgenol 1993; 160: 511–14.

40. John TG, Greig JD, Crosbie JL, Miles WFA, Garden OJ. Superior staging of liver tumors with laparoscopy and laparoscopic ultrasound. Ann Surg 1994; 220: 711–19.

41. Wexner SD, Cohen SM. Port site metastases after laparoscopic colorectal surgery for cure of malignancy. Br J Surg 1995; 82: 295–8.

42. Leveson SH, Wiggins PA, Giles GR, Parkin A, Robinson PJ. Deranged liver blood flow patterns in the detection of liver metastases. Br J Surg 1985; 72: 128–30.

43. Leen E, Goldberg JA, Robertson J et al. Detection of hepatic metastases using duplex color doppler sonography. Ann Surg 1991; 214: 599–604.

44. Leen E, Angerson WJ, Wotherspoon H, Moule B, Cook TG, McArdle CS. Detection of colorectal liver metastases – comparison of laparotomy, CT, US, and doppler perfusion index and evaluation of postoperative follow-up results. Radiology 1995; 195: 113–16.

45. Leen E, Angerson WG, Cooke TG, McArdle CS. Prognostic power of doppler perfusion index in colorectal cancer: correlation with survival. Ann Surg 1996; 223: 199–203.

46. Shuman WP. Liver metastases from colorectal carcinoma – detection with doppler US-guided measurements of liver blood flow – past, present, future. Radiology 1995; 195: 9–10.

47. Wagner JS, Adson MA, Vanheerden JA, Adson MH, Ilstrup DM. The natural history of hepatic metastases from colorectal cancer – a comparison with resective treatment. Ann Surg 1984; 199: 502–8.

48. Gayowski TJ, Iwatsuki S, Madariaga JR et al. Experience in hepatic resection for metastatic colorectal cancer – analysis of clinical and pathological risk factors. Surgery 1994; 116: 703–11.

49. Rougier P, Milan C, Lazorthes F et al. Prospective study of prognostic factors in patients with unresected hepatic metastases from colorectal cancer. Br J Surg 1995; 82: 1397–400.

50. Adson MA, Vanheerden JA, Adson MH, Wagner JS, Ilstrup DM. Resection of hepatic metastases from colorectal cancer. Arch Surg 1984; 119: 647–51.

51. Scheele J, Stangl R, Altendorfhofmann A. Hepatic metastases from colorectal carcinoma – impact of surgical resection on the natural history. Br J Surg 1990; 77: 1241–6.

52. Finlay IG, Meek D, Brunton F, McArdle CS. Growth-rate of hepatic metastases in colorectal carcinoma. Br J Surg 1988; 75: 641–4.

53. Woodington GF, Waugh JM. Results of resection of metastatic tumors of the liver. Am J Surg 1963; 105: 24–9.

54. Flanagan L, Foster JH. Hepatic resection for metastatic cancer. Am J Surg 1967; 113: 551–7.

55. Wilson SM, Adson MA. Surgical treatment of hepatic metastases from colorectal cancers. Arch Surg 1976; 111: 330–4.

56. Steele G, Bleday R, Mayer RJ, Lindblad A, Petrelli N, Weaver D. A prospective evaluation of hepatic resection for colorectal carcinoma metastases to the liver – gastrointestinal tumor study group protocol-6484. J Clin Oncol 1991; 9: 1105–12.

57. Schwartz SI. Hepatic resection for noncolorectal nonneuroendocrine metastases. World J Surg 1995; 19: 72–5.

58. Starzl TE, Iwatsuki S, Shaw BW et al. Left hepatic trisegmentectomy. Surg Gynecol Obstet 1982; 155: 21–7.

59. Cunningham JD, Fong Y, Shriver C, Melendez J, Marx WL, Blumgart LH. 100 consecutive hepatic resections – blood loss, transfusion, and operative technique. Arch Surg 1994; 129: 1050–6.

60. Hughes KS, Rosenstein RB, Songhorabodi S et al. Resection of the liver for colorectal carcinoma metastases – a multi-institutional study of long-term survivors. Dis Colon Rectum 1988; 31: 1–4.

61. van Ooijen B, Wiggers T, Meijer S et al.

Hepatic resections for colorectal metastases in the Netherlands – a multiinstitutional 10-year study. Cancer 1992; 70: 28–34.

62. Nordlinger B, Jaeck D, Guiget M, Vaillant JC, Balladur P, Schaal JC. Surgical resection of hepatic metastases: multicentric retrospective study by the French Association of Surgery. In: Nordlinger B, Jaeck D (eds) Treatment of hepatic metastases of colorectal cancer. Paris: Springer-Verlag, 1992, pp. 129–61.

63. Scheele J, Stang R, Altendorfhofmann A, Paul M. Resection of colorectal liver metastases. World J Surg 1995; 19: 59–71.

64. Doci R, Gennari L, Bignami P *et al.* Morbidity and mortality after hepatic resection of metastases from colorectal cancer. Br J Surg 1995; 82: 377–81.

65. Elias D, Detroz B, Lasser P, Plaud B, Jerbi G. Is simultaneous hepatectomy and intestinal anastomosis safe? Am J Surg 1995; 169: 254–60.

66. Soyer P, Roche A, Elias D, Levesque M. Hepatic metastases from colorectal cancer – influence of hepatic volumetric analysis of surgical decision making. Radiology 1992; 184: 695–7.

67. Fortner JG, Silva JS, Golbey RB, Cox EB, Maclean BJ. Multivariate analysis of a personal series of 247 consecutive patients with liver metastases from colorectal cancer. Treatment by hepatic resection. Ann Surg 1984; 199: 306–16.

68. Ekberg H, Tranberg KG, Andersson R *et al.* Determinants of survival in liver resection for colorectal secondaries. Br J Surg 1986; 73: 727–31.

69. Cobourn CS, Makowka L, Langer B, Taylor BR, Falk RE. Examination of patient selection and outcome for hepatic resection for metastatic disease. Surg Gynecol Obstet 1987; 165: 239–46.

70. Holm A, Bradley E, Aldrete JS. Hepatic resection of metastasis from colorectal carcinoma – morbidity, mortality, and pattern of recurrence. Ann Surg 1989; 209: 428–34.

71. Doci R, Gennari L, Bignami P, Montalto F, Morabito A, Bozzetti F. 100 patients with hepatic metastases from colorectal cancer treated by resection – analysis of prognostic determinants. Br J Surg 1991; 78: 797–801.

72. Rosen CB, Nagorney DM, Taswell HF *et al.* Perioperative blood transfusion and determi-

nants of survival after liver resection for metastatic colorectal carcinoma. Ann Surg 1992; 216: 493–505.

73. Sugihara K, Hojo K, Moriya Y, Yamasaki S, Kosuge T, Takayama T. Pattern of recurrence after hepatic resection for colorectal metastases. Br J Surg 1993; 80: 1032–5.

74. Adson MA. Resection of liver metastases – when is it worthwhile? World J Surg 1987; 11: 511–20.

75. Steele G, Ravikumar TS. Resection of hepatic metastases from colorectal cancer. Ann Surg 1989; 210: 127–38.

76. Hughes KS, Scheele J, Sugarbaker PH. Surgery for colorectal cancer metastatic to the liver optimizing the results of treatment. Surg Clin North Am 1989; 69: 339–59.

77. Hughes KS. Resection of the liver for colorectal carcinoma metastases – a multi-institutional study of indications for resection. Surgery 1988; 103: 278–88.

78. Yamamoto J, Sugihara K, Kosuge T *et al.* Pathologic support for limited hepatectomy in the treatment of liver metastases from colorectal cancer. Ann Surg 1995; 221: 74–8.

79. Scheele J, Stangl R, Altendorfhofmann A, Gall FP. Indicators of prognosis after hepatic resection for colorectal secondaries. Surgery 1991; 110: 13–29.

80. Lise M, Dapian PP, Nitti D, Pilati PL, Prevaldi C. Colorectal metastases to the liver – present status of management. Dis Colon Rectum 1990; 33: 688–94.

81. Bradpiece HA, Benjamin IS, Halevy A, Blumgart LH. Major hepatic resection for colorectal liver metastases. Br J Surg 1987; 74: 324–6.

82. Ekberg H, Tranberg KG, Andersson R *et al.* Pattern of recurrence in liver resection for colorectal secondaries. World J Surg 1987; 11: 541–7.

83. Nakamura S, Yokoi Y, Suzuki S, Baba S, Muro H. Results of extensive surgery for liver metastases in colorectal carcinoma. Br J Surg 1992; 79: 35–8.

84. Franco D, Smadja C, Kahwaji F, Grange D, Kemeny F, Traynor O. Segmentectomies in the management of liver tumors. Arch Surg 1988; 123: 519–22.

85. Iwatsuki S, Esquivel CO, Gordon RD, Starzl TE. Liver resection for metastatic colorectal-cancer. Surgery 1986; 100: 804–10.

86. Fong Y, Blumgart LH, Fortner JG, Brennan MF. Pancreatic or liver resection for malignancy is safe and effective for the elderly. Ann Surg 1995; 222: 426–37.

87. Stephenson KR, Steinberg SM, Hughes KS, Vetto JT, Sugarbaker PH, Chang AE. Perioperative blood transfusions are associated with decreased time to recurrence and decreased survival after resection of colorectal liver metastases. Ann Surg 1988; 208: 679–87.

88. Younes RN, Rogatko A, Brennan MF. The influence of intraoperative hypotension and perioperative blood transfusion on disease-free survival in patients with complete resection of colorectal liver metastases. Ann Surg 1991; 214: 107–13.

89. Cady B, Stone MD, McDermott WV et al. Technical and biological factors in disease-free survival after hepatic resection for colorectal cancer metastases. Arch Surg 1992; 127: 561–9.

90. Wanebo HJ, Chu QD, Avradopoulos KA, Vezeridis MP. Current perspectives on repeat hepatic resection for colorectal carcinoma: A review. Surgery 1996; 119: 361–71.

91. Elias D, Lasser P, Hoang JM et al. Repeat hepatectomy for cancer. Br J Surg 1993; 80: 1557–62.

92. Elias D, Lasser PH, Montrucolli D, Bonvallot S, Spielmann M. Hepatectomy for liver metastases from breast cancer. Eur J Surg Oncol 1995; 21: 510–13.

93. Jaques DP, Coit DG, Casper ES, Brennan MF. Hepatic metastases from soft tissue sarcoma. Ann Surg 1995; 221: 392–7.

94. Ochiai T, Sasako M, Mizuno S et al. Hepatic resection for metastatic tumors from gastric cancer – analysis of prognostic factors. Br J Surg 1994; 81: 1175–8.

95. Que FG, Nagorney DM, Batts KP, Linz LJ, Kvols LK. Hepatic resection for metastatic neuroendocrine carcinomas. Am J Surg 1995; 169: 36–43.

96. Ravikumar TS, Kane R, Cady B, Jenkins R, Clouse M, Steele GD. A 5-year study of cryosurgery in the treatment of liver tumors. Arch Surg 1991; 126: 1520–4.

97. Weaver ML, Atkinson D, Zemel R. Hepatic cryosurgery in treating colorectal metastases. Cancer 1995; 76: 210–14.

98. Preketes AP, King J, Caplehorn JRM, Clingan PR, Ross WB, Morris DL. CEA reduction after cryotherapy for liver metastases from colon cancer predicts survival. Aust N Z J Surg 1994; 64: 612–14.

99. Poston GJ, Walker SJ, Hartley MN, Sutton R. Phase II study of cryotherapy for hepatic tumours (abstract). Eur J Cancer 1995; 31A: S156.

100. Morris DL, Horton MD, Dilley AV, Walters A, Clingan PR. Treatment of hepatic metastases by cryotherapy and regional cytotoxic perfusion. Gut 1993; 34: 1156–7.

101. Cozzi PJ, Stewart GJ, Morris DL. Thrombocytopenia after hepatic cryotherapy for colorectal metastases – correlates with hepatocellular injury. World J Surg 1994; 18: 774–7.

102. Polk W, Fong YM, Karpeh M, Blumgart LH. A technique for the use of cryosurgery to assist hepatic resection. J Am Coll Surg 1995; 180: 171–6.

103. Preketes AP, Caplehorn JRM, King J, Clingan PR, Ross WB, Morris DL. Effect of hepatic artery chemotherapy on survival of patients with hepatic metastases from colorectal carcinoma treated with cryotherapy. World J Surg 1995; 19: 768–71.

104. Amin Z, Bown SG, Lees WR. Local treatment of colorectal liver metastases – a comparison of interstitial laser photocoagulation (ILP) and percutaneous alcohol injection (PAI). Clin Radiol 1993; 48: 166–71.

105. Vogl TJ, Muller PK, Hammerstingl R et al. Malignant liver tumors treated with MR imaging-guided laser-induced thermotherapy – technique and prospective results. Radiology 1995; 196: 257–65.

106. Armstrong JG, Anderson LL, Harrison LB. Treatment of liver metastases from colorectal cancer with radioactive implants. Cancer 1994; 73: 1800–4.

107. Burton MA, Gray BN. Adjuvant internal radiation therapy in a model of colorectal cancer-derived hepatic metastases. Br J Cancer 1995; 71: 322–5.

108. Petrelli NJ, Barcewicz PA, Evans JT, Ledesma EJ, Lawrence DD, Mittelman A. Hepatic artery ligation for liver metastasis in colorectal carcinoma. Cancer 1984; 53: 1347–53.

109. Scheithauer W, Rosen H, Kornek G-V, Sebesta C, Depisch D. Randomised comparison of combination chemotherapy plus supportive

care with supportive care alone in patients with metastatic colorectal cancer. Br Med J 1993; 306: 752–5.

110. Rougier P, Lasser P, Elias D. Chemotherapy of hepatic metastases of colorectal origin (systemic and local, in palliative or adjuvant treatment). In: Nordlinger B, Jaeck D (eds) Treatment of hepatic metastases of colorectal cancer. Paris: Springer-Verlag, 1992, pp. 109–28.

111. Kerr DJ, de Takats PG. Chemotherapy for gastrointestinal cancer: teaching old drugs new tricks. GI Cancer 1995; 1: 3–7.

112. Cunningham D, Zalcberg JR, Rath U et al. 'Tomudex' (ZD1694): results of a randomised trial in advanced colorectal cancer demonstrate efficacy and reduced mucositis and leucopenia. The 'Tomudex' Colorectal Cancer Study Group. Eur J Cancer 1995; 31A: 1945–54.

113. Bismuth H, Adam R, Farabos CH, Levi F. Resection of unresectable hepatic metastases from colorectal cancer with neoadjuvant chronotherapy. Eur J Cancer 1995; 31A: S209.

114. Ridge JA, Bading JR, Gelbard AS, Benua RS, Daly JM. Perfusion of colorectal hepatic metastases – relative distribution of flow from the hepatic artery and portal vein. Cancer 1987; 59: 1547–53.

115. Rougier P, Laplanche A, Huguier M et al. Hepatic arterial infusion of floxuridine in patients with liver metastases from colorectal carcinoma: long-term results of a prospective randomized trial. J Clin Oncol 1992; 10: 1112–18.

116. Allen-Mersh TG, Earlam S, Fordy C, Abrams K, Houghton J. Quality of life and survival with continuous hepatic artery floxuridine infusion for colorectal liver metastases. Lancet 1994; 344: 1255–60.

117. Wagman LD, Kemeny MM, Leong L et al. A prospective, randomized evaluation of the treatment of colorectal cancer metastatic to the liver. J Clin Oncol 1990; 8: 1885–93.

118. Kemeny N, Seiter K, Niedzwiecki D et al. A randomized trial of intrahepatic infusion of fluorodeoxyuridine with dexamethasone versus fluorodeoxyuridine alone in the treatment of metastatic colorectal cancer. Cancer 1992; 69: 327–34.

119. Kemeny NE. Regional chemotherapy of colorectal cancer. Eur J Cancer 1995; 31A: 1271–6.

120. Dasappa V, Ross WB, King DW, Clingan PR, Morris DL. Primary resection and synchronous regional hepatic cryotherapy or cryotherapy for colorectal cancer with liver metastases. Int J Colorectal Dis 1996; 11: 38–41.

121. Lang EK, Brown CL. Colorectal metastases to the liver – selective chemoembolization. Radiology 1993; 189: 417–22.

122. Pichlmayr R, Weimann A, Oldhafer KJ et al. Role of liver transplantation in the treatment of unresectable liver cancer. World J Surg 1995; 19: 807–13.

123. Penn I. Hepatic transplantation for primary and metastatic cancers of the liver. Surgery 1991; 110: 726–35.

124. Elias D, Farace F, Triebel F et al. Phase I–II randomized study on prehepatectomy recombinant interleukin-2 immunotherapy in patients with metastatic carcinoma of the colon and rectum. J Am Coll Surg 1995; 181: 303–10.

125. Welt S, Divgi CR, Scott AM et al. Antibody targeting in metastatic colon cancer: A phase I study of monoclonal antibody F19 against a cell-surface protein of reactive tumor stromal fibroblasts. J Clin Oncol 1994; 12: 1193–203.

126. Schlag P, Manasterski M, Gerneth T et al. Active specific immunotherapy with Newcastle-disease-virus-modified autologous tumor cells following resection of liver metastases in colorectal cancer – 1st evaluation of clinical response of a phase II-trial. Cancer Immunol Immunother 1992; 35: 325–30.

127. Qin Y, van Cauteren M, Osteaux M, Schally AV, Willems G. Inhibitory effect of somatostatin analogue RC-160 on the growth of hepatic metastases of colon cancer in rats: A study with magnetic resonance imaging. Cancer Res 1992; 52: 6025–30.

128. Konno H, Tanaka T, Matsuda I et al. Comparison of the inhibitory effect of the angiogenesis inhibitor, TNP-470, and mitomycin C on the growth and liver metastasis of human colon cancer. Int J Cancer 1995; 61: 268–71.

129. Geraghty PJ, Chang AE. Basic principles associated with gene therapy of cancer. Surg Oncol 1995; 4: 125–37.

5 Portal hypertension

Tom Diamond
Rowan W. Parks

Introduction Although uncomplicated portal hypertension does not require treatment, medical or surgical intervention is indicated once complications such as variceal haemorrhage or ascites, occur. Several treatment options are available, but the management will ultimately be tailored according to the medical fitness of the patient, and the medical facilities and local clinical expertise.[1] The availability of several non-operative therapies for variceal bleeding, including pharmacotherapy, balloon tamponade, endoscopic injection sclerotherapy, endoscopic variceal ligation and most recently transjugular intrahepatic portosystemic shunt (TIPSS) has relegated emergency surgery to a secondary, yet very important, role in most institutions. Following successful management of an acute variceal bleed, the patient should be considered for definitive long-term treatment. This chapter will outline the aetiology and pathophysiology of portal hypertension, the present methods of evaluation and the various therapeutic approaches available including those for management of acute variceal bleeding, for definitive long-term treatment of oesophageal varices and for management of ascites.

Aetiology Causes of portal hypertension can be categorised as prehepatic, intrahepatic and posthepatic. The intrahepatic causes can be further subdivided into presinusoidal, sinusoidal and postsinusoidal (Table 5.1). Prehepatic causes are usually due to portal vein thrombosis, the cause of which is unknown in the majority of cases, but may be secondary to sepsis, trauma or malignant obstruction. By far the most common intrahepatic cause of portal hypertension in the United States and Europe is cirrhosis.[2] This sinusoidal obstruction to portal flow has many different causes, the commonest being alcohol abuse, but others include viral hepatitis, primary and secondary biliary cirrhosis and haemochromatosis. World-wide, the most common cause of portal hypertension is probably schistosomiasis.[3] The importance of this presinusoidal block is that liver function is usually normal,[4] leading to a much improved

Table 5.1 *Causes of portal hypertension*

Prehepatic	Intrahepatic	Posthepatic
	Presinusoidal	
Portal vein thrombosis	Schistosomiasis	Caval abnormality
Splenic vein thrombosis	Early primary biliary cirrhosis	Constrictive pericarditis
Tropical splenomegaly	Congenital hepatic fibrosis	
Arteriovenous fistula	Chronic active hepatitis	
	Sarcoidosis	
	Toxins (e.g. vinyl chloride)	
	Sinusoidal	
	Cirrhotic	
	Post viral hepatitis (B,C,D)	
	Alcoholic	
	Cryptogenic	
	Metabolic (e.g. Wilson's disease, haemochromatosis)	
	Drugs (e.g. methotrexate)	
	Immunological	
	Non-cirrhotic	
	Acute alcoholic hepatitis	
	Cytotoxic drugs	
	Vitamin A intoxication	
	Postsinusoidal	
	Budd–Chiari syndrome	
	Veno-occlusive disease	

prognosis.[5] Postsinusoidal causes of portal hypertension result from hepatic vein thrombosis either as a major vein thrombosis (Budd–Chiari syndrome) or small vessel veno-occlusive disease.[6]

Patho-physiology

Normal portal pressure is 5–10 mm Hg with a portal flow in the range 1–1.5 l min^{-1}. Portal hypertension is present when portal pressure exceeds 12 mm Hg. The major changes associated with this rise in pressure are common to all causes of portal hypertension and are reduction in portal flow to the liver and the development of portal-systemic collateral channels. The sites of potential portal-systemic anastomoses are where the splanchnic and systemic venous circulations meet, such as: (1) gastro-oesophageal junction, (2) lower rectum, (3) peri-umbilical veins, (4) retroperitoneal veins of Retzius, (5) perihepatic veins of Sappey. The collateral circulation only partially decompresses the portal venous system. In some cases blood may be shunted through the collateral circulation in sufficient quantities that flow is reversed in the portal vein, i.e. hepatofugal or retrograde flow.[7]

Interestingly, it is usually only the lower oesophageal varices that bleed. Although increased portal pressure is essential for the development of varices, the raised hydrostatic pressure alone can not be the only factor responsible since there is a poor correlation between the height of portal pressure and the risk of bleeding.[8] It is probably a difference in the venous anatomy of the lower 4 cm of the oesophagus that accounts for the prevalence of bleeding from this site. Stelzner and Lierse[9] reported that, in the distal oesophagus of Rhesus monkeys, the submucosal veins pierced the muscularis mucosa to lie superficially, close to the overlying epithelium. Spence *et al.*,[10] using a computer image analysis system, demonstrated in humans an abrupt change in the vessel pattern at the gastro-oesophageal junction. A 7-fold increase in the area occupied by the veins in the lamina propria in this region was demonstrated. When these vessels are subjected to abnormal internal pressure they become markedly dilated. In addition, large intraepithelial channels develop from the underlying vessels in the lamina propria which may only be separated from the oesophageal lumen by a few epithelial cells.[11] Experiments have shown that large varices are more likely to rupture at lower transmural pressures than small varices.[12]

Varices may also occur in the gastric fundus, but are a source of bleeding in only 5% of cases. Dilatation of the gastric submucosal veins results in portal hypertensive gastropathy which affects mainly the fundus and body of the stomach and produces an erythematous appearance at endoscopy. An interesting, but rare, form of localised portal hypertension, known as left-sided, segmental, or 'sinistral' portal hypertension, occurs in patients with splenic vein thrombosis and should be suspected in patients with bleeding oesophageal varices and normal liver function.

Clinical features

Cirrhosis results in two major events; hepatocellular failure and portal hypertension. Patients with cirrhosis may have non-specific symptoms such as general malaise, anorexia or abdominal pain. The clinical signs of chronic liver failure include leuconychia, finger clubbing, palmar erythema, spider naevi, gynaecomastia (or breast atrophy in females), testicular atrophy and loss of secondary sexual hair. Portal hypertension is indicated by splenomegaly and abdominal wall venous collaterals (Caput Medusa).

The main complications of portal hypertension are variceal bleeding and ascites. Variceal bleeding is the most dramatic of these complications, but ascites also causes significant morbidity and can often be difficult to control. Variceal bleeding is also important in that it may precipitate hepatic failure which is a major determinant of survival.

Classification

Disease severity is assessed by a combination of clinical parameters and standard laboratory tests. The Child–Pugh classification is used to standardise disease stage. The combination of two clinical parameters

Table 5.2 *Child–Pugh classification*

	Number of points		
	1	2	3
Bilirubin (μmol l^{-1})[a]	<34	34–51	>51
Albumin (g l^{-1})	>35	28–35	<28
Prothrombin time prolonged by (s)	<3	3–10	>10
Ascites	None	Slight to moderate	Moderate to severe
Encephalopathy	None	Slight to moderate	Moderate to severe

Grade A 5–6 points; Grade B 7–9 points; Grade C 10–15 points.
[a]In primary biliary cirrhosis, the point scoring for bilirubin level is adjusted as follows: 1 = <68, 2 = 68–170, 3 = >170.

(ascites and encephalopathy), two biochemical criteria (bilirubin and albumin concentrations) and one haematological criterion (prothrombin time) is evaluated and scored (Table 5.2).[2] A total score from the five parameters classifies the patient as Child–Pugh grade A (score 5–6 points), B (score 7–9) or C (score 10–15).

Investigations

In the acute situation, emergency measurement of the haematocrit, haemoglobin, coagulation status and serum electrolytes should be performed. Liver function tests, serum albumin concentration and prothrombin time give an indication of liver function. Specific serological markers for hepatitis A, B and C may help to define the aetiology.[2] In addition, serological assessment of autoimmune disease and primary biliary cirrhosis are a routine part of evaluation.

Activity of the underlying liver disease may be apparent from standard biochemical and haematological tests, however, percutaneous needle biopsy may be used to demonstrate the presence of cirrhosis and assess its severity.

Upper gastrointestinal (GI) endoscopy is essential in the assessment of oesophageal varices. In a patient who is actively bleeding or has just stopped bleeding, it is important to establish the exact diagnosis and source of bleeding. It is important that adequate resuscitation and haemodynamic stability are accomplished before endoscopy is attempted. Of all patients presenting with upper GI haemorrhage in the Western world, oesophageal varices will be the cause of bleeding in only approximately 10%. In addition, in patients with known portal hypertension and oesophageal varices, or in those in whom the presence of portal hypertension is suspected from the history and examination, non-oesophageal variceal sources will be found in 10–25%. These include gastritis, peptic ulceration, Mallory–Weiss tears, gastric varices or portal hypertensive gastropathy. This is important in terms of further therapeutic strategy as some techniques (e.g. balloon tamponade, sclerotherapy) may be appropriate in patients with oesophageal varices but not in those with gastric varices or portal hypertensive gastropathy. When there is difficulty in identifying the exact cause of bleeding, repeat endoscopy should be undertaken.[13]

Radiological studies are an integral part of evaluation. Ultrasound combined with Doppler study of the vessels, computed tomography (CT) and angiography may be indicated.[14,15] The morphology of the liver can be assessed with ultrasound and CT. Ultrasound is also useful in demonstrating the portal and hepatic veins. When ultrasound is combined with Doppler flow measurements, directional flow may be depicted in these vessels. Arteriography may be used to demonstrate the venous anatomy (venous phase of superior mesenteric angiogram) and assess the degree and direction of portal venous flow.[16] This is essential prior to shunt surgery. If the patient's history and laboratory findings suggest cirrhosis secondary to extrahepatic biliary obstruction, cholangiography (ERCP) should be performed.

Management of bleeding varices

The management of bleeding oesophageal varices can be considered in two major categories; the emergency resuscitation and initial control of the bleeding episode and the long-term treatment of the patient who has varices which have bled and been controlled but where further treatment is necessary, to eradicate the varices and reduce the risk of further bleeding. In general, the emergency and long-term management of these patients is best carried out in a specialised centre where medical and nursing staff are experienced in routine observation and techniques related to the patient with liver disease and where recourse to specialised intervention is available if required.

Emergency control of an acute variceal bleed

Resuscitation

The initial resuscitation of a patient with bleeding oesophageal varices is similar to that for any patient with upper gastrointestinal (GI) haemorrhage. A wide-bore cannula (16 gauge) should be inserted. Central venous access is preferable, to record the venous pressure and monitor the response to administered fluids and blood. Colloidal fluids, packed red cells and coagulation factors (fresh frozen plasma) should be administered as required. Saline infusions should be avoided because of the risk of fluid retention and aggravation of ascites. Excessive transfusion or fluid administration should also be avoided as this may increase the risk of further bleeding by over expansion of the circulating blood volume. Comatose patients and those with massive haematemesis may require endotracheal intubation to prevent aspiration.

Pharmacotherapy

Several pharmacological agents are available for the emergency control of variceal bleeding. Most of these act by lowering portal venous pressure but others are thought to act by constricting the lower oesophageal sphincter, hence strangulating the varices and arresting haemorrhage.

Vasoactive drugs have been widely used in an attempt to control bleeding from oesophageal varices. Vasopressin was the first drug used to induce splanchnic vasoconstriction, however, it is only effective in half of the patients treated and its use is associated with the development of major complications in approximately 25% of patients.[17] Even the use of an analogue of vasopressin, triglycyl-lysine-vasopressin (Glypressin), or concomitant administration of the hormone with nitrates has failed to produce convincing benefits with respect to both the control of bleeding and reduction of side effects.[18]

The vasoactive peptide hormone somatostatin reduces oesophageal variceal pressure and has been shown to be beneficial in the treatment of bleeding varices. The results of several randomised trials suggest that variceal bleeding can be controlled in 65–70% of patients treated with no major complications being observed.[19] However, it has not been shown to reduce mortality significantly.[20]

Somatostatin has a half-life of less than 3 min, necessitating continuous intravenous infusion to achieve a therapeutic response. This short half-life together with its relatively non-specific effects and the rebound hormonal hypersecretion on cessation of infusion, have severely limited its clinical use. However, the more recently developed somatostatin analogue, octreotide, has a much more selective action than somatostatin, is longer acting and is also less expensive. Infusion of octreotide at 25 μg h^{-1} has been shown in one study to be as effective as balloon tamponade of the oesophagus in controlling variceal bleeding in the acute situation and has less associated morbidity and mortality.[21] In another recent study octreotide infused at 50 μg h^{-1} was as effective as injection sclerotherapy in achieving haemostasis and preventing rebleeding over a 48 h period.[22] Both somatostatin and octreotide have also been shown to be very effective in controlling early post-injection sclerotherapy bleeding, which can occur from the varices themselves, or from oesophageal ulceration or oesophagitis.[23] This observation would suggest that both somatostatin and octreotide are useful adjuvant treatments to injection sclerotherapy. Vasoactive therapy for control of variceal bleeding remains an attractive proposition since it is the only treatment which can be initiated, without specialist expertise, as soon as the patient enters hospital. Preliminary studies also suggest that octreotide is very effective in controlling severe gastric bleeding in patients with portal hypertensive gastropathy or gastric varices.[24] Octreotide should be administered intravenously as either 500 μg in 500 ml of 5% dextrose over 12 h, or 500 μg in 60 ml of 5% dextrose over 12 h via a syringe driver.

Agents which act by a constrictor effect on the lower oesophageal sphincter include pentagastrin and metoclopramide. Cisapride may possibly be effective via this mechanism but experience of its use in the management of bleeding varices is limited.

Therapy to reduce the risk of encephalopathy should also be instituted, including neomycin (250 mg–1 g qid), to reduce the number of ammonia-producing bacteria in the bowel and lactulose (10–30 ml tid) to increase gut motility and lower faecal pH, hence reducing ammonia absorption. Lactulose may also produce some benefit via an antiendotoxin effect.

Oesophageal tamponade

Balloon tamponade is very effective in achieving temporary control of variceal bleeding (70–90%),[12,24] but there is a high rate of recurrent bleeding (60%) after removal of the tube. In view of the high rate of recurrent bleeding, the use of balloon tamponade is indicated in selected cases only. These include control of massive bleeding from varices that cannot be sclerosed acutely, cases where acute sclerotherapy has failed and control of bleeding is necessary prior to surgical intervention and for transfer of a bleeding patient to a specialised centre where emergency sclerotherapy or surgical options are available.

In general it is unwise, and even hazardous, to insert a balloon tube in a patient before a definite diagnosis has been made by endoscopy. For example, attempts by an inexperienced clinician to insert a balloon tube in a patient with upper GI haemorrhage due to an oesophageal or gastric neoplastic lesion may result in inflation of the gastric balloon in the oesophagus and subsequent oesophageal rupture. With adequate resuscitation and use of pharmacological agents, particularly octreotide, insertion of a balloon tube prior to endoscopy is now rarely necessary. The one exception is possibly in a patient in whom there is a strong suspicion of oesophageal variceal bleeding (previous history of varices, or a history and examination strongly suggestive of portal hypertension), where there is massive bleeding and haemodynamic instability which cannot be controlled by resuscitation and pharmacotherapy.

The four-lumen (Sengstaken–Blakmore) tube is most commonly used (Fig. 5.1). The tube should be stored in a refrigerator prior to use to render it less pliable and facilitate insertion. A new tube is used for each patient and both balloons are tested for leaks prior to insertion. The nasal route for insertion is preferred as this is ultimately more comfortable for the patient. A lubricated Seldinger wire can be passed down the gastric aspiration channel if insertion proves to be difficult. Once in the stomach, the gastric balloon is filled with 200 ml of air and pulled back to impinge on the cardia. The oesophageal balloon is then inflated with air to obtain an intraluminal pressure of approximately 40 mm Hg (measured using a blood pressure manometer). The tube is strapped to the nares in this position but no traction is necessary. The gastric lumen allows test aspiration, which should be carried out approximately every 15 min to check for further bleeding. This lumen may also be used for administration of medication such as neomycin and lactulose. A fourth lumen

Figure 5.1 *Use of a four-lumen (Sengstaken–Blakemore) tube for oesophageal tamponade.*

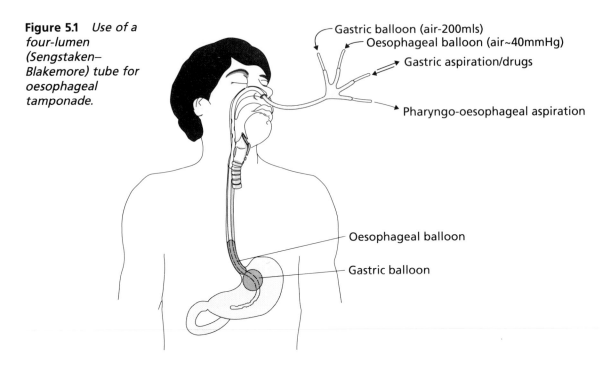

Gastric balloon (air-200mls)
Oesophageal balloon (air~40mmHg)
Gastric aspiration/drugs
Pharyngo-oesophageal aspiration
Oesophageal balloon
Gastric balloon

allows aspiration of the upper oesophagus and pharynx and reduces the risk of bronchial aspiration. In patients who are stuporose or comatose, the airway should be protected by an endotracheal tube. The use of oesophageal tamponade is a temporary holding measure until definitive therapy. The oesophageal balloon is generally deflated after 12–24 h to prevent oesophageal ulceration, but the gastric balloon position may be maintained. If bleeding recurs the oesophageal balloon may be reinflated but at this stage a more definitive therapy should be arranged. Those patients who do not rebleed within the subsequent 24 h can have the gastric balloon deflated and the tube removed, but these patients will also require definitive treatment.

Complications occur in about 10–20% of patients who require balloon tamponade.[25] Mechanical pressure effects may induce damage to the surface of the oesophagus with resulting mucosal ulceration. Oesophageal perforation and aspiration pneumonia may occur. In addition, patients may find the tube uncomfortable and often become distressed and agitated.

Injection sclerotherapy

Crafoord and Frenckner[26] first described injection sclerotherapy in 1939 in the management of acute bleeding in a patient with portal vein thrombosis. In 1973, Johnston and Rodgers[27] reported their 15-year experience of injection sclerotherapy in Belfast for acute bleeding of 195 admissions in 117 patients. Control of bleeding was obtained in 93%, and hospital mortality was 18%. Since then endoscopic injection sclerotherapy has become widely accepted and is now the most frequently used form of therapy for both emergency and long-term control of variceal haemorrhage.[28]

The technique relies on obliteration of varices by a process of sclerosis and fibrosis. Several methods are used to achieve this including intravariceal injection of sclerosant (the most widely used),[1,29] and paravariceal (submucosal) injection,[30] where the aim is to produce an area of fibrosis and thickening superficial to the varices. Some sclerotherapists use a combination of the intravariceal and paravariceal methods, in an attempt to combine the advantages of each.[31] Various sclerosing agents are used including ethanolamine oleate, sodium tetradecyl sulphate (STD), polidocanol, and more recently the tissue adhesive N-butyl-2-cyanoacrylate (Histoacryl).[32] The fact that several agents are available, and are effective, probably indicates that no one in particular is vastly superior to the others.

Injection sclerotherapy can be performed using either a rigid oesophagoscope or a fibreoptic endoscope. Both have advantages and disadvantages, although the latter is more commonly used nowadays. If one uses the rigid instrument, a general anaesthetic is required, but this gives the reassurance of a protected airway. The technique for the passage of the rigid instrument requires more training and skill. The advantages are that the tip of the rigid instrument can be used to compress any bleeding point and the wide-bore channel allows the passage of a large sucker for removal of blood or clot. Rotation of the instrument allows compression of the varix following injection of sclerosant. The flexible instrument is technically easier to pass, carries less risk of oesophageal damage and general anaesthesia is unnecessary. The main disadvantages are the problem of removing blood efficiently during active haemorrhage and the difficulty in providing adequate compression of the varix after injection to ensure the necessary intimal damage. This has been overcome by the use of a flexible outer sheath, or by the use of proximal or distal balloons.

Complications of injection sclerotherapy are generally minor and include low-grade fever, retrosternal discomfort and oesophageal ulceration or mucosal sloughing. More serious complications, which are generally rare, include oesophageal perforation, oesophageal stricture, pleural effusion and empyema. With repeated injection sclerotherapy sessions, complications become cumulative.[33] If oesophageal ulceration becomes a significant problem either somatostatin or omeprazole, or both, may be used.

In most centres, the initial sclerotherapy is performed at the time of diagnostic endoscopy. This will control acute variceal bleeding in the majority (>70%) of patients.[34] In the remainder, a second sclerotherapy session is necessary. After either one or two injection sessions, acute bleeding will be controlled in 90–95% of patients.[35] Failure of acute sclerotherapy is defined as failure to control acute bleeding after two emergency injection treatments during a single hospital admission.[36]

Such patients should be controlled with balloon tamponade and should undergo transjugular intrahepatic portal–systemic shunt (TIPSS) or one of the more major surgical options.

Results for sclerotherapy for the treatment of acutely bleeding gastric varices have generally been poor, although recent reports on the use of Histoacryl® glue have been very encouraging.[37] Injection sclerotherapy is not indicated in patients with bleeding due to portal hypertensive gastropathy. In these cases an emergency surgical procedure is indicated if pharmacotherapy fails. TIPSS or emergency surgical treatment may be indicated in the 5–10% of patients in whom emergency sclerotherapy fails. The available surgical options are portal–systemic shunt, oesophageal transection/devascularisation or liver transplantation.

Variceal ligation

Endoscopic variceal ligation (EVL) was introduced in 1988 by Stiegmann *et al.*[38] It is based on the same principle as banding of haemorrhoids. The varix is first sucked into a drum attached to the tip of the endoscope. An elastic 'O' band, mounted on the drum, is then released over the varix by pulling on a trip wire which runs through the working channel of the endoscope. The most important advantage of EVL is its simplicity. In contrast to endoscopic sclerotherapy, which requires intensive operator training in order to obtain good results, EVL is said to be relatively easy to learn and perform competently.[39]

The technique has been successful in the treatment of acute variceal bleeding and has proved particularly successful in the long-term management aimed at eradicating varices after a variceal bleed. This was confirmed in a prospective randomised trial comparing this technique with sclerotherapy.[40] The technique has also been used successfully in patients for whom injection sclerotherapy has failed.[41] Disadvantages of the technique include the tunnel vision produced by the application device on the tip of the endoscope, and the need to repeatedly withdraw the endoscope while loading a new elastic band, hence the use of an overtube in the pharynx is necessary. Complications of EVL are starting to appear as case reports. Several authors have reported overtube injury to the pharynx or oesophagus with resultant bleeding or perforation.[42,43] Massive bleeding from a band-induced ulcer and acute oesophageal obstruction due to occlusion of the lumen by banded oesophageal varices have also been reported.[44] A mechanism which allows repeated banding and obviates the need to use an overtube for repeated removal of the endoscope has recently been developed.

It has been the experience of some, that varices tend to recur within 3 to 6 months of initial eradication,[39] and therefore a combination of EVL and injection sclerotherapy may prove to be a useful option – using EVL to treat large varices followed by a course of injection sclerotherapy for small varices and to achieve fibrosis of the inner wall of the oesophagus.[45] The results of trials using this combined approach are eagerly awaited.

Portal–systemic shunts

Until the use of sclerotherapy became widespread in the early 1970s portal–systemic shunts were widely used for the emergency management of variceal bleeding. Shunt surgery has, however, been associated with a high operative mortality rate (7–30%), and a low 5-year survival, particularly in patients with marked hepatic functional decompensation. Therefore, in the vast majority of centres world-wide, routine portal–systemic shunting for acute variceal bleeding is not performed and shunts are reserved for the 5–10% of patients in whom bleeding is not controlled by pharmacotherapy and sclerotherapy. Shunts are, however, still a useful treatment in countries with a high incidence of non-cirrhotic portal hypertension, where the patients are in the second or third decade of life and they can be performed with lower mortality.[39]

Orloff, the main proponent of emergency shunt procedures, reported a 5-year survival rate of 64% in a series of 94 consecutive unselected patients who generally had their operations performed within 8 hours of admission to hospital.[46] The operative mortality rate was 20% in this series. A controlled comparison of routine emergency shunt versus conventional medical management followed by elective shunt by this same group showed better control of haemorrhage and improved early and late survival in the emergency shunt group.[47] Major criticisms of this trial are that endoscopic sclerotherapy, the 'gold standard' for treatment of acute variceal bleeding in most centres, was not used in the medical treatment arm and surgical crossover for patients who failed medical therapy was not allowed. The general view is that in Child–Pugh grade C patients, emergency shunt surgery carries a prohibitive mortality and it has no place in the management of these patients.

If the operation is to be performed in the acute situation, then the quickest and simplest procedure is probably the safest. Many surgeons therefore favour the end-to-side portacaval shunt or the interposition mesocaval shunt.[48] However, both these procedures completely divert portal flow away from the liver and thereby tend to cause more frequent episodes of encephalopathy than devascularisation procedures and selective shunts.[49] The trend away from portal–systemic shunts in recent years, despite the fact that they prevent recurrent variceal bleeding in virtually all patients, is related principally to the high mortality and high incidence of postoperative encephalopathy, which is often chronic and incapacitating.

Clear indications for emergency surgical intervention in many institutions include: (1) persistent variceal bleeding despite non-operative treatment with injection sclerotherapy, (2) failure of chronic sclerotherapy, (3) bleeding from gastric varices or portal hypertensive gastropathy that is unresponsive to acute pharmacotherapy. In our practice, we virtually never use emergency shunt procedures for acute variceal bleeding.

Transjugular intrahepatic portal–systemic shunts (TIPSS)

A method for producing an intrahepatic portal–systemic stent shunt via the transjugular route was first described in animals by Rosch *et al.* in 1969.[50] The first transjugular portal–systemic shunt procedures in humans were described in 1982 when balloon catheters were inflated to produce a tract between the portal and hepatic vein.[51] The subsequent use of metallic expandable stents to improve patency rates in humans was described in 1989 by Richter *et al.*,[52] and since then there has been a rapid increase in the use of this technique world-wide.

Internal jugular puncture is usually performed on the right side. A sheath is inserted and the right or middle hepatic vein is cannulated under radiological screening. A transjugular liver biopsy needle or sharp stylet is directed out of the hepatic vein, through the liver parenchyma and into a large branch of the portal vein. After passing a guide wire into the portal vein, an angioplasty balloon catheter is used to expand the tract before inserting a metallic stent (Palmaz® or Wallstent®) (Fig. 5.2).

Figure 5.2
Technique to create an intrahepatic portal–systemic stent shunt (TIPSS).

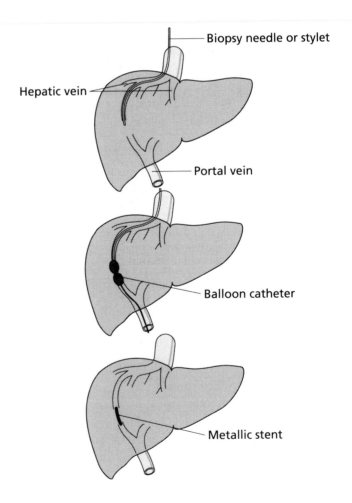

Biopsy needle or stylet

Hepatic vein

Portal vein

Balloon catheter

Metallic stent

At present, the main indication for this technique is to control and prevent variceal haemorrhage when endoscopic therapy has failed.[53] One advantage of TIPSS is that, being an intrahepatic procedure, the extrahepatic venous anatomy is not disturbed and subsequent liver transplantation can be more easily performed if required.[54] TIPSS has been used as first line management in the acute situation to control bleeding from gastric or oesophageal varices.[54] TIPSS can also be used before closure of a surgical portal–systemic shunt that is causing disabling encephalopathy and can be used to treat intractable ascites.

TIPSS can be successfully completed in more than 90% of patients with a procedure-related mortality of less than 1%, mainly from intraperitoneal bleeding.[55] Rebleeding occurs in 10–20% of patients,[56] and is usually associated with shunt-related complications, such as intimal hyperplasia, shunt migration, or thrombosis. If shunt occlusion occurs, a further shunt can be inserted or balloon dilatation of the existing shunt can be performed. New or worsened hepatic encephalopathy develops in about 10–20% of patients undergoing TIPSS.[56] In most cases the symptoms are mild and are readily treated with dietary protein restriction and lactulose therapy.[54]

Oesophageal transection/devascularisation

The alternative to portal–systemic shunting for surgical control of acutely bleeding oesophageal varices is transection of the oesophagus and end-to-end anastomosis using a stapling gun (Fig. 5.3a). The aim of

Figure 5.3
Oesophageal transection/ devascularisation procedures. (a) Oesophageal transection; (b) oesophageal transection and devascularisation; (c) Sugiura operation.

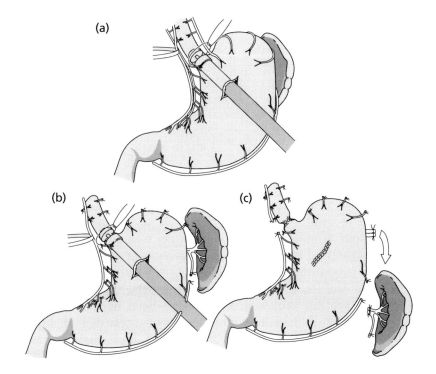

this procedure is to remove a segment of the lower 1–3 cm of the oesophagus, which is the most vulnerable in terms of variceal bleeding. Vankemmel[57] first reported the use of a circular stapling gun to perform oesophageal transection in 1974. It is a relatively simple operation, compared to portal–systemic shunting, but carries a similar mortality. As the portal circulation is not disturbed, postoperative encephalopathy is generally not a problem. However, the disadvantage of this procedure is that, although acute bleeding may be controlled in over 95% of patients, there is a significant rate of recurrent variceal bleeding (approximately 30% over the next 5–10 years) in contrast to shunt procedures.

The incidence of recurrent bleeding may be decreased by a combination of oesophageal transection and devascularisation of the lower oesophagus and upper stomach (Fig. 5.3b), but this may increase the operative risk. An even more extensive operation involves a thoraco-abdominal approach, with oesophageal transection and extensive devascularisation of the oesophagus and upper stomach, including a vagotomy, pyloroplasty and splenectomy (Sugiura operation) (Fig. 5.3c).[58] This was used extensively in Japan with excellent reported results in terms of operative complications and rebleeding.[59] However, it is now less popular in Japan and in Western practice the technique has never become widely established.

Long-term/definitive treatment of oesophageal varices

Approximately 70% of patients who bleed from varices are likely to have a further variceal bleed during their lifetime. The highest incidence is in the first few months following the variceal bleed and the highest mortality occurs during this initial phase, with the chance of survival returning to baseline thereafter.[60] There is general agreement that some form of specific long-term treatment is usually indicated.

The only form of treatment that cures both the underlying liver disease and the portal hypertension is liver transplantation. All patients with bleeding oesophageal varices should be considered for liver transplantation today.[61] Only a small percentage will ultimately receive a transplant, but management in possible transplant candidates should subsequently be directed to forms of therapy that will not interfere with any subsequent transplant procedure.

The alternative specific definitive procedures other than transplantation are long-term pharmacological management, repeated injection sclerotherapy, repeated variceal ligation, a transection and devascularisation operation, or a portal–systemic shunt procedure.[35]

Long-term pharmacotherapy

Although drugs have been used for the treatment of acute variceal bleeding for many years, pharmacotherapy has only recently (early 1980s) been investigated and used for the long-term prevention of recurrent variceal haemorrhage. The possible mechanism of action of long-term pharmacotherapy is by a reduction in portal pressure, probably via splanchnic arteriolar vasoconstriction. Beta blockade has been investigated in several clinical trials and a meta-analysis recently concluded that beta-blockers, principally propranolol, significantly reduced the incidence of recurrent bleeding and improved long-term survival when compared with placebo.[62] Subsequent reanalysis with more complete data and more strict criteria confirmed a significant reduction in rebleeding, but without a reduction in mortality.[63] Other agents currently being investigated for use in long-term pharmacotherapy include calcium channel blockers (verapamil), long-acting nitrates, serotonin antagonists and octreotide. Long-term drug therapy, however, has disadvantages, including the cost of lifelong therapy, problems with compliance in alcoholic patients, and potential side effects.

Repeated injection sclerotherapy

Repeated injection sclerotherapy is currently the most widely used technique for the treatment of recurrent oesophageal variceal bleeding. If a programme of repeated sclerotherapy is thought to be the most appropriate long-term therapeutic option, repeat injection sessions usually begin 1–2 weeks after the initial emergency session and are continued every 1–2 weeks until the varices have been completely eradicated. The interval between injection sessions varies in different centres; injections at weekly intervals produce earlier obliteration of varices but may be associated with a higher incidence of oesophageal mucosal sloughing and ulceration than injections at 2 or 3 weekly intervals. Once the varices have been eradicated, some centres advise follow-up endoscopy every 6 or 12 months and if there is any recurrence of varices further injection should be undertaken. However, we consider that repeat endoscopy is indicated only if rebleeding occurs after obliteration.

The efficacy of long-term sclerotherapy, in terms of ability to eradicate varices, prevent recurrent bleeding and ultimately improve survival, has been the subject of several controlled trials. In the majority of cases sclerotherapy is successful in eradicating varices completely and reducing the risk of subsequent bleeding. However, when patients are managed with injection sclerotherapy, 45–60% of them will rebleed at some time.[64] Many of these patients are successfully treated with subsequent sclerotherapy sessions, but the eventual failure rate of injection sclerotherapy is as high as 35% in some series.[65]

Failure of long-term sclerotherapy is defined as massive bleeding requiring resuscitation and blood transfusion, or two or more bleeding episodes during the injection programme. In this situation a shunt procedure or possibly a transection and devascularisation operation should be considered.[35,66] In terms of improvement of overall survival it is generally perceived that sclerotherapy, although effective in treating acute variceal bleeding and reducing the risk of recurrent bleeding, does not improve long-term survival. This is thought to be related to the fact that it is only a palliative procedure and does not alter the progression of the underlying disease process. However, a meta-analysis of the controlled trials, published in 1989, comparing chronic sclerotherapy with conventional medical therapy, shows a statistically significant survival advantage with the former technique.[67]

Repeated variceal ligation

This may be used alone, or in combination with sclerotherapy. It is currently being used in selected centres and world-wide experience is not nearly as great as with injection sclerotherapy, but if results of trials comparing it with sclerotherapy are favourable, its use will inevitably increase.

Elective portal–systemic shunts

Many types of portal–systemic shunts have been developed and surgical trainees often have difficulties understanding the differences between them. Basically they can be considered simply in two main categories; non-selective and selective. The non-selective shunts are those which decompress all of the portal system. Thus, the incidence of retrograde portal blood flow and risk of postoperative encephalopathy with these shunts is high. It is also thought that, by diverting portal flow away from the liver, they may result in deterioration of hepatocellular metabolism and function due to the loss of hepatotrophic factors in portal blood. Examples include the standard end-to-side portacaval shunt, the side-to-side portacaval shunt, the mesocaval shunt using a prosthetic graft, the portacaval prosthetic H graft and the central splenorenal shunt (Fig. 5.4).

One of the non-selective shunts, the portacaval prosthetic H graft, is worth further consideration. It has been suggested that by using a small diameter prosthesis (usually 10 mm) the resistance of the shunt could be

Figure 5.4 *Non-selective portal–systemic shunts. (a) End-to-side portacaval; (b) side-to-side portacaval; (c) mesocaval prosthesis; (d) portacaval prosthetic H graft; (e) central splenorenal.*

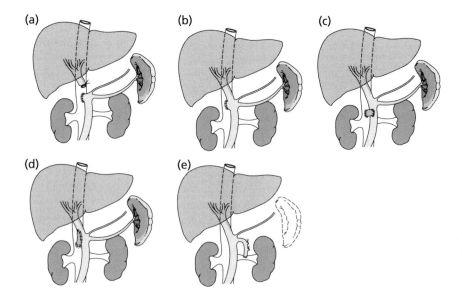

Figure 5.5 *Selective portal–systemic shunts. (a) Warren distal splenorenal; (b) Inokuchi left gastric–inferior venacaval.*

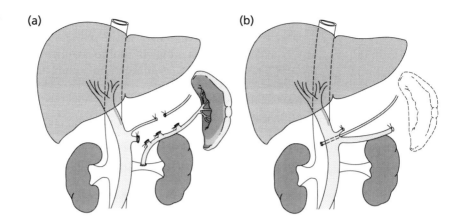

(a)　　　　　　　(b)

increased, thus decreasing the flux across the shunt and maintaining prograde (hepatopedal) portal flow. This should produce a 'partial' shunt which decompresses the portal system sufficiently to prevent recurrent variceal bleeding but maintains prograde portal flow, thus preventing encephalopathy and deterioration in hepatocellular function.[68] This shunt is currently being used in a few centres with encouraging results.[16,69] Other advantages are that it is a relatively easy shunt to construct and, as dissection in the area of the hepatic pedicle is minimal, the performance of subsequent orthoptic liver transplantation is not compromised.[16]

The selective shunts aim to decompress only a part of the portal system (the oesophagogastric venous network), thus preventing variceal bleeding, whilst maintaining portal venous pressure and prograde portal flow, thereby preventing encephalopathy.[70] Examples include the Warren distal splenorenal shunt and the Inokuchi left gastric–inferior vena caval shunt (Fig. 5.5). The Warren shunt is the most widely used and is reported to be associated with a much lower incidence of encephalopathy than the non-selective shunts.[71] However, not all patients, particularly alcoholic cirrhotics, maintain prograde portal perfusion after construction of the shunt.[72] Shunting continues to have a small but definite role for management of young patients who have minimal hepatic impairment and who do not have a history of diabetes, encephalopathy, active hepatitis or acute bleeding. It may also have a place in the treatment of patients with portal hypertensive gastropathy where reduction of portal pressure may be the only successful form of treatment.

Elective oesophageal transection/devascularisation
Transection/devascularisation procedures are being used less frequently for the elective or long-term management of patients with variceal bleeding. This is probably related to the fact that, although they have the advantages of being simple to perform and not associated

with encephalopathy, they are associated with a high incidence of recurrent variceal bleeding (approximately 30%). They may continue to have a limited role in some countries, where access to liver transplantation is not available and where the patient is unsuitable for a shunt procedure, namely, the elderly, patients with advanced liver disease, diabetics, patients with schistosomiasis and those with previous encephalopathy.

Liver transplantation

Since results of liver transplantation have improved and it has become more widely available it has become an option for some patients with recurrent variceal bleeding.[61] Because of economic factors and a limited supply of donor organs, transplantation is not available to all patients. In addition, a significant percentage of patients with variceal haemorrhage are not candidates for this procedure, because of advanced age, active alcohol or drug abuse or advanced disease in other organ systems. Likewise, patients with extrahepatic portal vein thrombosis and schistosomiasis are not transplant candidates because hepatic functional reserve is maintained indefinitely in these conditions. However, in patients who have end-stage liver disease, transplantation is the treatment of choice.[28] Bismuth *et al.*[73] have reported a 4-year survival rate of 73% in Child's grade C patients undergoing liver transplantation. By comparison, survival rates among comparable Child grade patients managed by primary shunt or sclerotherapy were 31% and 59%, respectively. This evidence suggests that patients with end-stage liver disease should undergo liver transplantation in the absence of any contraindications, and this has been confirmed by other investigators.[61,74] In patients whose disease is not end-stage but who are symptomatic, with a poor quality of life (e.g. encephalopathy, asthenia, fatigue), transplantation is also the treatment of choice. In patients with good hepatic function and static or slowly progressing disease early hepatic transplantation may not be necessary and they are best treated in the interim with an alternative technique (e.g. sclerotherapy, portal–systemic shunt (TIPSS). If future transplantation is anticipated, operative therapy should be considered carefully. In terms of technical considerations, non-shunt operations do not adversely affect subsequent transplantation and if a shunt is chosen, the distal splenorenal, the mesocaval or portacaval prosthetic H shunts, where dissection in the area of the hepatic pedicle is minimal, are most suitable. End-to-side and side-to-side portacaval shunts should be avoided in this situation. However, the use of these techniques has now largely been superseded by the use of a transjugular portal–systemic shunt (TIPSS).

Prophylactic therapy

The aim of prophylactic therapy is to prevent a first episode of variceal bleeding and hence reduce subsequent complications and mortality. It is thought that only 30% of cirrhotic patients with documented oesophageal varices will actually ever bleed from these.[34,75] For this reason most authors recommend observation until the first variceal bleed occurs. However, the high mortality at the time of the first bleed, over 50% in poor-risk Child–Pugh C patients, has led many investigators to consider prophylactic treatment. The options, all of which have been tested in controlled trials, include pharmacotherapy, injection sclerotherapy, portal–systemic shunt procedures and extensive transection and devascularisation operations.

The initial studies of prophylactic shunt procedures performed in the 1960s showed increased morbidity and mortality in the shunt groups[76–78] and were therefore abandoned. A more recent multicentre study from Japan comparing prophylactic portal non-decompressive surgery with conventional management, has shown significantly improved survival and reduced rebleed rates in the shunt group at 5 years.[79] This study has not been repeated in any other population and stands alone in this area. It must be remembered that there is a difference in aetiology of portal hypertension between Japan and most Western countries and therefore major prophylactic shunt surgery of this nature is currently unjustified outside controlled trials.

Many trials have compared prophylactic injection sclerotherapy with conventional medical management, but with conflicting results.[80–83] A meta-analysis of randomised controlled trials concluded that prophylactic sclerotherapy should not be widely applied at present owing to insufficient documentation of benefit.[84] There is even a danger that the injection treatment might precipitate the first variceal bleed and lead to the patient's death.[83]

The most widely used form of prophylaxis is pharmacotherapy, particularly beta-blockade with propranolol. Once again, the results of trials have been conflicting, although a number of studies have shown improved survival. A meta-analysis of seven prospective randomised trials has shown that the risk of the initial bleeding episode can be reduced to approximately 15%.[62] However, these trials have not shown a significant difference in the overall mortality rate and therefore, at present, prophylactic therapy in patients with varices which have not yet bled is not routinely practised.

Results/prognosis

The prognosis for an individual patient depends on the severity of the bleeding episode and the underlying liver function.[85] Patients with non-cirrhotic portal hypertension or cirrhosis with good liver function have a good short-term and long-term prognosis. In patients with established cirrhosis, the presence of alcoholic hepatitis, hepatocellular carcinoma and/or portal venous thrombosis may adversely affect prognosis. Operative mortality rates are also more dependent on the status of the liver disease at the time of surgery, rather than the procedure performed.

Summary of emergency and long-term management of bleeding oesophageal varices

The initial management of a patient with bleeding oesophageal varices is similar to that for any patient with upper GI haemorrhage and subsequent treatment follows a protocol with generally agreed indications for each therapeutic option (Fig. 5.6). Emergency endoscopy is necessary to confirm that the patient is bleeding from oesophageal varices. Pharmacotherapy, either with somatostatin or octreotide, may be used if necessary. Rarely, oesophageal tamponade may be necessary in a patient with massive variceal bleeding where acute sclerotherapy cannot be performed, in a patient in whom sclerotherapy has failed and who is waiting for surgery and for transport of an acutely bleeding patient to a specialised centre.

Figure 5.6
Algorithm for acute management of a patient with bleeding oesophageal varices. GI = gastrointestinal; TIPSS = transjugular intrahepatic portal–systemic stent shunt.

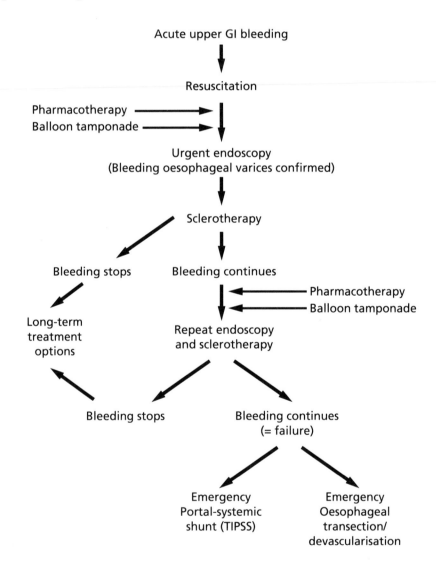

Once variceal bleeding has been confirmed immediate sclerotherapy should be performed. Using one or sometimes two injection sessions, acute variceal bleeding will be controlled in 90–95% of patients. Acute sclerotherapy is deemed to have failed when two injection sessions have been unable to control the acute bleeding episode.

In the 5–10% of patients in whom emergency sclerotherapy fails, an emergency surgical or radiological procedure is indicated. The available options are a portal–systemic shunt (including TIPSS) or oesophageal transection, with or without devascularisation. The indications for each of these options and their relative merits remain controversial. In general, emergency surgical portal–systemic shunting produces a definite arrest of haemorrhage and prevents recurrence, but is associated with a high incidence of encephalopathy and a high operative mortality. If an emergency portal–systemic shunt is contemplated, TIPSS is now the procedure of choice. On the other hand, oesophageal transection is associated with a significant incidence of recurrent bleeding, but encephalopathy is generally not a problem and the operative risk is less.

In general, therapeutic options for long-term control of variceal bleeding are palliative procedures, designed to prevent recurrent bleeding, and do not improve overall survival. The only treatment which addresses the underlying pathology and improves survival is liver transplantation. When considering which is the appropriate therapeutic option for each patient it is useful to first consider whether the patient is a candidate for transplantation (Fig. 5.7). Patients with advanced liver disease are best treated by transplantation. Patients with moderate liver dysfunction but who are symptomatic (e.g. encephalopathy, asthenia, fatigue), with a poor quality of life are also probably best treated by transplantation. Those awaiting a suitable liver graft should undergo sclerotherapy (or TIPSS if the bleeding is not controlled by sclerotherapy) in the interim period.

Long-term pharmacotherapy, particularly with beta-blocking agents, is currently being investigated but cannot, at present, be recommended for routine use. Prophylactic therapy (e.g. sclerotherapy, pharmacotherapy) to prevent a first episode of variceal bleeding is also being investigated but no significant benefit has been demonstrated.

Management of ascites

Background

In Western countries, the commonest cause for ascites is cirrhosis and portal hypertension. The exact mechanisms responsible for its development remain unclear but the primary factor in its initiation is renal sodium retention with subsequent water retention. There are two main hypotheses: the *underfill theory* postulates that a combination of factors, including hypoalbuminaemia and splanchnic vascular dilatation, results in hypovolaemia which leads to sodium and water retention, with consequent ascites formation; the *overflow hypothesis* contends that

Figure 5.7 *Long-term management algorithm for a patient with bleeding oesophageal varices. TIPSS = transjugular intrahepatic portal–systemic stent shunt.*

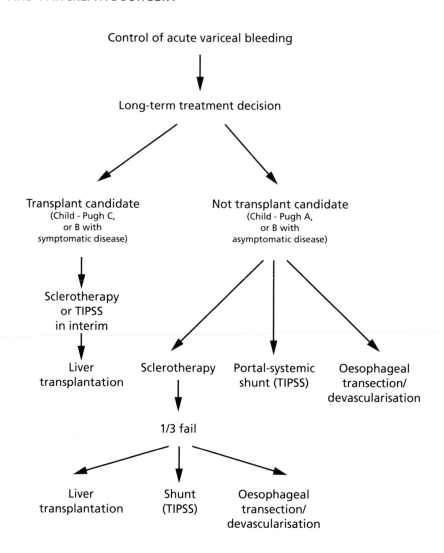

sodium retention is the primary event which induces ascites and leads to expansion of the plasma volume.[86,87]

The development of ascites in a cirrhotic patient is a sinister occurrence with a poor prognosis, with 20–50% of patients dying within one year. Precipitating factors, which should always be sought, include ongoing liver insult (e.g. due to alcohol), excessive sodium intake and development of spontaneous bacterial peritonitis (SBP), hepatocellular carcinoma or portal vein thrombosis.

Spontaneous bacterial peritonitis occurs in 15–20% of patients with ascites and is usually due to Gram-negative bacilli.[88] It is characterised by the sudden onset of abdominal pain and rebound tenderness with reduced or absent bowel sounds, but in some patients the signs may be more subtle. It occurs more frequently in patients who have had a variceal bleed and in those in whom the ascitic fluid protein content is low. Treatment involves immediate bacterial culture of blood and ascitic fluid and commencement of antibiotic therapy (e.g. a third generation cephalosporin).

The principal aim of treatment of ascites in the cirrhotic patient is to improve general comfort, appetite and quality of life. Treatment options range from simple dietary and medical measures to more complex surgical procedures, such as peritoneovenous or portacaval shunts.

Dietary restriction

A low sodium diet (40–60 mmol per day) is the most important initial measure in the control of ascites. This may be achieved with a 'no-added salt' diet and avoidance of obviously salty foods. This should precipitate a net sodium loss and, in patients with mild ascites, this alone may be sufficient. However, for the majority of patients this needs to be combined with diuretic therapy to ensure a negative fluid balance.

Diuretic therapy

Diuretic therapy aims to achieve a negative fluid balance of approximately 500 ml day^{-1}, although if the patient also has peripheral oedema, an initial daily loss of 1–2 litres is acceptable. Spironolactone is the mainstay of treatment as it inhibits the secondary hyperaldosteronism associated with ascites in these patients. The dose range is approximately 100–400 mg day^{-1}. It should be commenced at a low dose (e.g. 100 mg) and gradually increased every 2 or 3 days until a satisfactory diuresis is achieved. Addition of a loop diuretic (e.g. frusemide 40 mg day^{-1}) enhances the natriuretic effect of spironolactone and should be added when spironolactone alone does not produce a satisfactory diuresis.

It is important to remember that diuretics have important and significant side effects. Frusemide, if used alone, may induce hypokalaemia which can result in general muscle weakness and precipitate cardiac arrhythmias or gout. However, this effect is usually counteracted by the potassium-sparing effect of spironolactone, but this can lead to significant hyperkalaemia, which can be fatal. It is therefore important that the serum urea, electrolytes and creatinine are checked regularly – a rising serum potassium frequently limits the dose of spironolactone which can be used. Spironolactone may also exacerbate the gynaecomastia associated particularly with alcoholic cirrhosis, although this is usually reversible if the drug is discontinued and substituted with amiloride or triamterene.

Paracentesis

Paracentesis provides a rapidly effective method of treating the discomfort associated with tense ascites.[89] However, it may be hazardous, particularly if a large volume of fluid is removed, and can precipitate hepatic encephalopathy, hypokalaemia, systemic hypotension and renal failure. This is thought to be due to redistribution of intravascular fluid after removal of the ascites, with diffusion from the circulation into the peritoneal cavity resulting in hypovolaemia. However, large volume paracentesis does appear to be safe when performed in the presence of peripheral oedema as subcutaneous fluid may be mobilised into the circulation, thus preventing hypovolaemia. Other problems associated with paracentesis include damage to intra-abdominal viscera by the trocar and the risk of bacterial peritonitis if a strict aseptic technique and antibiotic prophylaxis are not used.

In view of the risk of hypovolaemia, intravenous salt-free albumin or a plasma expander, such as Dextran 70, may be given while performing paracentesis and this may allow a large volume of fluid to be removed each day (e.g. 4–6 litres). However, salt-free albumin is expensive and if paracentesis is performed on a periodic basis (e.g. 2–3 litres every 3–4 days), or in a patient with significant peripheral oedema, its use is probably not necessary.

Peritoneovenous shunt

Peritoneovenous shunting was first introduced in the early 1970s with the development of the Le Veen shunt (Fig. 5.8) and later, the Denver shunt, which has a pump which can be pressed by the patient to promote fluid flow. The theoretical basis for their use is that as ascites often accumulates rapidly following paracentesis a continuous system with a one-way valve which shunts fluid from the peritoneal cavity to the circulation may allow continuous excretion of excess fluid.

Peritoneovenous shunts are associated with well-recognised complications, such as local leakage of fluid around the shunt, infection and tube blockage.[90] More serious complications include disseminated intravascular coagulation (DIC) and expansion of the intravascular volume leading to pulmonary oedema or precipitation of bleeding from oesophageal varices.

The major indication for a peritoneovenous shunt is tense intractable ascites which, with the refinement of other management options, including diuretic therapy, paracentesis, TIPSS and liver transplantation, is now very rare. We have found it useful in two patients with alcoholic cirrhosis who had stopped drinking and had stable liver function, but whose ascites was not controlled by diuretic therapy, and repeated paracentesis resulted in significant inconvenience for them. There are definite contraindications to peritoneovenous shunting, including active bacterial peritonitis, systemic sepsis, congestive cardiac failure, recent variceal haemorrhage, significant encephalopathy and the presence of loculated or thick ascites.

Portal–systemic shunt

Traditional portal–systemic shunting is very effective at producing long-term relief of ascites, but this is achieved at the expense of a

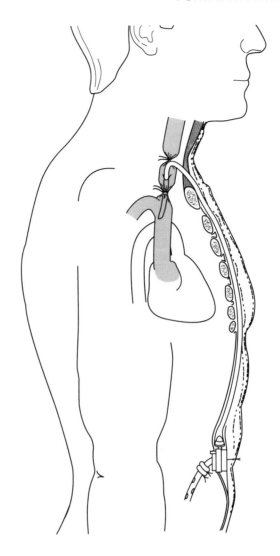

Figure 5.8 *A peritoneovenous shunt. A rise in intra-abdominal pressure forces fluid through the one-way valve into the superior vena cava.*

major surgical procedure and a significant risk of encephalopathy. This should not, therefore, be considered solely for the management of ascites. However, TIPSS provides a much less invasive technique and it is currently being evaluated in the treatment of refractory ascites. As most patients can be controlled with dietary restriction, diuretic therapy and paracentesis, the need for TIPSS, like peritoneovenous shunting, in the management of ascites is limited. However, it will probably have a small role and replace peritoneovenous shunting, particularly in the patient with intractable recurrent ascites who is awaiting liver transplantation.

References

1. Johnston GW. Bleeding from oesophageal varices. In: Imrie CW, Moosa AR (eds) Gastrointestinal emergencies. Edinburgh: Churchill Livingstone. 1987, pp. 24–45.
2. Henderson JM. Portal hypertension and shunt surgery. Adv Surg 1993; 26: 233–57.
3. Ryley NG, McGee JO'D. Cirrhosis and portal hypertension: pathological aspects. In: Blumgart LH (ed.) Surgery of the liver and biliary tract, 2nd edn. New York: Churchill Livingstone, 1994, pp 1589–602.
4. Warren KS, Reboucas G. Blood ammonia during bleeding from esophageal varices in patients with hepatosplenic schistosomiasis. N Engl J Med 1964; 271: 921–6.
5. Mohamed AE, al Karawi MA, al Otaibi R, Hanid MA. Results of sclerotherapy in 100 patients comparison of the outcome between schistosomiasis and hepatitis B. Hepatogastroenterology 1989; 36: 333–6.
6. Tilanus HW. Budd–Chiari syndrome. Br J Surg 1995; 82: 1023–30.
7. Rector WG, Hoefs JC, Hossack KF, Everson GT. Hepatofugal portal flow in cirrhosis; observations on hepatic hemodynamics and the nature of the arterioportal communications. Hepatology 1988; 8: 16–20.
8. Lebrec D, De Fleury P, Rueff B, Nahum H, Benhamou JP. Portal hypertension, size of esophageal varices and risk of gastrointestinal bleeding in alcoholic cirrhosis. Gastroenterology 1980; 79: 1139–44.
9. Stelzner F, Lierse W. Der angiomuskulare dehnverschlub der terminalen speiserohre langenbecks. Arch Klin Chir 1969; 321: 35–64.
10. Spence RAJ, Sloan JM, Johnston GW, Greenfield A. The venous anatomy of the lower oesophagus in normal subjects and in patients with varices: an image analysis study. Br J Surg 1984; 71: 739–44.
11. Spence RAJ, Sloan JM, Johnston GW, Greenfield A. Oesophageal mucosal changes in patients with varices. Gut 1983; 24: 1024–9.
12. Mahl TC, Groszmann RJ. Pathophysiology of portal hypertension and variceal bleeding. Surg Clin North Am 1990; 70: 251–66.
13. Bornman PC, Krige JEJ, Terblanche J. Management of oesophageal varices. Lancet 1994; 343: 1079–84.
14. Burns P, Taylor K, Blei AT. Doppler flowmetery and portal hypertension. Gastroenterology 1987; 92: 824–6.
15. Oliver TW, Sones PJ. Hepatic angiography: portal hypertension. In: Bernardino ME, Sones PJ (eds) Hepatic radiology. New York: Macmillan, 1984, pp. 243–75.
16. Adam R, Diamond T, Bismuth H. Partial portacaval shunt – renaissance of an old concept. Surgery 1992; 111: 610–16.
17. Westaby D. The management of active variceal bleeding. Intensive Care Med 1988; 14: 100–5.
18. Walker S. Vasoconstrictor therapy and bleeding oesophageal varices. Hepatogastroenterology 1990; 37: 538–43.
19. Jenkins SA, Shields R. Variceal haemorrhage after failed injection sclerotherapy: the role of emergency oesophageal transection. Br J Surg 1988; 76: 49–51.
20. Burroughs AK, McCormick PA, Hughes MD, Sprengers D, D'Heygere F, McIntyre N. Randomised, double-blind, placebo-controlled trial of somatostatin for variceal bleeding. Gastroenterology 1990; 99: 1388–95.
21. McKee R. A study of octreotide in oesophageal varices. Digestion 1990; 45 (Suppl): 60–5.
22. Jenkins SA, Copeland G, Sutton R, Kingsnorth AN, Shields R. Octreotide (SMS) versus sclerotherapy for bleeding varices: preliminary results. Br J Surg 1992; 79: 1224.
23. Jenkins SA, Shields R, Jaser N et al. The management of gastrointestinal haemorrhage by somatostatin after apparently successful endoscopic injection sclerotherapy for bleeding oesophageal ulcers. J Hepatol 1991; 12: 296–301.
24. Jenkins SA, Baxter JN, Rennie MJ. Acute and long-term treatment of oesophageal varices. Br J Intensive Care 1993; 3: 65–72.
25. Vlavianos P, Gimson AES, Westaby D, Williams R. Balloon tamponade in variceal bleeding: use and misuse. Br Med J 1989; 298: 1158.
26. Crafoord C, Frencker P. New surgical treatment of varicose veins of the oesophagus. Acta Otolaryngol 1939; 27: 422–9.
27. Johnston GW, Rodgers HW. A review of 15 years' experience in the use of sclerotherapy in the control of acute haemorrhage from oesophageal varices. Br J Surg 1973; 60: 797–800.

28. Terblanche J. Portal hypertension management. Surg Endosc 1993; 7: 472–8.

29. Rose JDR, Crane MD, Smith PM. Factors affecting successful endoscopic sclerotherapy for oesophageal varices. Gut 1983; 24: 946–9.

30. Paquet K-J, Oberhammer E. Sclerotherapy of bleeding oesophageal varices by means of endoscopy. Endoscopy 1978; 10: 7–12.

31. Terblanche J. Has sclerotherapy altered the management of patients with variceal bleeding? Am J Surg 1990; 160: 37–42.

32. Gottlib JP. Endoscopic obturation of oesophageal and gastric varices with a cyanoacrylic tissue adhesive. Can J Gastroenterol 1990; 4: 637–8.

33. Kahn D, Jones B, Bornman PC, Terblanche J. Incidence and management of complications after injection sclerotherapy: a 10 year prospective evaluation. Surgery 1989; 105: 160–5.

34. Terblanche J, Krige JEJ, Bornman PC. The treatment of esophageal varices. Ann Rev Med 1992; 43: 69–82.

35. Terblanche J, Burroughs AK, Hobbs KEF. Controversies in the management of bleeding oesophageal varices. N Engl J Med 1989; 320: 1393–8.

36. Bornman PC, Terblanche J, Kahn D, Jonker MA, Kirsch RE. Limitations of multiple injection sclerotherapy sessions for acute variceal bleeding. S Afr Med J 1986; 70: 34–6.

37. Mostafa I, Omar MM, Nouh A. Endoscopic control of gastric variceal bleeding with butyl cyanoacrylate. Endoscopy 1993; 25: A11.

38. Stiegmann G, Sun JH, Hammond WS. Results of experimental endoscopic esophageal varix ligation. Am Surg 1988; 54: 104–8.

39. Binmoellar KF, Vadeyar HJ, Soehendra N. Treatment of esophageal varices. Endoscopy 1994; 26: 42–7.

40. Stiegmann GV, Goff JS, Michaletz-Onody PA et al. Endoscopic sclerotherapy as compared with endoscopic ligation for bleeding esophageal varices. N Engl J of Med 1992; 326: 1527–32.

41. Saeed ZA, Michaletz PZ, Wincester CB et al. Endoscopic variceal ligation in patients who have failed endoscopic sclerotherapy. Gastrointest Endosc 1990; 36: 572–4.

42. Johnson PA, Campbell DR, Antonson CW, Weston AP, Shuler FN, Lozoff RD. Complications associated with endoscopic band ligation of esophageal varices. Gastrointest Endosc 1993; 39: 119–22.

43. Berkelhammer C, Madhav G, Lyon S, Robert J. 'Pinch' injury during overtube placement in upper endoscopy. Gastrointest Endosc 1993; 39: 186–8.

44. Saltzman JR, Arora S. Complications of esophageal variceal band ligation. Gastrointest Endosc 1993; 39: 185–6.

45. Hashizume M, Ohta M, Ueno K, Tanoue K, Kitano S, Sugimachi K. Endoscopic ligation of esophageal varices compared with injection sclerotherapy: a prospective randomized trial. Gastrointest Endosc 1993; 39: 123–6.

46. Orloff MJ, Orloff MS, Rambolt M, Girard B. Is portosystemic shunt worthwhile in Child's class C cirrhosis? Ann Surg 1993; 216: 256–66.

47. Orloff MJ, Bell RH, Greenberg AG. A prospective randomized trial of emergency portacaval shunt and medical therapy in unselected cirrhotic patients with bleeding varices. Gastroenterology 1986; 90: 1754.

48. Rikkers LF, Jin G. Surgical management of acute variceal hemorrhage. World J Surg 1994; 18: 193–9.

49. Rikkers LF, Jin G. Variceal hemorrhage: surgical therapy. Gastroenterol Clin North Am 1993; 22: 821–42.

50. Rosch J, Hanafee W, Snow H. Transjugular portal venography and radiologic portacaval shunt. An experimental study. Radiology 1969; 92: 1112–14.

51. Colapinto RF, Stronell RD, Birch SJ. Creation of an intrahepatic portosystemic shunt with a Gruntzig balloon catheter. Can Med Assoc J 1982; 126: 267–8.

52. Richter GM, Palmaz JC, Noeldge G, Rossle M. The transjugular intrahepatic portosystemic stent-shunt. A new nonsurgical percutaneous method. Radiology 1989; 29: 406–11.

53. Rossle M, Haag K, Ochs A et al. The transjugular intrahepatic portasystemic stent-shunt procedure for variceal bleeding. N Engl J Med 1994; 330: 165–7.

54. Ring EJ, Lake JR, Roberts JP et al. Using transjugular intrahepatic portosystemic shunts to control variceal bleeding before liver transplantation. Ann Intern Med 1992; 116: 304–9.

55. Rossle M, Ring EJ. Transjugular portosystemic shunts: current status. Progr Liver Dis 1994; 12: 177–89.

56. Jalan R, Redhead DN, Hayes PC. Transjugular intrahepatic portasystemic stent shunt in the treatment of variceal haemorrhage. Br J Surg 1995; 82: 1158–64.

57. Vankemmel M. Resection-anastomose de l'oesophage sus-cardial pour rupture de varices oesophagiennies. Nouv Presse Med 1974; 5: 1123–4.

58. Sugiura M, Futagawa S. A new technique for treating oesophageal varices. J Thorac Cardovasc Surg 1973; 66: 677–85.

59. Sugiura M, Futagawa S. Esophageal transection with para-esophagogastric devascularization (the Sugiura procedure) in the treatment of esophageal varices. World J Surg 1984; 8: 673–9.

60. Burroughs AK, Mezzanotte G, Phillips A, McCormick PA, McIntyre N. Cirrhotics with variceal hemorrhage: the importance of the time interval between admission and the start of analysis for survival and rebleeding rates. Hepatology 1989; 9: 801–7.

61. Iwatsuki S, Starzl TE, Todo S et al. Liver transplantation in the treatment of bleeding esophageal varices. Surgery 1988; 104: 697–705.

62. Hayes PC, Davis JM, Lewis JA, Bouchier IA. Meta-analysis of value of propranolol in prevention of variceal haemorrhage. Lancet 1990; 336: 153–6.

63. Pagliaro L, Burroughs AK, Sorensen TI, Lebrec D, Morabito A, Amico GD, Tine F. Beta-blockers for preventing variceal bleeding. Lancet 1990; 336: 1001–2.

64. Burroughs AK, McCormick PA. Prevention of variceal rebleeding. Gastroenterol Clin North Am 1992; 21: 119–47.

65. Rikkers LF, Jin G, Burnett DA, Buchi KN, Cormier TA. Shunt surgery versus endoscopic sclerotherapy for variceal hemorrhage: late results of a randomized trial. Am J Surg 1993; 165: 27–33.

66. Terblanche J, Kahn D, Borman PC. Long-term injection sclerotherapy treatment for esophageal varices: a 10-year prospective evaluation. Ann Surg 1989; 210: 725–31.

67. Infante-Rivard C, Esnaola S, Villeneuve JP. Role of endoscopic variceal sclerotherapy in the long-term management of variceal bleeding: a meta-analysis. Gastroenterology 1989; 96: 1087–92.

68. Rypins EB, Mason RG, Conroy RM, Sarfeh IJ. Predictability and maintenance of portal flow patterns after small-diameter portacaval H-grafts in man. Ann Surg 1984; 200: 706–10.

69. Sarfeh IJ, Rypins EB, Moussa R, Milne N, Conroy RM, Lyons KP. Serial measurement of portal haemodynamics after partial portal decompression. Surgery 1986; 100: 52–8.

70. Rikkers LF. Definitive therapy for variceal bleeding: A personal view. Am J Surg 1990; 160: 80–5.

71. Warren WD, Millikan WJ, Henderson JM et al. Ten years' portal hypertensive surgery at Emory. Results and new perspectives. Ann Surg 1982; 195: 530–42.

72. Maillard J, Flamant YM, Hay JM, Chandler JG. Selectivity of the distal splenorenal shunt. Surgery 1979; 86: 663–71.

73. Bismuth H, Adam R, Mathur S, Sherlock D. Options for elective treatment of portal hypertension in cirrhotic patients in the transplantation era. Am J Surg 1990; 160: 105–10.

74. Millikan WJ, Henderson JM, Stewart MT et al. Change in hepatic function, hemodynamics and morphology after liver transplantation. Physiological effect of therapy. Ann Surg 1989; 209: 513–25.

75. Grace ND. Prevention of initial variceal hemorrhage. Gastroenterol Clin North Am 1992; 21: 149–61.

76. Conn HO, Lindenmuth WW, May CJ, Ramsby GR. Prophylactic portacaval anastomosis. A tale of two studies. Medicine 1972; 51: 27–40.

77. Jackson FC, Perrin EB, Smith AG, Dagradi AE, Nadal HM. A clinical investigation of the portacaval shunt. ii Survival analysis of the prophylactic operation. Am J Surg 1968; 115: 22–42.

78. Resnick RH, Chalmers TC, Ishihara Am et al. A controlled study of the prophylactic portacaval shunt. A final report. Ann Intern Med 1969; 70: 675–88.

79. Inokuchi K, Cooperative Study Group of Portal Hypertension in Japan. Improved survival after prophylactic portal nondecompressive surgery for esophageal varices: a randomized controlled trial. Hepatology 1990; 2: 1–6.

80. Witzel L, Wolbergs E, Merki H. Prophylactic endoscopic sclerotherapy of oesophageal varices: a prospective controlled study. Lancet 1986; i: 773–5.

81. Sauerbruch T, Wotzka R, Kopcke W *et al.* Prophylactic sclerotherapy before the first episode of variceal haemorrhage in patients with cirrhosis. N Engl J Med 1988; 319: 8–15.

82. Piai G, Cipolletta L, Claar M *et al.* Prophylactic sclerotherapy of high-risk esophageal varices: results of a multicentric prospective controlled trial. Hepatology 1988; 8: 1495–500.

83. Santangelo WC, Dueno MI, Estes BL, Krejs GJ. Prophylactic sclerotherapy of large esophageal varices. N Engl J Med 1988; 318: 814–18.

84. Van Ruiswyk J, Byrd JC. Efficacy of prophylactic sclerotherapy for prevention of a first variceal hemorrhage. Gastroenterology 1992; 102: 587–97.

85. McCormick PA. Pathophysiology and prognosis of oesophageal varices. Scand J Gastroenterol 1994; 207: 1–5.

86. McCormick PA, McIntyre N. Pathogenesis and management of ascites in chronic liver disease. Br J Hosp Med 1992; 47: 738–44.

87. Gerbes AL. Pathophysiology of ascites formation in cirrhosis of the liver. Hepato-Gastroenterology 1991; 38: 360–4.

88. Garcia-Tsao G. Spontaneous bacterial peritonitis. Gastroenterol Clin North Am 1992; 21: 257–73.

89. Kellerman PS, Lines SL. Large volume paracentesis in the treatment of ascites. Ann Intern Med 1990; 12: 889–91.

90. Moskovitz M. The peritoneovenous shunt: expectations and reality. Am J Gastroenterol 1990; 85: 917–28.

6 Gallstones

Roger W. Motson
Donald Menzies

Introduction

Gallstones remain one of the commonest surgical problems in the developed world and although there have been major therapeutic advances in recent years, there has been no progress in the prevention of gallstone development. In the United Kingdom, it has been estimated from autopsy studies that approximately 12% of men and 24% of women of all ages have gallstones present.[1] The prevalence in North America is comparable to that in the United Kingdom and it is believed that 10–30% of gallstones become symptomatic. The high prevalence in American Indians, who have an incidence of 50% in men and 75% in women in the age group 25–44 years, points to the importance of genetic factors in the aetiology of gallstones.

In the United Kingdom, more than 40 000 cholecystectomies are performed each year,[2] whereas in the USA approximately 500 000 operations are performed annually.[3] The incidence of common bile duct stones found before or during cholecystectomy is 12%,[4] indicating that in the United Kingdom alone more than 4000 common bile ducts require stone clearance annually.

Composition and formation of gallstones

Gallstones are usually designated as cholesterol stones, mixed stones or pigment stones.[5] Pure cholesterol and pure pigment stones account for only 20% of gallstones and mixed stones are considered as variants of cholesterol stones as they usually contain over 50% cholesterol and account for about 80% of gallstones in Western countries. Chemical analysis shows a continuous spectrum of stone composition rather than three mutually exclusive stone types and 10–20% contain enough calcium to be rendered radio-opaque.

The two most important determinants of gallstone frequency in any population are age and gender; gallstones become more common with increasing age and are at least twice as common in women.[6] The increased frequency in women becomes manifest at puberty and an increased risk of gallstones is conferred by parity and by the ingestion of oral contraceptives.[7] Other factors related to the development of cholesterol gallstones include obesity, ileal disease or resection, cirrhosis, cystic fibrosis, diabetes mellitus, long-term parenteral nutrition and ingestion of clofibrate.[8] Little is known of the epidemiology and cause of bilirubin stones. They are especially common in the Far East and become more frequent with increasing age, although occur with equal frequency in men and women. They may be associated with haemolytic anaemia, cirrhosis and infection of bile with β-glucuronidase-producing bacteria such as *Escherichia coli* and *Bacteroides* species.

The metabolic mechanisms responsible for the formation of cholesterol gallstones centre on the solubility of the main constituents of bile.[9] The bile acid conjugates have detergent-like properties and form micelles in aqueous solution. Lecithin is incorporated into bile acids/lecithin mixed in micelles and these also incorporate cholesterol, thereby promoting its solubility in the aqueous environment of bile. The capacity of this solubilising system may, under certain circumstances, be exceeded and bile is then converted into a state of cholesterol supersaturate, thereby favouring the nidation of cholesterol microcrystals. There is evidence to suggest that factors responsible for cholesterol microcrystal nucleation and for its inhibition are present in bile.[10] Excessive secretion of cholesterol in the bile may account for the increased predisposition to gallstones in obese patients, those ingesting oestrogens and during pregnancy.

Biliary stasis, diminished gall bladder function and diet have similarly been implicated. Suture material has been identified in almost one-third of patients with ductal stones following cholecystectomy and may be an important nidus for stone formation.[11]

Presentation

Gallstones present with symptoms related to the site of gallstones and are therefore considered separately.

Cholecystolithiasis

Gallstones confined to the gall bladder may present with an acute episode of pain from acute cholecystitis, biliary colic, chronic recurrent abdominal discomfort from repeated episodes of mild biliary colic or from a vague collection of symptoms usually referred to as flatulent dyspepsia.

Pathophysiology

Impaction of a stone in the neck of the gall bladder is thought to result in gall bladder spasm which produces biliary colic. As the stone falls back, the gall bladder empties and the pain stops, whereas continuing impaction of the stone in the gall bladder neck produces continuing pain. The trapped bile becomes concentrated and sets up a chemical irritation producing local inflammation which creates a more constant pain and may take several days to resolve. The gall bladder contents may become secondarily infected or may be already contaminated since infected bile is present in approximately 30% of patients with gallstones.[12] This will add to the patient's toxaemia, and may lead to the development of empyema or possible gangrene and perforation. An empyema will produce pain, right upper quadrant tenderness and a swinging pyrexia. Urgent intervention is required since conservative measures rarely succeed in resolution. Increasing oedema and intramural vascular compromise may result in infarction of the gall bladder wall with consequent perforation of the organ.

The pathophysiology behind 'flatulent dyspepsia' is not understood. The gall bladder may be shrunken and contracted from episodes of subclinical inflammation but it is not unusual to find a normal looking gall bladder at cholecystectomy in patients with gallstones causing 'flatulent dyspepsia'. Contraction of the gall bladder against stones is the traditional explanation for postprandial discomfort but there is a poor correlation between such symptoms and the presence of gallstones in a general population. A mucocele may develop when a gallstone impacts in Hartmann's pouch in an empty gall bladder. The gall bladder secretes mucus behind the obstructing stone producing a steady increase in the size of the gall bladder which may be easily palpable.

Clinical features

There is a poor correlation between pathological findings in the gall bladder wall and the presenting clinical features. Typically, acute cholecystitis presents with sharp, constant right upper quadrant pain which frequently is of sudden onset but may have been preceded by years of postprandial epigastric discomfort. It will be worse on inspiration or movement and frequently radiates to the back or to the tip of the right shoulder blade. It may be associated with nausea, vomiting, loss of appetite and may persist for several days. Examination may reveal signs of toxaemia, the abdomen is tender in the right upper quadrant and classically a positive Murphy's sign is elicited. In more advanced cases, there may be a palpable inflammatory mass which is usually due to an enlarged oedematous gall bladder surrounded by adherent omentum. Clinical signs of toxicity and a swinging pyrexia should raise clinical suspicion of an empyema and the presence or development of diffuse upper abdominal peritonism is a sign of perforation of the gall bladder. The presence of jaundice suggests choledocholithiasis although the possibility of common bile duct compression from an inflamed and oedematous gall bladder may need to be considered (Mirizzi's syndrome).

Biliary colic presents in a similar fashion to acute cholecystitis but is usually not affected by movement and lasts only for several hours. It is often precipitated by ingestion of fatty foods but resolution is spontaneous. Chronic pain due to gallstones is attributed to the occurrence of 'flatulent dyspepsia' characterised by bouts of postprandial fullness, belching, nausea and a sensation of regurgitation of food. A family history of gallstone disease is not unusual and factors predisposing to the development of gallstones may be present. Patients presenting with flatulent dyspepsia or recurrent episodes of biliary colic have little to find on examination.

Choledocholithiasis

Pathophysiology

It is uncertain whether common bile duct (CBD) stones that are uncomplicated produce symptoms. It is traditionally held that the CBD cannot produce colicky pain as it does not contain smooth muscle, but pain in the right upper quadrant following cholecystectomy may be a sign of retained bile duct stones. A stone impacted in the lower end of the CBD may also be associated with nausea and vomiting.

Obstructive jaundice results when a stone becomes impacted within the common bile duct, usually in the ampulla. A stone may pass spontaneously or fall back into the CBD with spontaneous regression of the jaundice or it may remain impacted until it is removed. A stone at the lower end of the CBD may also cause pancreatitis by temporary obstruction of the pancreatic duct and this may be associated with transient jaundice (see Chapter 8). Ascending cholangitis results from infection within an obstructed or poorly draining biliary system. In patients with common bile duct stones, coliforms are identified within the bile in around 80% of cases.[12] The classic Charcot's triad of symptoms produced by bile duct stones consists of pain, obstructive jaundice and fever (with or without rigors). Acute cholangitis is occasionally associated with rapid development of septicaemic shock, a syndrome which has been named acute obstructive suppurative cholangitis.[13]

Clinical features

Presentation of a patient with right upper quadrant pain some time after cholecystectomy may indicate choledocholithiasis. However CBD stones are more likely to be either silent and found at the time of cholecystectomy or present due to one of the complications of obstructive jaundice, pancreatitis or ascending cholangitis. Pain is more frequently associated with obstructive jaundice due to gallstones as opposed to an underlying malignancy. In addition to the presence of bilirubin in the urine and pale stool, obstructive jaundice may be associated with pruritis and steatorrhoea. Examination will not normally reveal a palpable gall bladder and features of pancreatitis should be sought. Ascending cholangitis should be suspected in the presence of rigors and a swinging pyrexia associated with jaundice. The patient may demonstrate signs of bacteraemia or septicaemia with a flushed appearance, tachycardia and hypotension.

Investigations

The diagnosis of gallstone disease is suspected on clinical grounds but relies on the relevant laboratory or radiological investigations for confirmation. The differentiation between gallstone causes for pain and other intra-abdominal disease may require a plain radiograph of the abdomen but less than 10% of gallstones are radio-opaque and therefore the yield from abdominal radiographs is low. Occasionally, in cases of intestinal obstruction, air is seen in the biliary tree, suggesting a cholecyst–enteric fistula and gallstone ileus.

Blood tests

Liver function tests (LFTs) should be performed routinely in patients with suspected gallstones. Although these may not be affected by the presence of cholecystolithiasis, they may be abnormal in the presence of choledocholithiasis. Isolated elevation of unconjugated bilirubin is present in prehepatic jaundice such as is seen with excessive haemolysis. The biochemical picture of hepatic jaundice, as seen with hepatitis, is one of raised conjugated and unconjugated bilirubin, high aspartate (AST) and alanine (ALT) transaminase levels, but associated with a relatively normal or slightly raised alkaline phosphatase (ALP). Posthepatic (obstructive) jaundice is associated with a raised conjugated bilirubin only, high ALP and normal AST and ALT. In late cases of obstructive jaundice or in acute cholangitis, the transaminase levels will rise as hepatocellular damage proceeds.

Minor abnormalities in the LFTs occur with non-obstructing stones in the common bile duct. These minor abnormalities may prompt the undertaking of an operative cholangiogram at the time of surgery if a selective operative cholangiogram policy is being pursued.[14,15] In our experience, approximately 60% of patients with common bile duct stones (including asymptomatic stones) will have one or more abnormal liver function tests,[16] although a substantial number of patients with an abnormal liver function test will not have common bile duct stones.

In the acute situation, a serum amylase level should be ascertained to exclude a diagnosis of pancreatitis and an elevated white blood cell count may support a clinical diagnosis of acute cholecystitis.

Ultrasonography

Ultrasound is the investigation most widely used to confirm the diagnosis of cholelithiasis. It is easy to perform, causes little discomfort to the patient, avoids irradiation and potentially toxic contrast media and may be useful in demonstrating other structures in the upper abdomen. The gall bladder wall, as well as its contents, can be assessed and this may give additional information useful for planning management. The size of the common bile duct can be measured and stones identified within it.

Gallstones are seen as bright echoes within the gall bladder and large stones cast an acoustic shadow behind them. Their size and number can be assessed. CBD stones may be harder to identify, although the presence of a dilated common bile duct and small stones within the gall bladder give clues as to their presence.

The reliability of ultrasound in diagnosing gall bladder stones is very high. If the gall bladder cannot be identified, the presence of an echogenic focus in the gall bladder area is nearly as specific a finding as that of calculi in a distended gall bladder. With high quality ultrasound scanning, gallstones should be detected in at least 95% of patients with stones, but its reliability in detecting common bile duct stones may be as low as 23% in some jaundiced patients.[17] That the experience of the ultrasonographer may influence the result is aptly demonstrated by the fact that a further study detected common bile duct stones in 80% of jaundiced patients.[18]

Oral cholecystography

The use of oral cholecystography in the detection of gallstones has dramatically diminished with the increasing use of ultrasonography. The examination relies on a functioning gall bladder for concentration of the contrast media. False negative rates for small gallstones of 6–8% are reported.[19] Non-functioning gall bladders are common with cholelithiasis and although it may infer the presence of gall bladder stones, it is by no means definitive. Oral cholecystography may have a role in the identification of patients with biliary dyskinesia but has no part to play in the identification of common bile duct stones.

CT scanning

Computed tomography may be more accurate than ultrasound in identifying common bile duct stones, with a sensitivity of 75% for common bile duct stones causing obstructive jaundice.[20] However, the relatively low rate of gall bladder stone detection may be due, in part, to cholesterol stones being isodense with bile on CT scanning. The newer generation spiral CT scanners and MRI scanners may be better but their potential advantage over abdominal ultrasound scanning is not readily apparent.

Radio-isotope scanning

Technetium-labelled hydroxy imino-diacetic acid (HIDA) is excreted in the bile after intravenous injection. It may be useful for demonstrating the patency of the biliary tree or of biliary–enteric anastomoses but its use with gallstones is limited. Failure to demonstrate a gall bladder due to blocked cystic duct may assist in the diagnosis of acute cholecystitis but images are too poor to reveal common bile duct stones. HIDA scanning is of no value in cases of jaundice, since the isotope is not excreted into an obstructed system.

Intravenous cholangiography

The advent of laparoscopic cholecystectomy has ensured a revival in the use of intravenous cholangiography (IVC) as a means of identifying suspected common bile duct stones. Failure to opacify the biliary tree, however, arises in 3–10% of cases.[21,22] Although improvements in intravenous cholangiography make it a useful occasional alternative to ultrasonographic assessment of the bile duct, time, cost and occasional failure, together with a low risk of allergic reaction, make it less attractive. The adoption of infusional cholangiography improves the safety of the investigation and tomography improves imaging of the bile duct, though anatomical delineation is not as clear as peroperative cholangiography.[23] The use of IVC is therefore limited in that it cannot be employed in patients who are allergic to iodine or in those patients with biliary obstruction, as secretion of the contrast into the biliary tree does not occur.

Percutaneous transhepatic cholangiography

Percutaneous transhepatic cholangiography (PTC) is best performed in patients who have a dilated biliary tree, but is not routinely employed in patients with suspected gallstone biliary obstruction. Despite the use of a fine gauge needle, there is a risk of bile leakage and haemorrhage in patients with abnormal clotting.

Endoscopic retrograde cholangiopancreatography

Endoscopic retrograde cholangiopancreatography (ERCP) is considered the gold standard in preoperative common bile duct imaging. With direct visualisation of the papilla using a side viewing duodenoscope, the papilla can be selectively cannulated to provide images of both the pancreatic and common bile ducts. Water-soluble contrast medium is injected to outline the biliary tree and offers the advantage over other biliary tree imaging techniques of therapeutic intervention with sphincterotomy and stone extraction at the time of examination (Fig. 6.1).

There is general agreement that endoscopic removal of bile duct stones is preferable to surgery in postcholecystectomy patients, high risk surgical patients when the gall bladder is still present, patients with severe acute cholangitis and selected patients with acute biliary pancreatitis.[24–26] Duct clearance can be expected in 90–95% of patients undergoing successful sphincterotomy and this results in an overall success rate for endoscopic stone clearance of 80–95%, the highest success rates being recorded as experience increases.[24,25,27] Major complications occur in up to 10% of patients and include haemorrhage, acute pancreatitis, cholangitis and retroduodenal perforation, but the overall procedure-related mortality is less than 1%.[24] However, the 30-day mortality can reach 15%, reflecting the severity of the underlying disease. Difficulties in removing common bile duct stones endoscopically may be due to unfavourable or abnormal anatomy, such as periampullary diverticulum or previous surgery. Stones larger than 15 mm and those situated intrahepatically or proximal to a biliary stricture may be difficult to remove (Table 6.1). Adjuvant techniques include mechanical lithotripsy, extracorporeal shockwave lithotripsy and chemical dissolution.[28–30] Although successful stone fragmentation has been reported in up to 80% of patients, the major drawback is the need for multiple treatment sessions and at least one subsequent ERCP to extract stone fragments.

The establishment of ERCP in the prelaparoscopic era was based on the avoidance of an open exploration of the common bile duct, a procedure that was believed to have significant morbidity.[31] ERCP was,

Figure 6.1 (a) *A large stone has been demonstrated by endoscopic retrograde cholangiography within the common bile duct.*
(b) *The common bile duct stone has been snared by a Dormia basket ready for extraction.*

(a)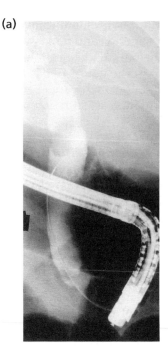

(b)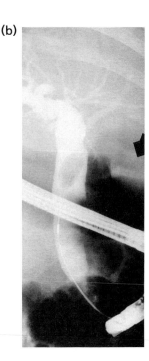

therefore, generally reserved for the high-risk surgical patients but open cholecystectomy and exploration of the common bile duct was reserved for the younger patient. In the laparoscopic era, management strategies vary considerably and are based on local endoscopic and laparoscopic resources and expertise.

For some, ERCP is the chosen method of preoperative CBD stone detection for any patient with suspected common bile duct stones. The advantage of this strategy is that duct clearance preoperatively removes the dilemma as to how to manage common bile duct stones found at operation. This management policy, however, will expose a substantial

Table 6.1 *Difficult bile duct stones at ERCP*

Stones greater than 15 mm
Intrahepatic stones
Multiple stones
Impacted stones
Stone proximal to a biliary stricture
Tortuous bile duct
Disproportionate size of the bile duct stone
Duodenal diverticulum
Billroth II reconstruction
Surgical duodenotomy

number of patients to an unnecessary endoscopic intervention. Since approximately 12% of patients undergoing elective cholecystectomy have common bile duct stones, it is therefore likely that more than 25% of cholecystectomies would require ERCP preoperatively with this strategy. In the UK, this would entail an additional 10 000 ERCPs per annum and if it were assumed that all these examinations were purely diagnostic, there would be approximately 100 major complications per year from this investigation.

If it is not the surgeon's practice to explore the common bile duct laparoscopically, preoperative ERCP would enable stone identification and duct clearance. This would also avoid the need for conversion to an open procedure. If, however, ductal stones are not suspected preoperatively, their presence can be determined at laparoscopic cholecystectomy by peroperative cholangiography. Common bile duct stones identified in this way could be referred for postoperative endoscopic clearance. Such a policy would reduce dramatically the number of ERCPs undertaken and in only a small proportion of patients in whom stones could not be cleared by ERCP, would a second operation be required. In those instances when the surgeon is trained in laparoscopic exploration of the common bile duct, ERCP could be reserved for the few patients in whom laparoscopic ductal clearance fails.

Prior to the establishment of laparoscopic cholecystectomy, preoperative endoscopic sphincterotomy had been suggested as a means of avoiding choledocholithotomy at the time of cholecystectomy. However, a randomised study had shown no significant advantage for patients treated by preoperative sphincterotomy as opposed to open cholecystectomy and exploration of CBD alone.[32] At the present time, the place of ERCP remains to be defined. A number of acceptable algorithms have been proposed to manage the laparoscopic cholecystectomy patients suspected of harbouring common bile duct stones.[33]

ERCP stent insertion

In the 5% or less of situations where extraction of common bile duct stones is incomplete or impossible, a nasobiliary tube or stent should be inserted to provide biliary decompression and prevent stone impaction of the distal common bile duct[34] (Fig. 6.2). Such manoeuvres may allow improvement of the patient's clinical condition until complete stone clearance can be achieved by further endoscopic manoeuvres or subsequent surgery. Temporary biliary endoprosthesis placement avoids accidental or intentional dislodgement of the nasobiliary catheter by a confused or unco-operative patient. The stent may become blocked after a few months, but bile drainage often continues around the stent and the presence of the stent alone may be sufficient to prevent stones from becoming impacted at the lower end of the common bile duct. In the surgically unfit patient, a change of stent may be required if jaundice recurs. Recurrent episodes of cholangitis may result in secondary biliary cirrhosis in the long term and careful consideration of the

Figure 6.2 *Multiple common bile duct stones lying above a mid-common bile duct stricture and not amenable to endoscopic extraction. Biliary drainage is maintained with two endoscopically placed stents.*

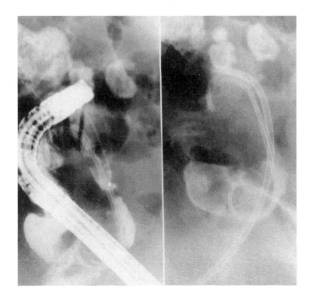

patient's level of fitness must be made before surgery is totally discounted.

Management of gall bladder stones

Asymptomatic stones

There has been much debate regarding the need for surgical intervention in patients with asymptomatic gallstones. In one American study which assessed the natural history of subjects with asymptomatic stones, individuals with gallstones were diagnosed by ultrasound scan on entry to a large University health care plan.[35] Only 2% of patients became symptomatic each year and presented with biliary colic or cholecystitis rather than the more serious complications of jaundice, empyema or cholangitis.[35] Only 10% of the asymptomatic patients, followed for a mean of almost five years by McSherry and colleagues, developed symptoms and only 7% required operation.[36] Although stones are undoubtedly associated with an increased risk of gall bladder cancer, only one of the 691 gallstone patients followed in this study were found eventually to have an incidental carcinoma at operation.

Non-operative treatments for gallstones

Dissolution

In the early 1970s there was great interest in the use of dissolution agents, principally chenodeoxycholic acid, in the treatment of gallstones.[37] Prerequisites for attempting dissolution therapy were a functioning gall bladder, multiple small stones (which have a greater total surface area for contact with the dissolution agent rather than a smaller number of larger stones) and radiolucency (indicative of pure cholesterol stones without a calcium or pigment matrix to impede dissolution). Success was slow to be achieved in most subjects, usually taking 6 to 12 months as judged by the disappearance of stones on ultrasound. Side effects of treatment included abdominal cramps, diarrhoea and occasional liver function test abnormalities. Despite the early encouraging results, gallstones often recurred when dissolution therapy was stopped. O'Donnell and Heaton[38] found that recurrence rates increased rapidly in the first few years, with rates of 13% at one year, 31% at three years, 43% at four years and 49% at 11 years. Although recurrent stones were readily re-dissolved, they generally recurred when therapy ceased.

Lithotripsy

Success with lithotripsy for renal stones led to the use of the same techniques for gall bladder stones. Early lithotriptors, with immersion in large water baths, were soon succeeded by smaller devices with a limited area of contact via a water-filled cushion. The biliary anatomy, however, did not lend itself to a repeat of the success observed with renal stones. The tidal flow of bile into and out of the gall bladder, along with the presence of multiple gallstones, were factors which contributed to the failure of the technique. Lithotripsy has therefore been retained only for the management of ductal stones resistant to endoscopic removal.[39]

Operative treatment of gall bladder stones

Open cholecystectomy

In the decade before the establishment of laparoscopic cholecystectomy, it did appear that the traditional practice of many surgeons was being eroded by alternative treatment for gallstones, including dissolution therapy and extracorporeal shockwave lithotripsy.

The operative mortality of open cholecystectomy for cholelithiasis had fallen in the years before the introduction of laparoscopic surgery, with many series reporting operative mortality rates of less than 1%.[40,41] Common duct exploration was regarded as increasing the risk of open cholecystectomy by 4–8-fold.[42] In a comparative study between a North American and European centre, 12–14% of patients developed complications and the bile duct was explored in 8.6% of the patients in Toronto as opposed to 17.9% in Geneva, the incidence of positive exploration being 61% and 73% respectively.[41] The factors increasing risk of postoperative mortality were advancing age, acute admission, admission to hospital within three months of the index admission and the number of discharge diagnoses.[42] Only 18% of postoperative deaths in this study were related to the gallstone disease or the surgery, with underlying cardiovascular or respiratory disease contributing to 48% of deaths.

There has been considerable uncertainty regarding the true incidence of bile duct injury at open cholecystectomy and the surveys available cite figures of one injury per 300–1000 operations.[43,44] At cholecystectomy, injury results from imprecise dissection and inadequate demonstration of the anatomical structures.[45] Although some patients do have anatomical anomalies or pathological changes which increase the risk of duct injury, it is noteworthy that in the extensive Swedish review, the patients most at risk appear to be young, slim females who have not undergone previous surgery.[43]

Given that the basis for symptoms before cholecystectomy often remains uncertain, it is not surprising that a substantial number of patients continue to experience problems after operation. In a detailed analysis of a consecutive group of patients undergoing cholecystectomy for presumed biliary pain in a District General Hospital between 1980 and 1985, Bates and his colleagues compared the outcome of an age and sex matched control group of surgical patients without gallstone disease.[46] Flatulent dyspepsia was more frequent in gallstone patients but operation markedly reduced these symptoms to an incidence almost identical to that of the control group (Table 6.2). However, within one year of cholecystectomy, no less than 34% of patients still suffered some abdominal pain and none of the 35 patients referred back to hospital for investigation had evidence of retained ductal stones. Multivariant analysis showed that preoperative flatulence and long durations of attacks of pain were risk factors for postoperative dissatisfaction.

Minilaparotomy cholecystectomy
There has been a resurgence of interest in open cholecystectomy through a small incision, the so-called minilaparotomy cholecystectomy, in recent years in an effort to reduce the trauma of open surgery to a similar level

Table 6.2 *Pattern of symptoms recorded by patients with gallstones before and after open cholecystectomy, and by age and sex match control surgical patients without gallstone disease*[46]

Symptoms	Controls (*n* = 278)	Gallstone Patients	
		Pre-op (*n* = 278)	One year post-op (*n* = 278)
Flatulence	30	66	44
Distention	33	57	37
Indigestion	38	71	43
Nausea	15	62	23
Vomiting	10	54	9
Fever	4	34	5
Rigor	4	30	5
Abdominal pain	0	100	34
Consulted GP for pain	0	100	23

Values are percentages.

now being achieved laparoscopically. There have been few controlled trials and those that have been performed have shown laparoscopic cholecystectomy to be superior in one and minilaparoscopic cholecystectomy superior in the other.[47,48] The technique relies on retractors to provide exposure for a fundus first cholecystectomy carried out without the surgeon's hands entering the abdominal cavity. Cholangiography is possible but not performed in most reports of the technique. The authors' limited first-hand experience of the technique has not persuaded them that the view of the cystic duct/common bile duct junction is comparable to that achieved by laparoscopic cholecystectomy.

Laparoscopic cholecystectomy

Initial scepticism that the technique of laparoscopic cholecystectomy would only be applicable to relatively few patients was followed by an enthusiasm to introduce the technique to a normally conservative surgical community. Surgeons were attracted by the excellent view of the gall bladder and biliary tree afforded by the laparoscope. Patients were attracted by an alternative to open cholecystectomy which carried a reputation for significant pain and a long recovery time. Similarly, the lack of major abdominal wounds and pain, the shorter hospital stay and the rapid return to full activity were considered advantageous. In addition, health providers and purchasers were attracted by the short hospital stay which appeared to offer significant cost savings.

The laparoscopic procedure could be offered to all patients with symptomatic gallstones, providing their cardiorespiratory status did not preclude laparoscopy. Of all patients presenting for operation 95% can be successfully completed laparoscopically. Obesity, acute inflammation, adhesions and previous abdominal surgery do not usually prevent a laparoscopic cholecystectomy, but may require some adaptations of technique to complete the procedure.[49–54] Techniques of laparoscopic cholecystectomy have been previously well described.[49,50] In difficult cases, improvement in the exposure of Calot's triangle may require additional or different positioning of the laparoscopic cannulae, the use of oblique viewing telescopes and placement of endoscopic retractors. Decompression of a distended or inflamed gall bladder may also improve access.

In a substantial audit of seven European centres,[51] 96% of procedures were successfully completed in the 1236 patients and only four bile duct injuries were reported. There were no postoperative deaths and a median hospital stay of three days with a median return to normal activities of only eleven days was observed. Fears that laparoscopic cholecystectomy in the management of acute cholecystitis could carry an unacceptable risk of disseminating infection or of perpetrating an injury to the bile duct appear unfounded.[54]

Anxieties regarding an increased incidence of bile duct injury with the introduction of laparoscopic cholecystectomy have not been substantiated by multicentre studies from Europe[51] and the United States,[52] with a reported incidence of injury to the common bile duct of between one in

200–300 cases. In a recent study in the West of Scotland, a prospective audit of laparoscopic cholecystectomy was undertaken.[55] A total of 5913 laparoscopic cholecystectomies undertaken by 48 surgeons and 37 laparoscopic bile duct injuries were reported. Major bile duct injuries were defined as those where laceration to more than 25% of the bile duct diameter occurred, where the common hepatic duct or common bile duct was transected or in those instances when a bile duct stricture developed in the postoperative period. Of the 37 injuries 20 were classified in this way, giving an incidence of 0.3%. Delayed identification of bile duct injury occurred in 19 patients and, although it was noted by the authors that cholangiography did not play a part in the identification of bile duct injuries it was noteworthy that imaging was used in only 8.8% of all laparoscopic procedures. During the course of this five-year study, the annual incidence of bile duct injury peaked at 0.8% in the third year but had fallen to 0.4% in the final year of audit. Although this incidence of ductal injury appears slightly greater than for open cholecystectomy, the true morbidity and mortality of laparoscopic cholecystectomy will only be known when multicentre prospective audit data become available from both specialist and non-specialist centres.

Cholecystostomy

For patients whose symptoms of acute cholecystitis do not settle, cholecystostomy was often undertaken in those cases where open cholecystectomy was thought to carry an unacceptable risk of injury to the biliary tree. The procedure could be undertaken under local anaesthesia and following decompression of the gall bladder and stone removal, a drain could be left *in situ*. With the demonstration that acute cholecystectomy could be undertaken safely,[54] cholecystostomy has become an infrequent surgical procedure. The technique can also be undertaken percutaneously under ultrasound guidance and may be of value during a difficult laparoscopic cholecystectomy when the risk of conversion to an open procedure may be considered unacceptable in the frail patient. In such instances, a drain can be inserted through one of the 5 mm cannulas which can be introduced directly into the gall bladder by re-insertion of a trocar.

Operative cholangiography

The advent of laparoscopic surgery has rekindled the debate over the potential benefit of operative cholangiography. Many surgeons who had previously performed the technique routinely at the time of open cholecystectomy abandoned cholangiography during laparoscopic cholecystectomy, since it was thought to be too difficult to undertake. Despite the availability of data supporting a selective approach to intraoperative cholangiography at open cholecystectomy,[15] this has yet to be determined for the laparoscopic procedure. The authors believe that operative cholangiography has an important role in laparoscopic cholecystectomy, not only to detect common bile duct stones but also to confirm, beyond doubt, the anatomy of the biliary tree, since the severity of bile duct injury appears far greater in laparoscopic surgery. The principal cause of damage is due to misidentification of the common bile duct as the cystic duct. Whereas the injury is usually immediately recognised at open surgery, the common bile duct is generally divided between clips at laparoscopic surgery and the gall bladder retracted to the right to open up Calot's triangle. At this point, an 'accessory duct' (in reality the common hepatic duct) is visualised, clipped and divided, resulting in resection of most of the extrahepatic biliary tree (Fig. 6.3). Peroperative cholangiography confirms beyond doubt that the structure thought to be the cystic duct is indeed that structure. In the situation previously described, the cholangiogram catheter would have been

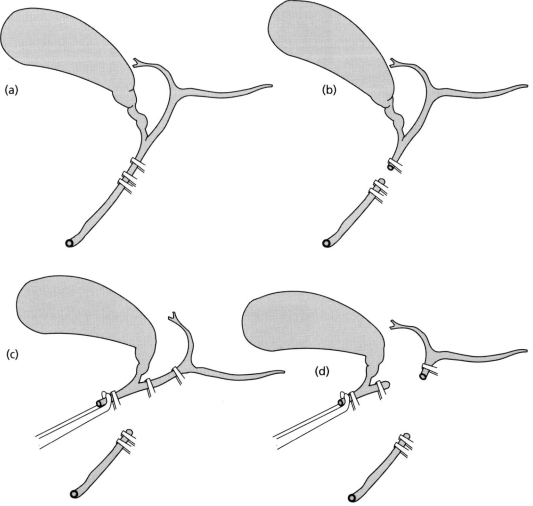

Figure 6.3.   *The 'classical' laparoscopic bile duct injury. (a) The common duct is misidentified as the cystic duct and is doubly clipped. (b) The common duct is then divided. (c) The gallbladder is retracted to the right, stretching the common hepatic duct and placing it in contact with the gallbladder. This is identified as an accessory duct, double clipped. (d) A high transection of the common hepatic duct results in the excision of most of the extrahepatic biliary tree.*

inserted mistakenly via an incision in the common bile duct (thought by the operator to be the cystic duct). If only the distal biliary tree is filled, the surgeon is alerted to the error before any duct is divided. Although critics of peroperative cholangiography will argue that the common bile duct has been injured by the incision through which the cholangiogram catheter is introduced, the injury at this point is recoverable, either by direct suture or insertion of a T-tube (Fig. 6.4). In the rarer situation when

Figure 6.4 (a) *The small diameter common bile duct has been mistaken for the cystic duct. Only the distal common bile duct and duodenum are shown with no proximal filling of the ducts. Recognition of the error at this stage averts a major injury to the common duct.*

(a)

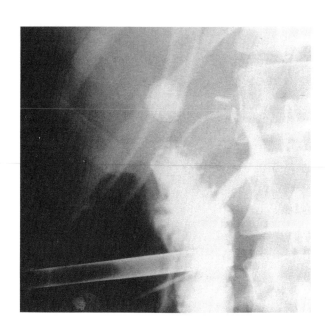

(b) *After further dissection, the cystic duct was identified and a T-tube placed in the incision in the common duct. A subsequent T-tube cholangiogram confirms the normal anatomy and laparoscopic cholecystectomy was completed successfully.*

(b)

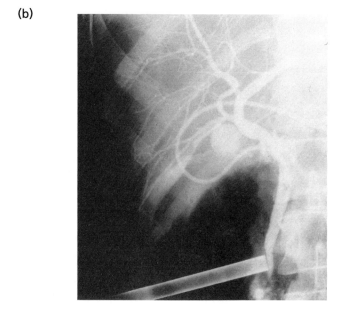

the cystic duct arises from the right hepatic duct, the latter can be very difficult to see as it lies behind the cystic duct and is often in the line with the viewing laparoscope. Cholangiography identifies such anomalies and helps to avert injury (Fig. 6.5).

The addition of cholangiography to the total dissection time of laparoscopic cholecystectomy is relatively short. On the basis that the time to learn operative cholangiography is not during the management

Figure 6.5
(a) *During what appeared to be a very straightforward laparoscopic cholecystectomy, the routine operative cholangiogram showed only the right hepatic duct and right intrahepatic biliary tree.*

(a)

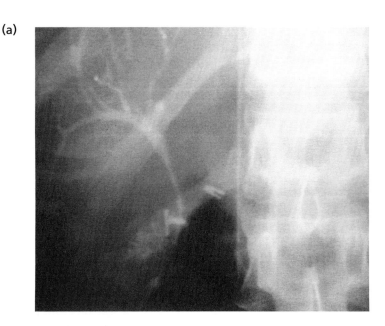

(b) *Repositioning of the catheter and the LigaClip showed the remainder of the biliary tree and made it clear that the structure initially thought to be the cystic duct was the distal right hepatic duct below an anomalous origin of the cystic duct.*

(b)

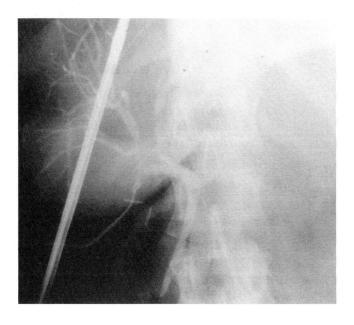

of a difficult case, such as following a failed preoperative ERCP in cases of suspected choledocholithiasis or when the biliary anatomy is difficult to identify, we recommend that it should be performed as a routine but should not be seen as a substitute to careful dissection of the infundibulum of the gall bladder and the cystic duct close to the gall bladder.[45] By dissecting these structures both anteriorly and posteriorly, the gall bladder is displaced (sometimes called the 'flag' technique) to enable the surgeon to see behind the gall bladder and thus minimise the risk of injury to the portal structures. In our own experience and despite strict adherence to these dissection techniques, cholangiography has, on two occasions, been the sole identifier of aberrant right hepatic ductal anatomy.

Numerous studies have examined risk factors for choledocholithiasis but, from multivariant analysis, it would appear that an increased diameter of the common bile duct and the presence of multiple (more than ten) gallstones are the only significant independent indicators.[14] During laparoscopic cholecystectomy, the surgeon may have difficulty in assessing common bile duct diameter and palpation of the extra-hepatic biliary tree, which some surgeons consider a useful adjunct in detecting common bile duct stones, cannot be undertaken.[56] Although percutaneous ultrasonography may be helpful in the assessment of common bile duct diameter, the emergence of ultrasound probes which can be passed down the laparoscopic ports will further improve on the accurate measurement of common bile duct diameter, as well as the stone load within the gall bladder. Both mechanical sectoral and linear array laparoscopic ultrasound probes have been shown to be as useful as cholangiography in the detection of common bile duct stones.[57–59] It remains to be seen whether the biliary anatomy can be as well demonstrated as with cholangiography, but it is possible that laparoscopic ultrasonography may facilitate a policy of selective cholangiography.

Operative treatment of common bile duct stones

Approximately 12% of patients undergoing surgery for symptomatic gall bladder stones will also have stones in the common bile duct. More than 90% of these patients will have preoperative indications such as a history of jaundice and abnormal liver function tests, but 5–10% have no indication of stones in the bile duct other than a positive finding (filling defect, absence of filling of the terminal segment of the common duct, delay or absence of flow into the duodenum) on the peroperative cholangiogram.

Choledochoscopy at open exploration of the common bile duct

The gradual adoption of operative choledochoscopy during the 1970s and 1980s saw a decline in the incidence of retained common bile duct stones following surgery from about 10% to 1.2%, with a number of surgeons reporting large series of patients with no retained stones.[16,60–62] Successful exploration of the common bile duct (ECBD) can only be achieved through an adequately-sized choledochotomy to facilitate both removal of any obvious stones and choledochoscopy. On initial examination of the proximal ducts, it is normally possible to visualise several generations of ducts when these are dilated. Once it has been ascertained that the upper ducts are clear, the distal biliary tree can be examined. It is mandatory to clearly visualise the rather ragged appearance of the ampulla of Vater and then withdraw the choledochoscope. If a stone is visualised it can be retrieved with a stone basket and the procedure repeated until the duct is clear. The common duct is closed with or without a T-tube. The latter is probably unnecessary for an experienced choledochoscopist but, for the less experienced surgeon, it allows access to the biliary tree for postoperative cholangiography to confirm ductal clearance and to allow re-exploration of the duct without the need for re-operation.

With the advent of laparoscopic cholecystectomy, ERCP and endoscopic sphincterotomy (ES) has become the usual procedure for treating common duct stones, since laparoscopic common duct exploration is not yet a widely practised technique. Moreover, cholecystectomy without cholangiography is commonly performed in the expectation that ERCP and ES will be effective in dealing with unrecognised retained common duct stones at a later date. Such a policy, however, does expose the patient to an additional and often unnecessary procedure. Laparoscopic common duct exploration has the advantage for the patient of being able to deal with both gall bladder and common bile duct stones at the same time.

Laparoscopic choledochoscopy

Laparoscopic ECBD has been described through the cystic duct or common duct using either fibreoptic instruments or radiologically guided wire baskets or balloons.[63–66] Instrumentation may also be undertaken employing a 'blind' approach. The laparoscopic approach to the common duct was developed initially by the transcystic route because of the ease of closure without the need for a suture technique. Unfortunately it may not always be possible to pass instruments down the cystic duct. The angle at which the cystic duct joins the common duct also reduces access to the common hepatic and intrahepatic ducts. An approach through the common bile duct is increasingly being advocated by the more experienced laparoscopic surgeons as larger calibre choledochoscopes and baskets can be readily passed up and down the common bile duct.

Where there is the facility for radiological screening in theatre, wire basket and balloon manipulation can be performed in a manner similar to that employed for ERCP. Balloons may be used not only to dilate the cystic duct to permit instrumentation with a choledochoscope, but also to dilate the ampulla of Vater. Stones may be pulled or pushed with balloons and stone-grasping baskets may be used to retrieve stones. Traditionally at open surgery, the common duct was decompressed postoperatively with a T-tube until it was known that the bile was draining satisfactorily through the ampulla and there was no bile leak. Most series of laparoscopic common duct explorations through the cystic duct do not report the routine use of drainage of the common duct but most recommend the placement of a T-tube or a subhepatic drain if a choledochotomy is performed. At present, the array of management strategies for common duct stones seems confusing and the techniques used depend on local circumstances. In hospitals with ready access to ERCP, a surgeon may see little need for ascending the learning curve of laparoscopic common bile duct exploration, whereas those units with less ready access to ERCP see many attractions in dealing with common duct stones by laparoscopic means. Heavy reliance on postoperative ERCP will, in a small proportion of patients, require the patient to undergo open choledochotomy.

With experience, the majority of common bile duct stones are treatable at the time of surgery provided a flexible approach is employed. No single technique will be applicable to the management of all stones. In general, if the stones are few in number, small (<1 cm) in size, and situated in the distal common duct, a transcystic choledochoscopy with a 3 mm choledochoscope is likely to be successful. If the stone, or stones, are large and numerous, or if the stones are situated in the common hepatic duct or intrahepatic biliary tree, a choledochotomy and exploration with the larger 5 mm choledochoscope is the preferred option. If laparoscopic transcystic exploration fails, the surgeon has three options: first, to ligate the cystic duct, complete the cholecystectomy and rely on postoperative ERCP; secondly, to perform a laparoscopic choledochotomy; or thirdly, to perform a laparotomy and formal exploration of the CBD. If laparoscopic choledochotomy fails, the two options are either insertion of a T-tube and subsequent extraction of the retained stone via the T-tube track, ERCP and sphincterotomy; or conversion to laparotomy. Individual circumstances will dictate which option is the most suitable.

After successful choledochotomy, the authors prefer to close the common bile duct, leaving a subhepatic drain. A T-tube, or a straight tube via the cystic duct, can be useful if it is known or suspected that clearance of the duct is incomplete. By leaving such a tube *in situ*, access to the biliary tree is maintained for subsequent confirmatory postoperative cholangiography and, if necessary, postoperative choledochoscopy (see below).

There are no data at present to indicate which of these strategies is the most effective in terms of stone clearance, lack of complications or costs. We believe that most patients with common duct stones can be treated at the time of laparoscopic cholecystectomy, in the same manner as in the open cholecystectomy era. It remains to be proven whether this or one of the strategies involving ERCP proves to be the most efficient or cost-effective technique.

Postoperative choledochoscopy and radiologically guided stone retrieval

It usually takes approximately six weeks for the T-tube track to mature, at which time percutaneous radiologically guided stone extraction or percutaneous choledochoscopy can be performed. A cholangiogram is obtained immediately prior to the procedure as a proportion of stones will have passed spontaneously. The T-tube is removed and either a steerable catheter or a choledochoscope is advanced down the track and into the common bile duct. With choledochoscopy, the remainder of the technique is identical to that carried out at open operation.[67] With the steerable catheter technique, fluoroscopy and further cholangiograms are taken as the stones are retrieved with a stone basket.[68,69] If there is uncertainty as to the completeness of clearance, a straight tube may be inserted to keep the track open for a further attempt a few days later. Both techniques are successful in more than 95% of cases and carry less risk of complications such as pancreatitis or haemorrhage than ERCP. Providing there are no time constraints and the patient is happy to be managed as an outpatient with a T-tube, this is the preferred technique for patients with a T-tube *in situ*.

Transhepatic stone retrieval

A few patients, particularly those who have previously undergone a Polya gastrectomy, will not have their ampulla accessible for ERCP. Access to the common duct can be achieved using a percutaneous transhepatic technique. Over a percutaneously inserted guidewire, a series of dilators are advanced into the biliary tree, so as to develop a transhepatic track. Following insertion of a sheath, a choledochoscope or steerable catheter can be inserted and stones retrieved.[70]

Acalculous biliary pain

Given the poor understanding of the mechanisms of pain production in patients with acalculous biliary disease, the outcome for patients following cholecystectomy is uncertain. There is gathering evidence that some patients have abnormal motility of the sphincter of Oddi, in addition to the gall bladder. Some authors have reported improvement in symptoms in as many as 85–95% of patients with acalculous biliary pain after cholecystectomy[71] but it is conceivable that surgery confers a placebo effect. Controversy exists on the use of cholecystokinin (CCK) provocation tests as a means of reproducing symptoms and predicting which patients might benefit from cholecystectomy. In one study, all 26 patients with positive CCK tests showed improvement after removal of the gall bladder,[72] whereas ten of the 16 patients with negative tests were found to have other pathology accounting for their pain. Despite these encouraging results, other investigators have failed to demonstrate differences in outcome in patients with positive CCK tests when compared to those with negative tests.[73] Objective criteria on which to base the decision to recommend cholecystectomy in such patients are difficult to define. It is clear, however, that, despite the minimally

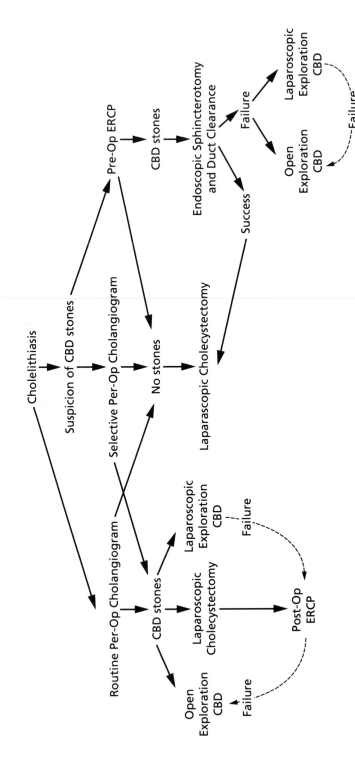

Figure 6.6   *Algorithm showing the available strategies for management of common bile duct stones.*

invasive nature of laparoscopic cholecystectomy, there should be no relaxation in the indications for cholecystectomy with patients with acalculous biliary pain.

Current recommen-dations
The standard treatment for symptomatic gallstones is now laparoscopic and there are few exceptions to a trial of a laparoscopic approach in all comers. Previous abdominal surgery may not have produced sufficient adhesions to obscure a satisfactory view of the gall bladder and biliary tree. All surgeons undertaking cholecystectomy, by whatever technique, should be capable of performing operative cholangiography. It may, on occasion, be necessary to perform a cholangiogram when technical difficulties arise and the surgeon should therefore be proficient at rapid cannulation of the cystic duct.

An algorithm for the management of common bile duct stones is shown in Fig. 6.6. The management strategy chosen will depend on personal experience, equipment availability, time, and the availability of other departmental expertise. There is no consensus as to the ideal approach. There is no doubt, however, that the common bile duct can be explored by laparoscopic means with a low incidence of retained stones, minimal increase in hospital stay, and few complications. It remains to be seen whether this technique establishes itself as the standard approach to common bile duct stones or whether ERCP in the pre- or postoperative period proves to be more widely accepted.

References

1. Godfrey PJ, Bates T, Harrison M, King MB, Padley NR. Gallstones and mortality: a study of all gallstone related deaths in a single health district. Gut 1984; 25: 1029–33.
2. Hospital In-patient Inquiry, 1980: Main tables. Department of Health and Social Security/ Office of Population Census and Surveys, London: HMSO, 1989.
3. Socio-economic fact book for surgery. Socio-economic Affairs Department, American College of Surgeons, 1988.
4. Motson RW. Operative cholangiography. In: Motson RW (ed.) Retained common duct stones. Prevention and treatment. London: Grune and Stratton, 1985, pp. 8–9.
5. Neoptolemos JP, Hofmann AF, Moossa AR. Chemical treatment of stones in the biliary tree. Br J Surg 1986; 73: 515–24.
6. Bennion LJ, Grundy SM. Risk factors for the development of cholelithiasis in man. N Engl J Med 1978; 299: 1161–221.
7. Scragg RKR, McMichael AJ, Seamark RF. Oral contraceptives, pregnancy and endogenous oestrogen in gallstone disease – a case controlled study. Br Med J 1984; 288: 1795–9.
8. Scragg RKR, McMichael AJ, Paghurst PA. Diet, alcohol and relative weight in gallstone disease: a case controlled study. Br Med J 1984; 288: 1113–18.
9. Smith BF, LaMont JT. The central issue of cholesterol gallstones. Hepatology 1986; 6: 529–31.
10. Burnstein MJ, Ilson RG, Petrunka CN, Taylor RD, Strasberg SM. Evidence for important nucleating factor in the gallbladder bile of patients with cholesterol gallstones. Gastroenterology 1983; 85: 801–7.
11. Wosiewitz U, Schenk J, Sabinski F, Schmack B. Investigations on common bile duct stones. Digestion 1983; 26: 43–52.
12. Keighley MRB. Micro-organisms in the bile. A preventable cause of sepsis after biliary

surgery. Ann R Coll Surg, Engl 1977; 59: 328–34.

13. Glenn F, Moody FG. Acute obstructive suppurative cholangitis. Surg, Gynecol Obstet 1961; 113: 265–73.

14. Taylor TV, Torrance B, Rimmer S, Hillier V, Lucas SB. Operative cholangiography: is there a statistical alternative? Am J Surg 1983; 145: 640–3.

15. Wilson TG, Hall JC, Watts JM. Is operative cholangiography always necessary? Br J Surg 1986; 73: 637–40.

16. Menzies D, Motson RW. Operative common bile duct imaging by operative cholangiography and flexible choledochoscopy. Br J Surg 1992; 79: 815–17.

17. Pasen P, Partanen K, Pikkarainen P, Alhava E, Pirinen A, Janatuinen E. Ultrasonography, CT, and ERCP in the diagnosis of choledochal stones. Acta Radiol 1992; 33: 53–6.

18. Lindsel DRM. Ultrasound imaging of pancreas and biliary tract. Lancet 1990; 335: 390–3.

19. Berk RN, Cooperberg PL, Gold RP, Rohrmann CA, Forrucci JT. Radiography of the bile ducts. A symposium on the use of new modalities for diagnosis and treatment. Radiology 1982; 145: 1–9.

20. Baron RL. Common bile duct stones. Reassessment of criteria for CT diagnosis. Radiology 1987; 162: 419–24.

21. Hammerstrom L-E, Holmin T, Stridbeck H, Ihse I. Routine preoperative infusion cholangiography at elective cholecystectomy: a prospective study in 694 patients. Br J Surg 1996; 83: 750–4.

22. Bloom ITM, Gibbs SL, Keeling-Roberts CS, Brough WA. Intravenous infusion cholangiography for investigation of the bile duct – a direct comparison with ERCP. Br J Surg 1996; 83: 755–7.

23. Joyce WP, Keane R, Burke GJ et al. Identification of bile duct stones in patients undergoing laparoscopic cholecystectomy. Br J Surg 1991; 78: 1174–6.

24. Leese T, Neoptolemos JP, Carr-Locke DL. Successes, failures, early complications and their management: results of 394 consecutive patients from a single centre. Br J Surg 1985; 72: 215–19.

25. Vaira D, Ainley C, Williams S et al. Endoscopic sphincterotomy in 1000 consecutive patients. Lancet 1989; ii: 431–34.

26. Rosso PG, Kortan P, Haber G. Selective common bile duct cannulation can be simplified by the use of a standard papillotome. Gastrointest Endosc 1993; 39: 67–9.

27. Lambert ME, Betts CD, Hill J et al. Endoscopic sphincterotomy – the whole truth. Br J Surg 1991; 78: 473–6.

28. Birkett DH. Biliary laser lithotripsy. Surg Clin North Am 1992; 72: 641–52.

29. Webber J, Ademak HE, Riemann JF. Extracorporeal piezo-electric lithotripsy for retained bile duct stones. Endoscopy 1992; 24: 239–43.

30. Shaw MJ, Mackie RD, Moore JP et al. Results of a multi-centre trial using a mechanical lithotriptor for the treatment of large bile duct stones. Am J Gastroenterol 1993; 88: 730–3.

31. Leese T, Neoptolemos JP, Baker AR, Carr-Locke DL. Management of acute cholangitis and the impact of endoscopic sphincterotomy. Br J Surg 1986; 73: 988–92.

32. Neoptolemos JP, Carr-Locke DL, Fossard DP. A prospective randomised study of preoperative endoscopic sphincterotomy versus surgery alone for common bile duct stones. Br Med J 1987; 294: 470–4.

33. Lichtenstein D, Carr-Locke D. Closed treatment of choledocholithiasis. In: Paterson-Brown S, Garden J (eds) Principles and practice of surgical laparoscopy. London: WB Saunders, 1994, pp. 105–40.

34. Leung JWC, Cotton PB. Endoscopic naso-biliary catheter drainage in biliary and pancreatic disease. Am J Gastroenterol 1991; 86: 389–94.

35. Gracie WA, Ransahoff DF. The natural history of silent gallstones: the innocent gallstone is not a myth. N Engl J Med 1982; 307: 798–800.

36. McSherry CK, Glenn F. The incidence and causes of death following surgery for non-malignant biliary tract disease. Ann Surg 1980; 191: 271–5.

37. Iser JH, Dowling RH, Mok HYI, Bell GD. Chenodeoxycholic acid treatment of gallstones. N Engl J Med 1975; 293: 333–78.

38. O'Donnell LDJ, Heaton KW. Recurrence and re-recurrence of gallstones after medical dissolution: a long-term follow-up. Gut 1988; 29: 655–8.

39. Sauerbruch T, Stern M. Fragmentation of bile duct stones by extracorporeal shockwaves. A new approach to biliary calculi after failure of

routine endoscopic measures. Gastroenterology 1989; 96: 146–52.

40. Herzog U, Messmer P, Sutter M, Tondelli P. Surgical treatment for cholelithiasis. Surg Gynecol Obstet 1992; 175: 238–42.

41. Clavien PA, Sanabria JR, Mentha G et al. Recent results of elective open cholecystectomy in a North American and a European centre – comparison of complications and risk factors. Ann Surg 1992; 216: 618–26.

42. Bredesen J, Jorgensen T, Andersen TF et al. Early post-operative mortality following cholecystectomy in the entire female population of Denmark – 1977–1991. World J Surg 1992; 16: 530–5.

43. Andren-Sandberg A, Alinder A, Bengmark S. Accidental lesions of the common bile duct at cholecystectomy: pre- and per-operative factors of importance. Ann Surg 1985; 201: 328–33.

44. Banting S, Carter DC. Expectations of cholecystectomy. In: Paterson-Brown S, Garden J (eds) Principles and practice of surgical laparoscopy. London: WB Saunders, 1994, pp. 53–66.

45. Garden OJ. Iatrogenic injury to the bile duct. Br J Surg 1991; 78: 1412–13.

46. Bates T, Ebbs SR, Harrison M, A'Hern RP. Influence of cholecystectomy on symptoms. Br J Surg 1991; 78: 964–7.

47. MacMahon AJ, Russell IT, Baxter JN et al. Laparoscopic versus minilaparotomy cholecystectomy: a randomised trial. Lancet 1994; 343: 135–8.

48. Majeed AW, Troy G, Nicholl JP et al. Randomized, prospective, single-blind comparison of laparoscopic versus small-incision cholecystectomy. Lancet 1996; 347: 989–94.

49. Dubois F, Icard P, Berthelot G, Levard H. Coelioscopic cholecystectomy. Ann Surg 1990; 211: 60–2.

50. Nathanson LK, Shimi S, Cuschieri A. Laparoscopic cholecystectomy: the Dundee technique. Br J Surg 1991; 78: 155–9.

51. Cuschieri A, Dubois F, Mouiel J et al. The European experience of laparoscopic cholecystectomy. Am J Surg 1991; 161: 385–7.

52. The Southern Surgeons Club. A prospective analysis of 1518 laparoscopic cholecystectomies. N Engl J Med 1991; 324: 1073–8.

53. Wilson P, Leese T, Morgan WP, Kelly JF, Brigg J. Elective laparoscopic cholecystectomy for 'all comers'. Lancet 1991; 338: 795–7.

54. Unger SW, Rosenbaum G, Unger HM, Edelman DS. A comparison of laparoscopic and open treatment of acute cholecystitis. Surg Endosc 1993; 7: 408–11.

55. Richardson MC, Bell G, Fullarton GM and The West of Scotland Laparoscopic Cholecystectomy Audit Group. Incidence and nature of bile duct injuries following laparoscopic cholecystectomy: an audit of 5913 cases. Br J Surg 1996; 83: 1356–60.

56. Cassey GP, Kapadia CR. Operative cholangiography or extraductal palpation: an analysis of 418 cholecystectomies. Br J Surg 1981; 68: 516–17.

57. Windsor JA, Garden OJ. Laparoscopic ultrasonography. Aust NZ J Surg 1993; 63: 1–2.

58. John TG, Banting SW, Pye S, Paterson-Brown S, Garden OJ. Preliminary experience with intracorporeal laparoscopic ultrasonography using a sector scanning probe. A prospective comparison with intraoperative cholangiography in the detection of choledocholithiasis. Surg Endosc 1994; 8: 1176–81.

59. Greig JD, John TG, Mahadaven M, Garden OJ. Laparoscopic ultrasonography in the evaluation of the biliary tree during laparoscopic cholecystectomy. Br J Surg 1994; 84: 1202–6.

60. Finnis D, Rowntree T. Choledochoscopy in exploration of the common bile duct. Br J Surg 1977; 64: 661–4.

61. Grange D, Maillard J-N. La choledochoscopie peroperatoire. Gastroenterol Clin Biol 1981; 5: 857–65.

62. Griffin WT. Choledoschoscopy. Am J Surg 1976; 132: 697–8.

63. Khoo D, Walsh CJ, Murphy C, Cox M, Motson RW. Laparoscopic common bile duct exploration: evolution of a new technique. Br J Surg 1996; 83: 341–6.

64. Rhodes M, Nathanson L, O'Rourke N, Fielding G. Laparoscopic exploration of the common bile duct: lessons learned from 129 consecutive cases. Br J Surg 1995; 82: 666–8.

65. Petelin JB. Clinical results of common bile duct exploration. Endosc Surg Allied Technol 1993; 1(3): 125–9.

66. Berci G, Morgenstern L. Laparoscopic management of common bile duct stones. A multi-institutional SAGES study. Society of Ameri-

can Gastrointestinal Endoscopic Surgeons. Surg Endosc 1994; 8: 1168–74.

67. Menzies D, Motson RW. Percutaneous flexible choledochoscopy: a simple method for retained common bile duct stone removal. Br J Surg 1991; 78(8): 959–60.

68. Burhenne HJ. The technique of biliary duct stone extraction. Radiology 1974; 113: 567–72.

69. Mason R. Percutaneous extraction of retained gallstones via the T–tube track – British experience of 131 cases. Clin Radiol 1980; 31: 587–97.

70. Nussinson E, Cairns SR, Vaira D, Dowsett JF, Mason RR. A 10 year single centre experience of percutaneous and endoscopic extraction of bile duct stones with T-tube *in situ*. Gut 1991; 32: 1040–3.

71. Nathan MH, Newman MA, Murray DJ, Camponovo R. Cholecystokinin cholecystography. Four years evaluation. Am J Roentgenol 1970; 110: 240–51.

72. Lennard TWJ, Farndon JR, Taylor RMR. Acalculus biliary pain: diagnosis and selection for cholecystectomy using the cholecystokinin test for pain reproduction. Br J Surg 1984; 71: 368–70.

73. Sunderland GT, Carter DC. Clinical application of the cholecystokinin provocation test. Br J Surg 1988; 75: 444–9.

7 Benign and malignant lesions of the biliary tract

Irving S. Benjamin

Since gallstones have been considered in a previous chapter this account will concentrate on intrinsic lesions of the biliary tract. These can best be considered under the headings shown in Table 7.1.

Since many biliary tract lesions share a number of features in common, it will be helpful to look at the relevant features of biliary anatomy and physiology, and the presentation and investigation of the biliary tract as a whole before considering the specific details of each lesion.

General considerations

Biliary anatomy

The segmental anatomy of the biliary tract and the anatomy of the extrahepatic biliary tree have been considered in Chapter 1. Biliary segments may be considered as independent entities, and alteration of the biliary drainage and blood supply (particularly portal blood) of each segment will have a variable effect on that segment and on the liver as a whole. Segmental changes may be asymptomatic, and yet produce functional and radiological abnormalities. Table 7.2 shows a classification of biliary tract obstruction and some commonly associated lesions. Complete, intermittent and chronic incomplete obstruction (types I–III) can occur to the whole liver or to one or more segments (type IV). For example, a cholangiocarcinoma arising in a segmental or lobar duct will cause progressive segmental obstruction, but as long as there is no infection this process may be asymptomatic. Measurement of liver function tests will reveal elevation of alkaline phosphatase, which is a sensitive indicator of obstruction, but the patient will not become jaundiced until the tumour has involved the confluence. By this stage there will be long-term effects of segmental biliary tract obstruction, with associated fibrosis and atrophy. This has a critical impact on management of biliary tumours, and the mechanisms and clinical presentations have been reviewed in detail by Hadjis.[1]

Table 7.1 *Benign and malignant lesions of the biliary tract*

Congenital anomalies	Biliary atresia
	Choledochal cyst
	Spontaneous perforation of bile duct
Calculous disease	Choledocholithiasis
	Biliary fistula
	Internal
	External
	Mirizzi syndrome
Inflammatory lesions	Cholangitis
	Acute suppurative
	Parasitic infestation
	Ascaris
	Clonorchis
	Hydatid
	Primary sclerosing cholangitis
	Secondary sclerosing cholangitis
	Idiopathic inflammatory strictures
Benign strictures and biliary strictures	Idiopathic inflammatory strictures
	Traumatic
	Postcholecystectomy
	Other
Tumours	Benign
	Adenoma
	Papillomatosis
	Rare varieties
	Malignant
	Ampullary tumours
	Cholangiocarcinoma
	Carcinoma of gall bladder
	Secondaries
	Others
Functional disorders	Gall bladder dyskinesia
	Papillary stenosis
	Sphincter of Oddi dysfunction

Variants in the extrahepatic biliary anatomy are also considered elsewhere in this volume. Their main importance lies in vulnerability of the extrahepatic bile ducts at cholecystectomy. The 'normal' arrangement with a single confluence occurs in only 57% of cases according to Couinaud.[2] In more than 25% the right anterior or posterior sectoral ducts joins the left hepatic duct separately, and in a small proportion there is a common junction between the right posterior sectoral duct and the cystic duct with the common hepatic duct.

Table 7.2 *A classification of biliary tract obstruction and commonly associated lesions*

Complete biliary tract obstruction	Tumours, especially of the pancreatic head Ligation of the common bile duct Cholangiocarcinoma Parenchymal liver tumours primary or secondary
Intermittent obstruction	Choledocholithiasis Periampullary tumours Duodenal diverticula Papillomas of the bile duct Choledochal cyst Polycystic liver disease Intrabiliary parasites Haemobilia

Chronic incomplete obstruction	Strictures of the common bile duct
	    Congenital
	    Traumatic (iatrogenic)
	    Sclerosing cholangitis
	    Postradiotherapy
	Stenosed biliary–enteric anastomoses
	Chronic pancreatitis
	Cystic fibrosis
	Stenosis of the sphincter of Oddi
	Dyskinesia (sphincter of Oddi dysfunction)

Segmental obstruction	Traumatic (including iatrogenic) Hepatodocholithiasis Sclerosing cholangitis Cholangiocarcinoma

The portal venous anatomy is relatively constant and usually easily defined, but in almost a quarter of cases the right hepatic artery takes its origin from the superior mesenteric artery, and may be vulnerable during operations on the pancreas or bile duct. Also of importance is the blood supply of the bile duct, which runs in two longitudinal '3 o'clock and 9 o'clock' vessels to the left and right of the duct, with the predominant source of blood supply running cephalad.[3] These arteries may be injured during dissection of the ductal system, and may be vulnerable to thermal damage at laparoscopic cholecystectomy.

Biliary physiology

Some 0.5–1.5 l of bile are excreted per day, and most of the constituents are reabsorbed in the distal ileum. Hepatic bile is diverted into the gall bladder as a function of hepatic secretory pressure, sphincter of Oddi tone and cystic duct resistance. During fasting the gall bladder absorbs fluid and concentrates the bile, which is expelled from the normal gall bladder by intermittent contractions, either spontaneous or produced by the stimulus of cholecystokinin released from the postprandial duodenum and small bowel mucosa. The human common bile duct does contain a small amount of smooth muscle, but has little propulsive function. However, the sphincter of Oddi is a complex muscular structure which produces a basal pressure some 3 mmHg above the pressure in the common bile duct and pancreatic duct, and a series of antegrade phasic contractions which proceed distally producing a peristaltic effect. Cholecystokinin or its analogues inhibit these phasic contractions and reduce basal sphincter pressure allowing flow of bile into the duodenum. The clinical evidence for functional disorders of the sphincter of Oddi and their management will be considered briefly later in this chapter.

Presentations of biliary tract disorders

The commonest presentation of biliary tract lesions are biliary obstruction, pain due to organic or functional lesions in the biliary tract, cholangitis, and fistula formation, and there are also some rarer phenomena such as haemobilia.

Biliary tract obstruction (Table 7.2)

Total biliary obstruction will increase pressure within the biliary tract, and effective bile production ceases when this exceeds the secretory pressure of bile (20 cm H_2O). This pressure is usually, but not always, sufficient to cause dilatation of the extrahepatic and intrahepatic biliary tree. In one series of cases of biliary obstruction 8% showed no evidence of ductal dilatation.[4] Absence of dilatation should raise the suspicion of secondary biliary cirrhosis or of coexisting hepatic disease such as alcoholic or post-hepatitic cirrhosis. Partial or segmental obstruction may not cause dilatation. Most patients will present with jaundice, and a systematic approach to diagnosis is essential. Numerous algorithms have been described, and one such scheme is shown in Fig. 7.1. However, this is only a guide to investigation of the jaundiced patient, and many variations may have to be applied to individual situations.

Cholangitis

This ranges from severe acute suppurative cholangitis associated with complete biliary obstruction to chronic low-grade sepsis in a partially obstructed biliary tree. Normal bile is sterile, but colonisation is common in the presence of stones in the gall bladder or bile duct. In malignant biliary obstruction without stones, organisms are found in the bile in only one-third of cases, but after previous instrumentation this rate becomes much higher.[5] In benign biliary strictures, there may be up to 80% positive cultures. Acute cholangitis produces oedema and neutrophil infiltration and intrahepatic microabscesses may form, which may

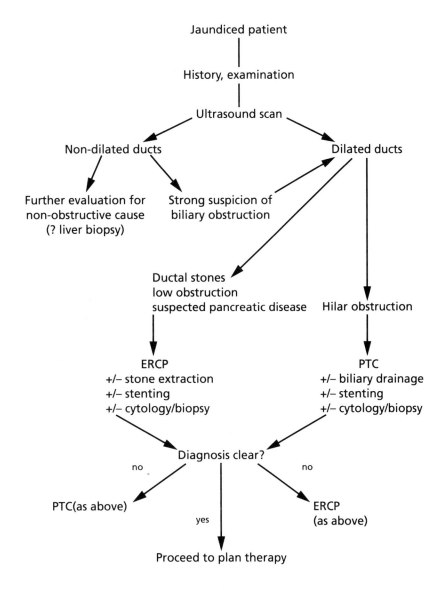

Figure 7.1 *Schematic diagram of an algorithmic approach to diagnosis in suspected obstructive jaundice.*

not resolve until adequate biliary drainage is restored (Fig. 7.2). The fibrotic changes associated with long-standing biliary obstruction become more marked in the presence of infection.

The combination of bacterial colonisation and stasis may promote formation of intraductal stones, by deconjugation of bilirubin by bacterial betaglucuronidase to form calcium bilirubinate precipitates.[6]

The classical Charcot's triad (fever, right upper quadrant pain and jaundice) is present in only 50–60% of patients with acute cholangitis. Bacteraemia due to cholangiovenous or cholangiolymphatic reflux occurs when the ductal pressure is raised to 25 cm H_2O.[7] The organisms found in bile and blood are usually enteric organisms, such as *Escherichia*

Figure 7.2
Intrahepatic abscess associated with chronic low-grade biliary obstruction due to a plastic stent. Change of the stent allowed resolution of the abscess.

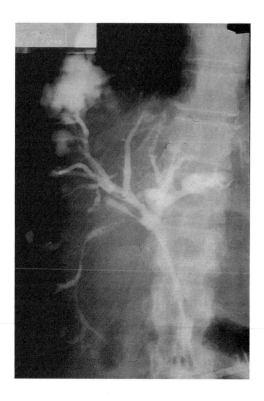

coli, Klebsiella and *Enterococcus*. Anaerobes occur in less than one-third of patients without previous biliary instrumentation. Cholangitis may follow endoscopic retrograde cholangiopancreatography (ERCP) in up to 5% of patients with obstructed ducts, and antibiotic prophylaxis is recommended in these patients.

Haemobilia

This is an uncommon but sometimes life-threatening complication. The majority of cases are due to trauma, including liver biopsy. Persistent haemorrhage is generally of arterial origin, or associated with arteriovenous aneurysm or fistula. It may sometimes present as chronic obscure gastrointestinal bleeding (90% with malaena), often intermittent. Occasionally blood can be seen issuing from the papilla on endoscopy. Clots may form within the biliary tree and cause colic, and may be mistaken for common duct calculi on cholangiography. Treatment will depend on the cause of haemorrhage, and arteriography and arterial embolisation may combine diagnosis and therapy.[8]

Investigation of the biliary tract

Clinical

A careful history and physical examination are essential. In the past history, gallstones, previous biliary surgery, risk factors for liver disease (alcohol, hepatitis exposure, drugs, blood transfusion etc.), and features suggestive of pancreatic disease (alcohol, steatorrhoea, chronic pain, diabetes) are all important. If there has been previous biliary surgery then the patient should be asked about the postoperative course, the length of stay in hospital, infective complications or prolonged drainage.

On examination, apart from obvious features such as jaundice and palpable abdominal masses, stigmata of chronic liver disease should be sought. An abdominal mass may not represent a large liver tumour but be due to a hyperplastic liver lobe following contralateral obstruction.

Laboratory investigations

Tests of liver function may not always distinguish 'surgical' from 'medical' jaundice. While different patterns of liver enzymes (in particular alkaline phosphatase) may suggest an intrahepatic or extrahepatic cause, in long-standing biliary obstruction, the cytoplasmic enzymes (aspartate transaminase (AST) and alanine transaminase (ALT)) may also be elevated due to chronic obstruction and infection. Gamma glutamyl transpeptidase activity is high in biliary obstruction, but it is also acutely raised following alcohol intake.

It is not necessary to undertake serological tests for hepatitis and autoimmunity unless these features are specifically suspected. It may be important, however, to screen for hepatitis in patients who have had previous exposure from hepatitis endemic areas before considering surgery.

Tumour markers have limited value. CA19-9 may be helpful in distinguishing cholangiocarcinoma from sclerosing cholangitis, and has proved useful in screening for tumours in primary sclerosing cholangitis patients under consideration for liver transplant.

Some authors have found dynamic liver function tests useful to evaluate functional hepatic reserve for liver resection. Clearance of aminopyrine and antipyrine (minor analgesics) is dependent on function of the cytochrome *P*450, which is impaired in the presence of biliary obstruction, and was shown by one group to be a good predictor of outcome in surgery for obstructive jaundice.[9]

Biliary imaging

Plain abdominal X-ray

This is of limited value, though radio-opaque gallstones may occasionally be visualised. Air within the biliary tree indicates biliary-enteric communication. This is most commonly found after surgical anastomosis or sphincterotomy, and its absence after such a procedure may suggest inadequacy of the anastomosis. Aerobilia is also found in the presence of a spontaneous biliary–intestinal fistula due to gallstones, and more rarely as a result of gas-forming organisms in severe cholangitis.

Oral cholecystogram

This has been largely superseded by ultrasound which has a very high sensitivity for gall bladder stones and sludge.

Intravenous cholangiography

In combination with tomography this procedure has undergone something of a resurgence for detecting choledocholithiasis before laparoscopic cholecystectomy. However, it remains insensitive and carries a significant incidence of toxic reaction and rarely death.

Endoscopic retrograde cholangiopancreatography (ERCP)

The scope of this investigation is considered in greater detail elsewhere. In the diagnosis of jaundice it is particularly valuable when distal bile duct obstruction is suspected, because it will allow precise definition of the distal biliary tree and pancreatic duct, and may allow cytological and histological examination. In the case of choledocholithiasis it may of course be used for endoscopic sphincterotomy and stone extraction.

In the presence of a very tight biliary stricture only the distal bile duct may be filled at ERCP even with the use of a balloon catheter and high pressure injection, and if there is a complex hilar stricture it may not be possible to outline both right- and left-sided hepatic ductal systems. The same is true of endoscopic stenting, and precise placement of a stent in such cases may require percutaneous transhepatic assistance.

Percutaneous transhepatic cholangiography (PTC)

When ERCP is not possible (for example after previous biliary diversion or sometimes after Billroth II gastrectomy) this may be the only means of accessing the upper biliary tract. PTC carries a higher risk of bile leakage and bleeding. Delineation of all separated intrahepatic segments can be obtained by separate needle punctures. A guidewire can often be placed across the stricture for transhepatic stenting, or be passed down to the duodenum where it is grasped for endoscopic stenting in a combined procedure. The availability of self-expanding metallic stents which can be placed using a 7Fr gauge introducer has allowed safe single-stage percutaneous stenting. If a stricture cannot be traversed, then external transhepatic biliary drainage can still be used for preoperative preparation of the jaundiced patient, though its value has remained unproven.[10]

Radio-nucleide scans

Technetium-99m-labelled derivatives of iminodiacetic acid (HIDA, DISIDA, PIPIDA) not only allow imaging of the biliary tree but also calculation of parameters which reflect liver blood flow, hepatocyte function, and the dynamics of biliary excretion. It can also be valuable in showing differential segmental liver function, and in demonstrating external or internal biliary fistulae, and can be of special value in following patients who have had biliary-enteric bypass for stricture repair (Fig. 7.3).

(a)

(b)

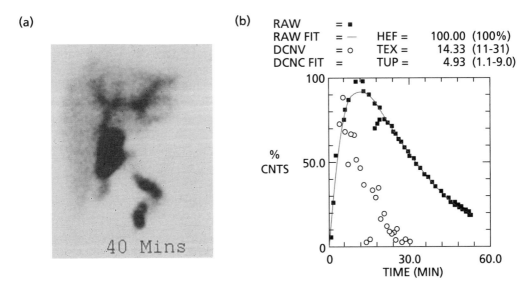

```
RAW       = ■
RAW FIT   = ┄┄    HEF =    100.00  (100%)
DCNV      = ○     TEX =     14.33  (11-31)
DCNC FIT  =       TUP =      4.93  (1.1-9.0)
```

Figure 7.3 *HIDA scan after a biliary–enteric bypass, (a) Showing good excretion into the Roux limb. (b) The derived parameters of hepatic perfusion, extraction and biliary flow.*

Scanning

The role of the various scanning modalities for each of the biliary lesions will be discussed in the relevant sections, but it should be noted that ultrasound, computed tomography (CT) and magnetic resonance imaging (MRI) scanning are complementary rather than competitive, and on occasions more than one method may be needed.

Congenital anomalies

Problems of development within the biliary tract may present in infancy or may not become evident until later in childhood or even in adult years. The most important of these are considered in this section.

Biliary atresia

This occurs in approximately one per 10 000 live births, with a slight female preponderance. The extrahepatic bile ducts are destroyed to a variable extent by an inflammatory process which begins before birth, and whose aetiology remains uncertain. A congenital origin is suggested by the association with other anomalies. Howard[11] found associated anomalies in approximately 20% of 237 cases, including cardiac anomalies, malrotation or situs inversus, and anomalies of the portal vein, inferior vena cava or spleen. The splenic anomalies (16% of cases) include polysplenia and asplenia, some with an associated preduodenal portal vein. These workers have suggested that this should be recognised as a specific biliary atresia–splenic malformation syndrome. There are a number of reports of biliary atresia in twins and families. An infective origin has also been suggested, but although experimental models of intrauterine viral infection have produced some of the features, the complete syndrome has not been reproduced, and no viral particles have been isolated in infants with biliary atresia. Metabolic factors may include bile acid toxicity within the hepatobiliary system.[12] Finally, abnormal anatomical arrangements have been found, as in patients with choledochal cysts, with an abnormal biliary and pancreatic ductal junction.

Pathology

Three types are described:

Type I: atresia of the common bile duct, with a common hepatic duct remnant;

Type II: atresia of the common hepatic duct and bile duct with right and left duct remnants;

Type III: atresia of the whole of the extrahepatic ductal system.

Histology of excised hilar tissue shows fibrosis and inflammation and some vestigial duct structures. Kasai made the important observation in 1959 that excision of this tissue permitted a flow of bile from the porta hepatis, and described small channels which communicate with the intrahepatic ducts.[13] The size of these channels (up to 300 μm) may have a significant effect on restoration of bile flow. The liver proximal to biliary atresia shows changes of large duct obstruction, which may progress to secondary biliary cirrhosis.

Presentation

There are rarely any specific prenatal features, and the presentation is with prolongation of the normal physiological neonatal jaundice with pale stools and failure to thrive. Occasionally the onset may only become apparent after several weeks. Delay in referral for surgery is very common[14] and early diagnosis is essential for successful management. It is important to exclude infections and congenital metabolic disorders such as α_1-antitrypsin deficiency. Liver function tests are non-specific. Ultrasound should exclude a choledochal cyst. Percutaneous liver biopsy shows characteristic but non-specific changes associated with biliary obstruction. ERCP is possible in infants, and may be diagnostic.[11]

Management

The introduction of the portoenterostomy which now carries Kasai's name was a major advance. The gall bladder is mobilised and dissected down to the fibrous hepatic duct remnant, which is then excised together with its thickened overlying peritoneum, to remove all the tissue lying in front of the hilar vessels.[11] A Roux loop of jejunum is anastomosed to the cut edges with a fine absorbable suture. The use of a cutaneous stoma in the Roux loop has now largely been abandoned.

If this procedure does not succeed in restoring bile flow and curing jaundice, reoperation is successful in less than one-third of patients.[15]

Biliary atresia is the commonest indication for transplantation in children and is used when diagnosis and treatment has been unduly delayed or when portoenterostomy fails. Results are good, with a greater than 60% five-year survival.[16] Re-transplant may be necessary in some cases.

Results

Portoenterostomy has revolutionised the results, and success is highly dependent on early surgery. Neonatal jaundice should be assumed to be due to biliary atresia until there is good evidence for an alternative diagnosis. The King's College Hospital group[14] reported restoration of bile flow in 86% of infants treated before eight weeks of age, but only 36% in older children, and reported a probability of 60% of survival (without need of transplantation) at five years in a series of 147 cases.[11] A further 20 children in this series underwent transplantation before the age of three. Results such as these can only be achieved in the hands of a paediatric surgeon skilled in the management of these patients. Many children develop late problems, with persistent biliary fibrosis and portal hypertension and varices in the oesophagus or in ectopic sites, and follow-up must be into adult years with careful surveillance and endoscopic sclerotherapy when indicated.[17]

Choledochal cysts

The incidence of this anomaly in the West is between one in 100 000 and one in 150 000 live births.[11] In Japan, it accounts for one in 1000 admissions to hospital, compared to one in 13 000 in the USA. There is a 3 or 4:1 female preponderance.

Aetiology

These are true congenital lesions, and some are now diagnosed by antenatal ultrasound. A more or less constant finding is an anomalous junction between the bile duct and the pancreatic duct, with a common channel from a few millimetres to several centimetres in length. This results in free reflux of pancreatic juice into the bile duct. Experimental reproduction of this lesion leads to common bile duct dilatation with weakening of the duct wall and inflammatory changes in the endothelium.[18]

Classification

The classification by Alonso-Lej[19] is generally used (Fig. 7.4). The commonest is type 1 which has been subdivided into a cystic or a fusiform dilatation of the common bile duct. Large cysts are easy to identify, but subtle forms of fusiform dilatation are being recognised increasingly, in association with low-grade obstruction or recurrent pancreatitis. The clue may lie in the anomalous pancreatic–bile ductal junction. Type 2 is a simple diverticulum and type 3 a choledochocele in the distal duct. Type 4 is the second most common, with extra- and intrahepatic cysts. Type 5 is confined to the intrahepatic ducts, and may

Figure 7.4
Classification of choledochal cysts (after Alonso-Lej[19]).

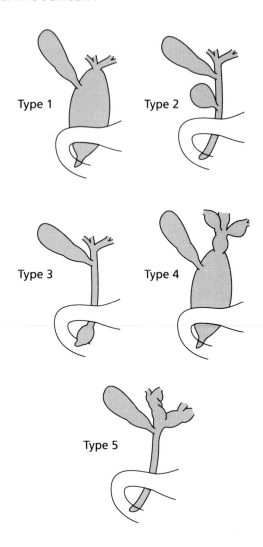

Type 1

Type 2

Type 3

Type 4

Type 5

merge into the syndrome of Caroli's disease which in turn is associated with congenital hepatic fibrosis.

Pathology

The duct shows progressive chronic inflammation, with ulceration and areas of loss of biliary epithelium. The wall may be thickened and fibrotic. Most contain high levels of biliary amylase and/or lipase.

An important feature is the propensity to malignant change. Precursor areas of dysplasia may be seen in the duct epithelium. The mechanism is unclear, and its relationship to pancreatic reflux has not been defined. Biliary stasis predisposes to formation of secondary bile acids, which are mutagenic. The risk increases with duration of exposure: malignancy is hardly ever seen in cysts removed in infancy, and the mean age of presentation is 32 years.[20] Voyles *et al.*[21] showed an age-related incidence, increasing from 0.7% in the first decade of life to more than 14% after 20 years of age.

Presentation

The classical presentation in infancy is a triad of jaundice, pain and mass in the right hypochondrium. In adulthood cholangitis is more common, and both children and adults may present with recurrent pancreatitis. It is important to be aware of the possibility of a subtle fusiform dilatation of the bile duct in patients with otherwise unexplained recurrent acute pancreatitis. Perforation has been reported, and a number of patients have presented with jaundice in pregnancy, presumably due to distortion or compression of the cyst causing distal obstruction.

Investigations

There are no specific laboratory tests, and the initial diagnosis is usually made by ultrasound. Biliary imaging is essential, and usually ERCP or PTC allows definition of the cyst and of the anomalous ductal junction (Fig. 7.5). ERCP must be undertaken with caution to avoid infection of the cyst or precipitation of pancreatitis.

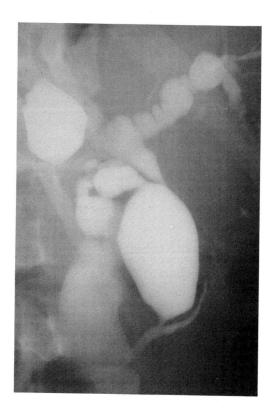

Figure 7.5 *ERCP of a choledochal cyst, showing the anomalous pancreatobiliary ductal junction.*

Management

The old treatment of cyst-duodenostomy relieves jaundice but does not eradicate biliary stasis nor remove the risk of malignancy. Endoscopic sphincterotomy may also fail to reduce the rate of complications. The type 3 cyst (choledochocele) may be so treated, or is occasionally removed by a transduodenal approach. For the other extrahepatic cysts the ideal treatment is excision of the entire dilated extrahepatic biliary tree from the confluence down to the biliary–pancreatic ductal junction, taking care to avoid pancreatic damage. It is generally possible to lift the whole extrahepatic biliary tree off the portal vein safely, and reconstruct the hepatic duct by an hepatico-jejunostomy Roux-en-Y. When the upper limit of the cyst involves the hepatic duct confluence, it is reasonable to compromise, and leave a very small cuff of the confluence intact to allow a safe and durable anastomosis.

Spontaneous perforation of the bile ducts

Davenport and Howard[22] have collected 70 cases of this rare occurrence from the literature over the last 65 years. The majority occur at between one and eight weeks, at the junction of the cystic duct. There are no associated antenatal features, and the infant presents with jaundice, abdominal distension, and sometimes vomiting. Laparotomy is mandatory, and it is important to exclude any distal bile duct obstruction by means of cholangiography. The perforation may be due to inspissated bile found in the distal duct. Insertion of a T-tube through the perforation seems perfectly safe, though a number of cases have been repaired by biliary diversion, using the gall bladder.

Inflammatory lesions

Acute cholangitis

The general features and pathology of this condition have already been described in the section on the presentation of biliary disease, and the management options are discussed in Chapter 6 on gallstones, the commonest cause. Some special categories require specific treatment here.

Parasitic infestation

Ascariasis

The round worm *Ascaris lumbricoides* is common in tropical and subtropical regions, particularly in Asia, Africa and Central America, where it may afflict around one-third of the population. The worm may grow to 10–20 cm in length in the small intestine, where ova are excreted and transmitted to other subjects. Larvae released in the duodenum enter the portal system and traverse the liver to the lungs from where they are able to travel up the respiratory tract and back into the intestine where they mature to adulthood. Adult worms enter the bile duct through the ampulla, where they can cause cholangitis, particularly if secondary bacterial contamination occurs. Live worms move in and out of the biliary tree and can sometimes be seen on endoscopy, and dead worms may form a nidus for stones in the bile duct.

Biliary ascariasis may be asymptomatic, or may present with acute suppurative cholangitis, strictures of the bile duct and acute pancreatitis. The condition may be diagnosed on plain radiology, and ultrasound may show long linear filling defects of the worms within the biliary tree, sometimes moving. Endoscopy and ERCP are diagnostic, and endoscopic extraction of worms and biliary decompression may abort an attack of cholangitis.

After the acute stage of biliary obstruction and cholangitis have resolved, anthelmintics have a very high cure rate. The stools must be examined after treatment to confirm eradication, and ultrasound or ERCP should be performed to ensure that no worms are left in the ducts. Papillary stenosis may be treated by endoscopic sphincterotomy. Re-infestation occurs in up to one-third of patients, and is usually symptomatic. The end result of recurrent re-infections is one form of the syndrome of recurrent pyogenic cholangitis.[23]

Clonorchis sinensis

This organism is a flat worm 10–25 mm in length common in China and South East Asia. They are generally acquired by eating raw infected fish, and the larvae migrate from the duodenum up the common bile duct where they become fixed by two large suckers, and continue to lay eggs which are excreted in the faeces. A freshwater snail and certain types of carp may form intermediate hosts.

Clonorchis sinensis is classically associated with recurrent pyogenic cholangitis (cholangiohepatitis), though the aetiological role has not been entirely proven. The infested biliary epithelium becomes inflamed and undergoes adenomatous hyperplasia, leading to fibrosis and the formation of intrahepatic stones. There is a strong association with cholangiocarcinoma. The features of recurrent pyogenic cholangitis are considered below, and there are no other specific features of clonorchiasis. Drug treatment is with praziquantel, and surgical management depends on the degree of ductal damage.

Hydatid disease

Echinococcus is endemic in many Mediterranean and Far Eastern countries, and in other sheep-farming areas. The life cycle involves sheep and dogs, and transmission from man to man does not occur. The ingested parasites enter the portal circulation from the duodenum and implant in the liver. The biliary tract can become invaded and daughter cysts may cause biliary obstruction and cholangitis. It is important to recognise such a communication because the use of toxic scolicidal agents in the treatment of hepatic hydatid cysts may induce caustic lesions of the biliary epithelium. A preoperative ERCP and sphincterotomy to release the cysts may avoid the need for choledochotomy at the time of surgery.

The main treatment is surgical, but albendazole and praziquantel may be used both pre- and postoperatively.

Recurrent pyogenic cholangitis

This syndrome in Far Eastern patients is also known as oriental cholangiohepatitis. It is commonest in South East Asia and Hong Kong and is characterised by gross irregular dilatation and intrahepatic stricture formation with repeated attacks of bacterial infection, pus formation and intrahepatic stones. As noted above, an association with ascariasis and *Clonorchis sinensis* has been noted, but the causative association is unproven. The intraductal changes vary from copious stone formation to thick inspissated biliary sludge, and the stricture formation incarcerates stones within the hepatic ducts. The left duct is more frequently and severely affected. There may be associated fibrosis and atrophy and ultimately biliary cirrhosis. Chronic abscess formation may ensue, and there is an association with intrahepatic cholangiocarcinoma.

The clinical presentation is often in young adults with the characteristic Charcot's triad. Deep jaundice is unusual and fever may be recurrent and low grade rather than acute. There will be a high index of suspicion in endemic areas, but the condition should also be suspected in an immigrant population in the west. Laboratory investigations are non-specific, with leucocytosis and obstructive liver function tests with a very high serum alkaline phosphatase. Ultrasound is virtually diagnostic and CT scanning may provide complementary information. ERCP is the method of choice for cholangiography but PTC may be required if a stone or stricture prevents filling of the intrahepatic duct.

Immediate treatment of the cholangitis is with broad spectrum antibiotics, but surgery is virtually always required except for patients with very minor and localised strictures, which may be amenable to endoscopic dilatation. Occasionally surgery is required as an emergency because of septic shock, and the objective is to clear the common bile duct of the stones, ideally using flexible choledochoscopy, and placing a large T-tube. This emergency procedure will not provide a definitive solution to the problem, and biliary drainage must be secured. A supraduodenal choledochoduodenostomy generally leads to continuing symptoms of cholangitis, perhaps aggravated by distal 'sump syndrome'.

Whereas transduodenal sphincteroplasty may be more satisfactory from this point of view, the best procedure is disconnection of the extrahepatic biliary tree and hepaticojejunostomy Roux-en-Y. A direct approach to ducts in the left liver to remove stones and drain obstructed segments may be necessary, and hepatic resection is sometimes indicated (Fig. 7.6). Some authors have advocated a cutaneous stoma following a hepaticojejunostomy to allow repeated ductal exploration by choledochoscopy and instrumentation.[24] There is a high recurrence rate on long-term follow-up despite aggressive management.[25]

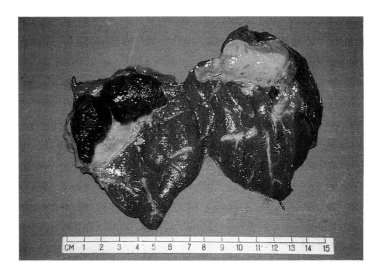

Figure 7.6 *Left hepatectomy specimen in a patient with cholangiohepatitis: the left hepatic ducts are distended with intrahepatic stones.*

Primary sclerosing cholangitis (PSC)

This fibrosing diffuse inflammatory process may affect any or all the parts of the biliary tree. The spectrum of disease varies from apparently localised, solitary, non-progressive extrahepatic biliary strictures to intrahepatic disease afflicting all segments of the liver and causing irregular narrowing and intervening relative dilatation. There is diffuse chronic inflammatory cell infiltrate with supervening neutrophil infiltration during acute attacks, and thickening of the duct walls with intense periductal fibrosis and obliteration of small ductules. Peripheral areas of the liver show features of large duct obstruction with cholestatic changes, and the whole may progress to secondary biliary cirrhosis. The features on liver biopsy are characteristic through not always diagnostic.[26]

Aetiology

The evidence for an autoimmune aetiology is now very strong. Chapman *et al.*[27] demonstrated a preponderance of tissue type HLA-B8 (60% versus 25% in controls), a genotype associated with other immunological disorders including primary biliary cirrhosis and ulcerative colitis. Infection may be the trigger, and in ulcerative colitis there may be loss of integrity of the intestinal mucosal barrier to gastrointestinal organisms. The incidence of PSC may be as high as 5% in patients with extensive colitis, and the incidence of inflammatory bowel disease in patients with PSC has been reported between 25 and 100%.

Presentation

The condition may be asymptomatic for many years, and the onset of symptoms may be insidious, with pruritus, jaundice, ill-defined upper abdominal pain, and intermittent fever and chills, and commonly weight loss. Physical signs may be absent, but jaundice, hepatomegaly and splenomegaly may be found in up to half the patients.

The course of the disease is extremely variable, and is characterised by relapses and remissions. Many cases are diagnosed in the course of investigation of inflammatory bowel disease, which is often the dominant feature.

Investigation

Alkaline phosphatase may be elevated even in the presymptomatic stage, and is out of proportion to the serum bilirubin. The transaminases may be normal. Antimitochondrial antibodies are absent, and if present should suggest primary biliary cirrhosis rather than PSC. Eosinophilia may be found, and copper metabolism may be abnormal.

Radiology is the cornerstone of diagnosis, mainly by ERCP and sometimes PTC, which show multifocal strictures of the intrahepatic and/or extrahepatic bile ducts. The ducts may show a beaded appearance with irregular strictures and occasional areas of focal dilatation. Liver biopsy is frequently performed, but findings are characteristic rather than diagnostic.

Management

Expectant

Asymptomatic patients are treated expectantly, despite extensive changes on cholangiography and liver biopsy. The response to medical treatment has long been disputed and trials of steroids have had variable results. The combination of steroids and azothiaprine was found to increase the death rate from supervening pyogenic infection. Ursodeoxycholic acid may improve symptoms and liver functions, and trials of other agents including methotrexate and colchicine are in progress. Most therapy has little effect on modulating the course of this highly variable disease, and treatment tends to be supportive until there is need for mechanical or surgical intervention.

Endoscopic and radiological

The objective is to eradicate significant dominant strictures and improve drainage from obstructed segments. This may be performed by ERCP or less commonly by PTC using balloon dilators, and some success may be achieved when strictures are short and localised. There is a danger of worsening the condition by adding bacterial cholangitis to the inflammatory process, and stenting should be avoided because this introduces a foreign body into the biliary tract. The combination of endoscopic sphincterotomy and proximal biliary strictures is a particularly undesirable one, and usually results in intrahepatic abscess formation. Transhepatic intubation with a permanent indwelling catheter has been used in some centres, but gives rather poor palliation. Some of these patients will come to transplantation, and procedures which increase septic complications are to be avoided at all costs.

Operative

This is largely restricted to treatment of dominant extrahepatic strictures by biliary disconnection and hepaticojejunostomy. Provision of an access loop may make dilatation of more proximal strictures feasible, and as long as this can be achieved without creating too much adhesion and sepsis then it should not prejudice transplantation. It was thought that proctocolectomy might improve PSC, but experience has shown that this is not so. By contrast, ulcerative colitis symptoms have been shown to improve following liver transplantation, probably as a consequence of the immunosuppression.[28]

Transplantation is used in patients whose liver function is deteriorating relentlessly. The results are good with actuarial survival rates at one and three years of 71 and 57%, respectively.[29] Unexpected cholangiocarcinomas were discovered in 8.6% of livers resected for transplantation in this series.

Cholangiocarcinoma and PSC

There is a strong association among inflammatory bowel disease, cholangiocarcinoma and PSC, and the radiological features of PSC and cholangiocarcinoma may be indistinguishable. Cytology may be useful with endoscopic or percutaneous brushings, though the sensitivity is not high. Biopsy of suspicious lesions by choledochoscopy or cholangioscopy may be preferable, but again not always diagnostic. The use of the tumour marker CA19-9 has helped to distinguish some cases of cholangiocarcinoma. However, none of these is sufficiently reliable in isolation, and it is necessary to have a high index of suspicion of this complication or differential diagnosis.

Benign strictures

Inflammatory

Localised inflammatory masses of unknown origin have been reported in both adults[30] and children.[31] The features are those of chronic inflammation, with epithelial loss and subepithelial fibrosis with areas of epithelial hyperplasia and regeneration. Hadjis[32] reported a benign aetiology in almost 10% (8/104) of suspected cholangiocarcinomas: some of these proved, on postresection histology, to be primary sclerosing cholangitis with a localised, dominant, extrahepatic stricture.[33] Others, however, showed the non-specific features above.

Traumatic

Postcholecystectomy

The majority of benign bile duct strictures are sustained during cholecystectomy. Although severe inflammation ('dangerous pathology') or anatomical variations ('dangerous anatomy') may be responsible for some,[34] in most cases there appear to be no such circumstances, and the injury is due to operative errors ('dangerous surgery') in dissecting the gall bladder and cystic duct.[35,36]

Since the introduction of laparoscopic cholecystectomy (LC) there have been many reports of bile duct injuries[37–40] and some authors[41–43] have suggested that the incidence might be significantly increased, perhaps as much as 10-fold, over open cholecystectomy. There have still been no randomised studies which address this issue directly, but there is now a growing body of evidence regarding the true incidence of biliary complications following LC.

A large questionnaire survey in 1750 hospitals in the United States, which included almost 78 000 laparoscopic cholecystectomies, revealed a bile duct injury rate (excluding cystic duct injuries) of 0.6%.[44] The rate was significantly lower in institutions that had performed more than 100 cholecystectomies. Larson[45] reported on almost 2000 cases by a group of surgeons all trained at one centre, and found a bile duct injury rate of 0.25%, similar to that for the open operation. Much higher rates have been reported, as high as 1% in one series of 600 patients in an American regional hospital.[46] There are two valuable series, one from the UK[47] and one from Holland.[48] The first was a prospective study carried out in the West of Scotland over a two-year period after the introduction of laparoscopic cholecystectomy, the value of which lies in its almost complete collection rate. These authors reported a 0.7% bile duct injury rate in 1683 laparoscopic procedures. A further study from this group over 5 years showed that during the later period the injury rate was significantly less.[49] The Dutch study[48] was conducted in a similarly closed population, and produced a figure of 0.8% in over 6000 laparoscopic cholecystectomies in two years. Most authors now believe that the injury rate diminishes dramatically after a 'learning curve' and may eventually be not much higher than that for the open procedure. Davidoff[38] has discussed the mechanisms of biliary injury at LC in detail.

These observations all serve to emphasise the need for all surgeons performing cholecystectomy (either 'open' or laparoscopic) to be familiar with the potential for bile duct injury and the possible approaches should this occur.

Classification

The classification generally accepted for biliary strictures is that of Bismuth[50] (Fig. 7.7). Since the advent of laparoscopic cholecystectomy a number of injury classifications as opposed to stricture classifications have been devised[48,49] but there is no standard classification yet.

Presentation

The presentation and management of laparoscopic and open bile duct injuries are similar: some are identified and treated intraoperatively[51] but many are not discovered until the early postoperative period or even weeks to months after the procedure when the patient develops jaundice

Figure 7.7 *Bismuth classification of biliary strictures.*

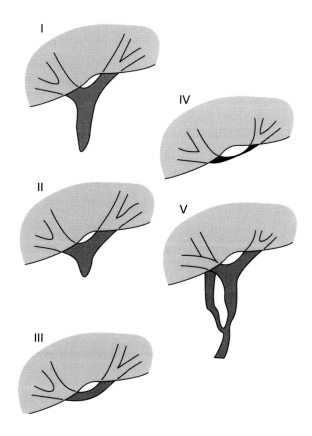

or cholangitis.[37,38] In one study of open cholecystectomy injuries, only 18% of injuries were recognised during the operative procedure.[52] It has long been proposed that the routine use of intraoperative cholangiography would prevent bile duct injuries, but despite many years of controversy this hypothesis remains unproven for either open[34,36] or laparoscopic cholecystectomy.[53,54] However, cholangiography may allow immediate identification of such injuries when they do occur, and the level and severity of biliary injury incurred may be less.[55]

Patients whose injury is not recognised at operation may present in several ways. If the duct is clipped or ligated then there will be a rapid onset of obstructive jaundice. If the ductal obstruction is partial then there may be gradual onset, or the patient may present days to weeks later with cholangitis. Some patients with presumed ischaemic or thermal injury do not present for months or even years after the original injury (Fig. 7.8). If a sectoral duct has been ligated but the main duct remains patent, this may result in silent atrophy of a sector of liver unless there is proximal sepsis, in which case the patient may present with fever and liver abscess. If there is a lateral injury to the main duct or a sectoral duct, or division of a sectoral duct, then the patient may present with biliary peritonitis or with external biliary drainage. The range of presentations is thus limited, and the rule of thumb should be that any

Figure 7.8 *A tight stricture at the level of the cystic duct which did not present until 18 months after cholecystectomy. The presumed mechanism for this is a gradually progressive ischaemic stenosis.*

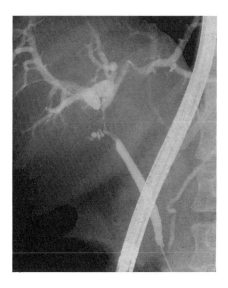

patient who presents with abdominal distension, unexpected abdominal pain or fever in the postoperative period should be suspected of having a biliary injury until proven otherwise.

Investigative techniques

The initial investigation is ultrasound, which may show a subhepatic collection or ductal dilatation according to the injury. Laboratory investigations are of value only in confirming jaundice with a raised alkaline phosphatase, and there is usually an associated leucocytosis. Biliary imaging is mandatory, and usually performed by ERCP. If there is external biliary drainage through a well-established fistula or tube, then cholangiography by this route may show the site of the injury. In the case of a transected sectoral duct a combination of ERCP and fistulogram or percutaneous cholangiogram may be necessary. HIDA scanning may also be useful in this situation.

Management options

Surgical

The direct sutured anastomosis between the biliary duct and a Roux-en-Y limb of jejunum remains the 'gold standard' for treatment of biliary strictures. There may be a few cases in which the injury is recognised at the time of primary operation, and in which circumstances are favourable for direct end-to-end repair of the duct with fine absorbable sutures, usually over a T-tube introduced through a separate choledochotomy (Fig. 7.9). For such a repair to succeed there must be no significant damage to the wall of the duct, no impairment of its blood supply from extensive dissection or use of diathermy, no surrounding collection of

Figure 7.9 (a)
Repair of a biliary injury over a T-tube. The patient presented with biliary peritonitis 24 h after laparoscopic cholecystectomy, and was re-explored and a side injury of the duct repaired.
(b) *Stricture after removal of the T-tube. This was initially stented endoscopically, but the patient came to repair by hepaticojejunostomy some months later.*

(a)
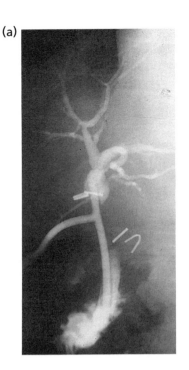

(b)
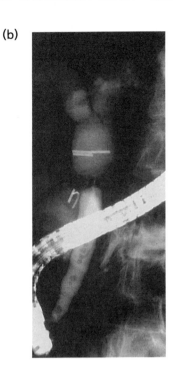

infected bile, and no loss of length producing tension in the repair. Few patients fulfil these criteria, and it is not possible to say what the true restricture rate is under these ideal circumstances, but the overall long-term success rate for such repairs is no more than 50%.[56]

The temptation to re-explore the patient with a suspected bile duct injury immediately should be resisted and imaging studies obtained to define the location and nature of the injury, while the patient is stabilised. In patients with intra-abdominal abscesses or bile collections, control of sepsis is of primary importance, and it may be necessary to perform preliminary CT or ultrasound guided drainage, and perform the biliary procedure at a later date. If portal hypertension is suspected the patient should undergo endoscopy and sometimes angiography prior to bile duct repair.

The operative approaches are considered at the end of this chapter, but it should be noted that a directly sutured hepatico-jejunostomy can be used in almost all patients, even those with hilar strictures. The mucosal graft procedure[57,58] gained some popularity in the UK because of the difficulty of accessing the hilar ducts. However, by using the left duct approach of Bismuth[50] based on the work of Hepp and Couinaud,[59] most hilar strictures can be successfully approached and a direct anastomosis performed. We have reported a series of 21 patients who had previously undergone 28 mucosal grafting procedures for strictures judged 'too high' for a sutured anastomosis. In 20 of these 21 patients a satisfactory sutured anastomosis could be achieved.[52]

Non-operative methods

Percutaneous balloon dilatation[60,61] and metal stenting[62] have been suggested as a primary means of treating benign bile duct strictures. Although some reports have suggested limited success in follow-up,[63] there has been a significant selection bias in choosing patients and in analysing results. Since the majority of patients who are able to undergo a direct sutured repair of their bile duct stricture will have good long-term results (see below),[64–67] it is the author's practice to reserve the use of radiological dilatation for those patients who are not suitable for a direct repair or in whom there are severe general risk factors such as severe secondary liver disease and portal hypertension.[34] In our operative series the mortality in patients without portal hypertension was 2%, rising to 23% in patients with portal hypertension.[34] In this group of patients radiological intervention and variceal sclerotherapy should be considered as primary treatment. However, careful consideration should be given to employing such a non-operative approach, since the development of recurrent cholangitis and secondary biliary cirrhosis may require a liver transplant. The use of trans-anastomotic tubes is considered below (Operative Approaches). The evidence for the value of long-term stenting in preventing stenosis is somewhat anecdotal,[68] with some authors suggesting a long duration of tube splinting[64,65] whereas others suggest only a short duration or no tube placement at all.[34] It is the author's practice to place a fine catheter across the anastomosis to allow for postoperative cholangiography on about the 7th day, after which it may be removed (Fig. 7.10). However, there is no strong argument against omitting a tube altogether if a wide anastomosis has been created and there is no suspicion of likely difficulties.

Figure 7.10
Postoperative tubogram at 7 days after hepaticojejunostomy for a hilar stricture. All hepatic ducts are filled and there is no leak of contrast, and the tube was removed immediately. The radiological marker on the end of the access loop is visible at the bottom right (see text).

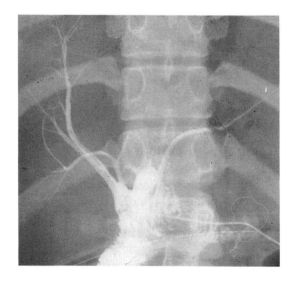

Results

General

The success rate for repair of the strictures is related to the severity and level of the injury, but a success rate of about 80% during long-term follow-up is reported from very many series, with the majority of re-strictures occurring within five years.[65]

In assessing the outcome of bile duct stricture repair, a 2–3 year minimum follow-up is essential,[35] and some have suggested a minimum of 7–10 years.[50]

The experience at Hammersmith Hospital in 130 post-cholecystect-omy biliary strictures followed-up for a mean of 7.2 years, showed a good or excellent outcome in 80% of 106 patients after a single sutured stricture repair. Of the 20% of patients who required a subsequent intervention (operative or radiological) half have had a good outcome without subsequent biliary symptoms, so that an overall good or excellent outcome was reported in 90%. The principal factors which predict a poor outcome after stricture repair include a Bismuth grade IV stricture and three or more previous attempts at stricture repair.[52] This supports the need for early referral to a specialist centre since repeated suboptimal repair attempts lead to a progressively higher level of stricture and risk the development of biliary cirrhosis and portal hypertension.

Tumours   Benign tumours

Compared to malignancy of the bile ducts, benign tumours are uncom-mon; in one report they were found in only two of 4200 biliary operations.[69] The classification of benign biliary tumours (according to the second edition of the WHO histological classification of tumours of the gall bladder and extrahepatic bile ducts[70]) is shown in Table 7.3, together with a number of other benign lesions which may present as suspected tumours. The more important of these lesions are considered in more detail below.

Presentation

The presentation of benign biliary tumours may be insidious, mimicking gallstones or sphincter of Oddi dysfunction, but may present like biliary tract cancer, with persistent or intermittent obstructive jaundice with or without abdominal pain. Periampullary tumours may be slow-growing and well-differentiated, and even endoscopy and biopsy may fail to distinguish the benign from the malignant lesion.

Investigative techniques

Although liver function tests, tumour markers, and other non-invasive investigations have their place in the initial investigation, radiology is the mainstay of diagnosis, and also the best guide to therapy.

Table 7.3 *Benign tumours and pseudotumours of the biliary tract*

Benign epithelial tumours	Adenoma
	  Tubular
	  Papillary
	  Tubulopapillary
	Cystadenoma
	Papillomatosis (adenomatosis)

Benign non-epithelial tumours	Granular cell tumour Ganglioneurofibromatosis Lipoma Haemangioma Lymphangioma Neurofibroma
Pseudotumours	Regenerative epithelial atypia Papillary hyperplasia Adenomyomatous hyperplasia Intestinal metaplasia Pyloric gland metaplasia Squamous metaplasia Heterotopias Xanthogranulomatous cholecystitis Cholecystitis with lymphoid hyperplasia Inflammatory polyp Cholesterol polyp Malacoplakia Congenital cyst Amputation neuroma Primary sclerosing cholangitis

A preoperative tissue diagnosis is valuable, and biopsies may be obtained under direct vision or using endoscopic forceps at ERCP, or cytological brushings obtained from within the duct. Similar techniques can be used at percutaneous cholangiography. Alternatively, ultrasound or CT-guided fine needle aspiration cytology or biopsy may be obtained (see under cholangiocarcinoma below), though results from large numbers of patients with benign disease have not been reported.

Ultrasound will usually define the level of biliary obstruction, but more sophisticated information requires specific expertise in hepatobiliary ultrasound. Dilatation of the intrahepatic biliary tree may be absent when there is intermittent obstruction from periampullary lesions or bulky, soft intraductal tumours. Many bile duct tumours can actually be visualised on ultrasound as thickening of the duct or intraductal filling defects.[71]

CT scanning offers little advantage over ultrasound for benign tumours.

Angiography is rarely indicated, but it often used when malignancy is suspected. Complete **cholangiography** should usually be obtained. It can be difficult to determine the site of origin of bulky intraductal tumours. ERCP may be adequate, or a combination of ERCP and PTC may be necessary.

Specific tumour types
Adenoma
There are three histological types: tubular, papillary and tubulopapillary. The common tubular adenoma is similar to intestinal adenomas, with Paneth cells and some serotonin-immunoreactive endocrine cells, and may show severe dysplasia or carcinoma in situ.

Bile duct adenomas (BDA) are usually asymptomatic liver nodules discovered incidentally during intra-abdominal surgery or at autopsy, and their importance lies in distinguishing them from malignant neoplasms. They are usually subcapsular, well circumscribed but non-encapsulated, spheroidal or ovoid, ranging in size from 1 to 20 mm (mean 5.8 mm), and greyish-white to yellow or tan in colour. Cho et al.[72] reported 13 patients with BDA among 2125 autopsies.

Some authors believe that BDA is a developmental anomaly or hamartoma.[73] However, BDA is distinct from the von Meyenburg complex; only two patients have been described under 20 years of age and it is not associated with other malformations, and is therefore probably a true neoplasm.

Ductal adenomas (in common with papillomas) are commonest in the distal third of the duct, close to the papilla. They are often soft and may be difficult to palpate. These lesions may be premalignant,[74] and should be completely excised whenever possible.

Biliary papilloma and papillomatosis
Only 27 cases of intrahepatic or diffuse intra- and extrahepatic biliary papillomatosis were described between 1959 and 1991.[75] This benign epithelial tumour consists of multiple soft fragile papillary lesions from 2 mm to 2 cm composed of a delicate fibrovascular stalk with a single layer of cuboidal or columnar mucus-secreting epithelial cells which stain positively with mucicarmine and PAS stains.[75-77] They may secrete abundant mucus, and occasionally produce diarrhoea and electrolyte depletion as well as obstructive jaundice.[78] They appear histologically benign, with regular papillary fronds without nuclear atypia or mitoses, and may become very bulky, and shed tumour fragments, leading to distension of the ducts (Fig. 7.11).

The tumours appear to be more frequent in women,[69] in the sixth or seventh decade.[75] Most patients with biliary papillomatosis present with partial and intermittent obstruction of the bile duct by secretory material or fragments of tumour.[77,79] The history may extend for more than 20 years, with chronic blood loss and anaemia, right upper quadrant pain, biliary colic, obstructive jaundice and pruritus.[80]

Figure 7.11
Ultrasound scan showing a bulky filling defect in the extrahepatic bile ducts due to biliary papillomatous tumour.

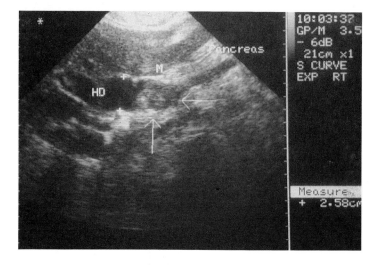

Most are diagnosed initially as bile duct obstruction due to stones or malignancy. Ultrasonography may show distended intra- and/or extrahepatic bile ducts, or an intraluminal filling defect. Cholangiography shows multiple filling defects in normal or distended bile ducts (Fig. 7.11). Flexible choledochoscopy is useful in intraoperative diagnosis.[75]

Treatment is both controversial and difficult. Radical excision, possibly including hepatectomy, offers the only certainty of a cure, because local recurrence is very frequent.[75,77,80,81] However, most have been treated by palliative techniques such as choledochotomy and repeated curettage with an internal or external drainage procedure.[81–83] Internal drainage by a biliary–enteric anastomosis with an access loop results in better palliation. External drainage should be avoided because of the large fluid and electrolytes losses.

The role of chemotherapy remains unproven.[77] Local radiotherapy by iridium needles has also been used.[75]

The long-term prognosis for biliary papillomatosis is poor. Hubens *et al.*[75] reported a mean survival of 36 months in 13 patients with adequate follow-up. Five patients (38%) survived for more than five years, two lived for 6 years after curettage and external T-tube drainage,[84,85] one underwent internal drainage[82] and two underwent resections. However, the majority died after two or three years, due to episodes of recurrent obstruction and cholangitis.

Biliary cystadenoma

This represents less than 5% of non-parasitic biliary cysts.[86–88] The majority arise from intrahepatic ducts, but 15% arise from the extrahepatic ducts and gall bladder. Their cause remains largely unknown although the presence of aberrant bile ducts in cystadenoma suggests a congenital origin.[86,87] Although usually benign, the biliary cystadenoma tends to recur after excision and there may be progression to cystadenocarcinoma.[86,89] The intrahepatic tumours may reach 5–27 cm in diameter and consist of multiloculated cysts containing mucinous, serous, bile-stained or brownish fluid without cells,[90] lined with tall columnar epithelium similar to the lining of normal bile ducts.[89] The cystadeno-carcinoma typically consists of hyperchromatic columnar cells with prominent nucleoli and frequent mitoses, forming disordered papillary projections and pleomorphic glands.

Biliary cystadenoma occurs predominantly in women, with a wide age range.[88] The clinical picture is non-specific with abdominal pain, a palpable abdominal mass, cholangitis, nausea or vomiting ranging from 2 weeks to 5 years.[88,90,91]

Diagnosis relies largely on ultrasound and CT findings, with fluid-filled masses with internal echoes of multiple septa and papillary projections.[92] Calcification may be detected on CT, and may be more common in cystadenocarcinoma than cystadenoma.[90,92] Intrahepatic biliary cystadenomas must be differentiated from simple hepatic cysts, polycystic liver, mesenchymal hamartoma, liver abscess, haematoma and hydatid cyst. Because differentiation of cystadenocarcinoma may not be possible, total surgical excision is the preferred treatment. Other procedures such as aspiration, external or internal drainage, mar-supialisation and enucleation leave the patient at significant risk for progressive enlargement, secondary infection, and malignant transformation.[91,93,94] Long-term follow-up with ultrasound or CT scan of the abdomen is indicated.[95,96]

Granular cell tumour of the biliary tree

These constitute less than 10% of all benign biliary tumours, with only 45 cases reported since 1952.[97] They are usually yellow–tan, non-encapsulated lesions less than 3 cm in diameter, containing nests or sheets of large rounded granular eosinophilic cells with small, centrally located vesicular nuclei, and large PAS-positive cytoplasmic granules. Their histogenesis is controversial, but Schwann cells and primitive mesenchymal cells have been proposed.[98,99]

Presentation is with biliary obstruction, usually in young patients, with a mean age of 35 years, and a curious predominance in black females (65%),[97] but there are no specific features. The majority of tumours occur near the junction of the cystic, hepatic and common bile ducts, and the treatment of choice is excision and Roux-en-Y hepatico-jejunostomy.

Neural tumours

These are extremely rare. One case of biliary obstruction in von Recklinghausen's neurofibromatosis and one paraganglionoma has been reported.[100,101] Amputation neuroma following previous surgery has also been reported as a cause of biliary obstruction.

Leiomyoma

Only four have been reported, all of them arising in the distal portion of the duct.[69]

Tumour-like lesions

Some 'pseudo-tumours' of the biliary tract are included in Table 7.3. Heterotopic tissue is usually gastric mucosa, but is extremely rare. The process may be developmental. An even rarer finding is that of heterotopic pancreatic tissue in the bile ducts.

Management options

The treatment for most benign biliary tumours is surgical. Even if malignant disease can be excluded, the main aim is to relieve and prevent biliary obstruction. This is often best achieved by surgical excision and hepaticojejunostomy. Long-term biliary stenting is generally to be avoided. The use of an access loop may be of value when benign lesions with a propensity for local recurrence have been incompletely excised. For lesions in the region of the papilla, radical excision is not generally indicated, and transduodenal wide local excision can be performed and followed-up endoscopically.

Ampullary tumours

Pathology

Many of these tumours have in the past been wrongly classified along with cancer of the head of the pancreas, leading to the erroneous identification of five-year survivors following bypass for 'pancreatic cancer'.[102] Most are adenocarcinomas though a number of other tumours such as carcinoids, other neuroendocrine tumours and sarcomas may arise from the ampulla. An important variant is benign villous adenoma, which may be part of an adenomatous syndrome such as Gardner's syndrome. There may be a true adenoma–carcinoma sequence. Spread of the tumours is by local extension to involve the pancreas and duodenum, and metastasis to regional lymph nodes.

Presentation

Most patients present with biliary obstruction in the sixth or seventh decades. Jaundice may be intermittent due to repeated necrosis and sloughing, and associated with anaemia due to chronic gastrointestinal bleeding. A classic but rare occurrence is of grey or silvery stools as a result of biliary obstruction combined with melaena. Familial adenomatous polyposis may result in periampullary adenomas and carcinomas one to two decades after the associated colon cancers.

Investigation

Laboratory tests showing intermittent biliary obstruction and a microcytic hypochromic anaemia are characteristic. As with most other tumours of the biliary tract tumour markers are variable, with carcinoembryonic antigen (CEA) and CA19-9 often elevated.

Imaging is important, and simultaneous bile duct and pancreatic duct dilatation on ultrasound (the 'double-duct' sign) suggests a possible periampullary cancer. Endoscopy will make the diagnosis in the majority of cases, missing only small intra-ampullary tumours. Biopsies should be obtained in every case, but false negatives may occur because of difficulty in accurate placement of the biopsy. CT scanning produces information complementary to ultrasound. The classic appearance of the 'inverted 3' sign in the duodenum used to be reported in barium meals, but these are now rarely used. For localised tumours angiography is not commonly indicated, unlike the situation with proximal biliary cancers and cancers of the head of pancreas.

Cholangiography is usually obtained by ERCP unless there is an impassable tumour at the ampulla. In this case PTC may show the ductal anatomy and demonstrate the extent of duct involvement.

Management

This depends on the stage of the tumour and the condition of the patient. Very elderly and frail patients who are not considered suitable for surgical exploration are often well palliated by endoscopic stenting, or even simply by sphincterotomy, which may have to be repeated. For patients fit for surgery, resection offers excellent palliation and a significantly higher cure rate than that for cancer of the head of pancreas. The choice lies between local excision and pancreatoduodenectomy. In patients with very small tumours local excision may be curative, but pancreatoduodenectomy is the procedure of choice. Transduodenal radical excision of a bulky ampullary cancer may, in fact, be more hazardous than resection of the head of pancreas. The main hazards are pancreatitis and duodenal or pancreatic fistula formation. Pylorus-preserving pancreatoduodenectomy[103] may be particularly applicable to these tumours. Fear that this procedure would compromise radicality has not been borne out by experience.[104,105]

Patients unsuitable for resection can be treated by palliative bypass (hepaticojejunostomy) though this leaves the potential problems of future bleeding or gastric outlet obstruction.

Adjuvant therapy

There is no good evidence regarding the role of chemotherapy or radiotherapy in surgically resected ampullary cancers. Studies of unresected tumours generally include both ampullary and pancreatic cancers, so conclusions are impossible for this tumour type.

Results

The overall 5-year survival rates reported for radical resection and for local excision are rather similar, ranging from 25 to 55%. Results from the Mayo Clinic[106] in 104 patients over 24 years revealed a hospital mortality of 6% and a 5-year survival of 34%. This is in stark contrast to the generally poor results for patients with cancer of the pancreatic head.

Cholangiocarcinoma

Hilar cholangiocarcinoma was first described clinically by Altemeier *et al.* in 1957,[107] but for almost two decades the diagnosis was rarely made during life, and often missed at laparotomy. Improvements in diagnostic techniques have changed this situation, and most of these tumours are now recognised preoperatively.

Incidence

This tumour is uncommon in the West with some 6000 new cases per annum in the USA, and around 400 in England and Wales. The reported autopsy incidence is 0.01 to 0.5%.[108] There is a marked geographic variation. The age-standardised annual incidence in France was 1.7 and 0.5 per 100 000 for males and females, respectively,[100] whereas in North-East Thailand, the rates were 135.4 and 43.0 per 100 000.[110] This may relate to parasitic infestation (see below).

Pathogenesis

A number of factors have been implicated. There is a strong association with inflammatory bowel disease and with sclerosing cholangitis (PSC). Aflatoxin exposure in farm workers in Denmark,[111] and methylene chloride[112] and vinyl chloride monomer[113] in factory workers in the USA have been implicated as chemical carcinogens. The incidence of gall bladder (GB) cancer is increased 14.7-fold 20 years after surgery for gastric ulcer, but there is no increase in the incidence of tumours in the rest of the biliary tract.[114]

The risk of malignancy in choledochal cysts has been noted earlier,[21] and is related to an anomalous junction between the pancreatic and biliary ductal systems (APBDJ). Two types of APBDJ have been defined: type I (pancreatic duct joins bile duct) is associated with GB cancer, whereas the type II APBDJ (bile duct joins pancreatic duct) is associated with biliary cysts. Suda *et al.*[115] found an APBDJ in 14.2% of cases of biliary tract carcinoma, and in 4/4 cases of congenital biliary dilatation. The biliary amylase level is extremely high in both types. Ohta *et al.*[116] showed epithelial mucosal atypia with papillary proliferation and epithelial hyperplasia in patients with both anomalies. Kato *et al.*[117] examined the mutagenicity of the bile in type I patients, and showed positive results in 6/12 patients, with a high incidence of polyploid DNA in the gall bladder epithelium in 2/4 patients, both of whom had mutagenic bile.

Pathology

The tumours are mucus-secreting adenocarcinomas arising from the epithelium of any part of the biliary tract, morphologically similar to intrahepatic cholangiocellular carcinoma. The gross appearance varies with the site.[118] Periampullary tumours are generally papillary, those in the mid-duct nodular, and tumours of the hepatic duct confluence generally stenosing. For some reason the confluence is the site of predilection: attention was first drawn to this group of tumours in a report of 13 patients by Klatskin,[119] and cholangiocarcinoma at the hilus continues to bear his name. These tumours can be very highly differentiated, and it may be difficult for the pathologist to distinguish between cancer and inflammation, especially on frozen section. Many express CEA on histochemical staining, and this may help to identify foci of malignancy in small biopsy specimens.[120]

The tumours produce a dense sclerotic reaction and show a strong tendency to longitudinal subepithelial growth and to perineural invasion, which is a negative prognostic feature.[121] Multicentricity is frequently described but may be due to retrograde seeding. It is not easy to ascertain the limits of tumour invasion on gross inspection. The tumour invades both adjacent liver tissue and vessels (portal vein and hepatic artery). Lymphatic spread is via the periductal nodes to the coeliac nodes.

Staging

Formal pathological staging is by the TNM system (Table 7.4), but such complete staging can only be made after surgery and pathological examination of the resected specimen. There is no universally accepted clinical staging system for hilar cholangiocarcinoma but any such staging system must take account of both biliary and vascular involvement. The available techniques for preoperative staging have been reviewed by Adam and Benjamin.[122] The scheme proposed by Bismuth describes Type I tumours, entirely below the confluence, Type II tumours, affecting the confluence, and Type III tumours extending to the first order right or left intrahepatic ducts,[123] but this classification does not describe the origin and mode of spread. Many originate eccentrically in the right or left duct and subsequently involve the confluence, so that some lesions require major hepatic resection for their eradication.[124] Such resections must take account of a possible atrophy/hyperplasia complex and must leave adequately functioning liver tissue, and not an atrophic and possibly infected lobe.[1]

Presentation

Obstructive jaundice is the rule and the disease may be extensive before jaundice develops: lymph node or visceral metastases were present at diagnosis in 77% of patients with gall bladder cancers and in 83% of those with extrahepatic biliary tumours in one series.[109] Of the patients with biliary cancer seen at Hammersmith Hospital 40% had episodes of ill-defined **pain** for some time before diagnosis.[125] **Fever** may occur, due to cholangitis in obstructed biliary segments, especially if there has been radiological or other intervention. The **systemic effects** of malignancy are often evident at presentation. Weight loss is common. A history of inflammatory bowel disease should be sought.

Table 7.4 *TNM definitions for extrahepatic bile duct cancer*

Primary tumour (T)

TX: Primary tumour cannot be assessed
T0:   No evidence of primary tumour
Tis: Carcinoma in situ
T1:   Tumour invades the mucosa or muscle layer
  T1a: Tumour invades the mucosa
  T1b: Tumour invades the muscle area
T2:   Tumour invades perimuscular connective tissue
T3:   Tumour invades adjacent structures: liver, pancreas, duodenum, gallbladder, colon, stomach

Regional lymph nodes (N)

NX: Regional lymph nodes cannot be assessed
N0:   No regional lymph node metastasis
N1:   Metastasis in cystic duct, pericholedochal and/or hilar lymph nodes (i.e., in the hepatoduodenal ligament)
N2:   Metastasis in peripancreatic (head only), periduodenal, periportal, coeliac, and/or superior mesenteric lymph nodes

Distant metastasis (M)

MX: Presence of distant metastasis cannot be assessed
M0:   No distant metastasis
M1:   Distant metastasis

Stage grouping

Stage 0   Tis, N0, M0
Stage I   T1, N0, M0
Stage II   T2, N0, M0
Stage III   T1, N1, M0
            T2, N1, M0
Stage IVA   T3, any N, M0
Stage IVB   any T, any N, M1

From Extrahepatic bile ducts. In: American Joint Committee on Cancer: manual for staging of cancer, 4th edn. Philadelphia: JB Lippincott, 1992, pp. 99–103.

Investigative techniques
Laboratory

Liver function tests are useful only in defining the degree of obstructive jaundice. Elevated alkaline phosphatase may be an early isolated abnormality in a symptomatic but anicteric patient.

Tumour markers are of limited value: CEA is expressed in the cells of bile duct cancer,[120] and may be elevated in the serum. CA19-9 and CA50 are frequently elevated, but this is not specific.[126] CA19-9 has been found to be useful in detecting cholangiocarcinoma in patients with PSC awaiting liver transplant.

Haematological tests should include measurement of coagulation status. Many patients are chronically anaemic on presentation, and leucocytosis may be a significant adverse prognostic factor in obstructive jaundice.

Nutritional status has a major impact on surgical risk. Low haemoglobin may be regarded as a nutritional index, but the most significant parameters are low serum albumin and history of recent weight loss.[127]

Radiological

Ultrasound can identify the level of obstruction in practically all cases.[71] The presence of gall bladder stones should be readily identified, and abnormalities of the gall bladder wall may raise suspicion of gall bladder cancer. Ultrasound can identify tumour masses in many cases of bile duct cancer, and duplex scanning may show portal venous invasion. Masses within the liver may indicate secondaries, or microabscesses secondary to biliary obstruction.

CT may have some advantages over ultrasound in the diagnosis of malignant biliary tumours, especially in detecting intrahepatic spread of tumour or local lymphadenopathy. Engels et al.[128] detected lymphadenopathy in three-quarters of patients with gall bladder or bile duct cancer at presentation. CT is of specific value in defining lobar or segmental hepatic atrophy.

Cholangiography should be used to delineate the full extent of tumour involvement, including definition of all hepatic segmental ducts; examinations carried out before referral to a specialist centre are often incomplete. The choice between PTC and ERCP has been discussed earlier, and may be dictated by local availability and expertise. Arguably ERCP is the procedure of first choice for distally placed tumour whereas for suspected upper biliary tract lesions, PTC is preferable, because the proximal extent of disease is important in staging and planning of treatment. Both procedures may be required for complete diagnosis.[129]

Nimura et al.[130] have extended the use of complete cholangiography to map all segmental ducts prior to surgery by PTC with drainage and percutaneous cholangioscopy, with a 96% positive rate on cholangioscopic biopsy. By contrast some surgeons regard complete cholangiography before operation as undesirable because of the risks of introducing infection, and rely on intraoperative cholangiography and/or ultrasound. This is a minority view, and most prefer to enter operative management with maximum anatomical information. Broad-spectrum antibiotic prophylaxis and careful, low-pressure cholangiography should minimise the risks of infection. The possibility of interventional procedures should be considered before the diagnostic manoeuvre is undertaken; there should be close consultation between radiologist and endoscopist and the surgeon at the time of the procedure.

Angiography is used selectively. Arterial encasement is virtually diagnostic of malignant tumour. Information about the portal vein can often be satisfactorily obtained at ultrasound, especially with the use of duplex Doppler scanning. However, when there remains doubt with potentially operable lesions then visceral angiography remains the gold standard. It may be difficult to differentiate between compression and invasion of the portal vein and ultrasound may actually be superior in this regard. With very few exceptions involvement of the main stem of the portal vein precludes resection (see below).

A preoperative **tissue diagnosis** may often be obtained by biopsy or cytological brushings at ERCP or PTC. We found only one false positive result (reported as 'highly suspicious') in over 200 such examinations,[131] with predictive value of positive and negative results of 98% and 53%, respectively. The diagnostic value relies heavily on accurate targetting of the biopsy and an experienced cytopathologist.

Laparoscopy can detect small peritoneal nodules missed on ultrasound and CT, and may eliminate an unnecessary laparotomy. Warshaw et al.[132,133] found such additional metastatic lesions at laparoscopy in 17 of 40 patients with pancreatic cancer, and reported an overall accuracy of 93% for laparoscopy with a complication rate of 1% and a mortality rate of 0.5%. More recently the combination of laparoscopy and laparoscopic ultrasound has been reported to be of value in the staging of pancreatic neoplasms and assessment of resectability.[134] Similar results have not yet been reported for bile duct tumours, but a strong case may be made for its use.[135]

Management options
Overview
It is important to keep in mind the aims of treatment of cholangiocarcinoma. The first is relief of biliary obstruction, followed by long-term prevention of cholangitis. The final objective, eradication of tumour, is less often achieved and occupies third place in this hierarchy of treatments. On these principles a judgement must be made between the complementary forms of therapy – endoscopic, radiological or operative. These decisions may be very subtle, and because of the infrequency of these tumours most should be referred to specialist centres.

Operative intubation
This has been largely supplanted by the use of endoscopic or radiological methods. The procedure may not be easy, requiring opening of the bile duct below the tumour, operative dilatation, and the insertion of a suitable stent, which may be either entirely intraductal or may exit through the common duct with or without a jejunal loop. The transhepatic tube first described by Praderi was popularised by Terblanche and his colleagues.[136] A metal instrument is passed through the tumour from the duct below, and railroaded through the dilated intrahepatic ducts onto the liver surface. A tube is then drawn through the liver with holes above and below the tumour, allowing bile to drain internally into the distal duct. A Roux limb of jejunum may be attached over the choledochotomy. Both ends are brought out through the skin, in a 'U' configuration. The ends of the tube can be closed off, or joined together outside the body as an external conduit, and the tube is easy to change without

anaesthesia. However, placing a U-tube is a major operation, and also patients may suffer recurrent attacks of cholangitis, bile leakage and infection around the tube sites. Though some authors[137] continue to favour the use of long-term transhepatic tubes, the palliation may be relatively poor compared with that of internal bypass. If such tubes are used, it is probably wise to replace them electively at intervals (perhaps three months), rather than waiting for the onset of cholangitis.

Surgical bypass

Biliary–enteric bypass for proximal biliary cancer is more difficult than for distally placed tumours, but it is often possible to carry out a hepaticojejunostomy to the left duct. If the confluence has not been disconnected by the tumour, the right liver will also be drained by this procedure. Even in the absence of such a communication effective palliation will still be obtained provided there is no sepsis within the right liver. When the left duct is involved by tumour it is possible to gain access to an intrahepatic duct within the left liver. In the Longmire procedure part of the left lobe is resected to locate an intrahepatic duct.[138] This procedure has now been superseded by a bypass to the duct of segment III, accessed by splitting the liver just to the left of the umbilical fissure.[139] These authors reported left duct or segment III bypass in 96 patients with an operative mortality of 7%. No internal or external tube is necessary, and the duration of palliation may be excellent. Similar techniques for biliary–enteric bypass have been described to the duct of segment V.

Resection

World-wide experience of resection for hilar cholangiocarcinoma has remained relatively small. Resectability rates reported from specialist units vary widely. The majority of Western series report a resectability rate of 15–20%.[125,140–142] Adoption of a more aggressive policy, including the use of liver transplantation, leads to higher resectability rates of 35–60%.[143–145] The resectability rate described in Japanese series, some with large numbers of patients, has been consistently higher than in Western reports (52–92%.[146–148]). It is not absolutely clear why this should be so, but it reflects in part an increased readiness to undertake extensive resections in these patients, including resections of the portal vein, radical lymphadenectomy, and major hepatic resections.

Some authors believe that resection should be confined to patients in whom cure is a realistic goal, but it may be that debulking of tumour with a good internal biliary–enteric bypass provides palliation which may have useful advantages over intubation or even over simple bypass. One must distinguish between local ductal resection and resection involving hepatectomy, which may be required for tumours which involve second order ducts in the right or left liver. Local resections carry a very low mortality and morbidity, but the addition of major hepatectomy raises mortality considerably (10–30% in recent series). Some surgeons feel that the caudate lobe (segment I) should routinely be removed when removing bile duct cancers, because of the risk of leaving residual tumour (see below).[148,150,151] Resection of the nodes and lymphatics along the hepatoduodenal ligament may also be important for survival. Relatively few authors recommend excision and reconstruction of the portal vein. If a short segment of the portal vein is involved by tumour it is perfectly feasible to resect and re-anastomose it end-to-end,[124] but there is no evidence that more extended resections and vascular reconstruction confer any survival benefit.[151]

Assessment of resectability
Preoperative staging and cytological evaluation should have been carried out before operation is undertaken. The extent of ductal and vascular involvement will determine local resectability, or the need for hepatic resection. The following criteria would suggest an irresectable tumour:

1. Involvement of bilateral second order intrahepatic ducts, or multifocal tumour on cholangiography;
2. Extensive involvement of the main stem of the portal vein;
3. Involvement of major vessels or ducts on opposite sides of the liver;
4. Liver atrophy or infection inconsistent with a viable liver remnant after resection.

The validity of these criteria was examined in a series of 37 consecutive patients studied at Hammersmith Hospital, London.[152] Resection was possible in 23 of 24 patients thought to be potentially resectable before operation. Lymph node involvement and intraperitoneal spread may be difficult to determine preoperatively: laparoscopy may help in this situation. Intraoperative ultrasound may be of value in assessing resectability.[153] Metastatic tumours can appear very well differentiated, and it can be difficult for the pathologist to determine clearance at a resection margin, especially on frozen section, so that this must often await definitive histological examination.

If the tumour is not locally resectable, then the patient may be evaluated for major liver resection in order to gain tumour clearance.[124] This may frequently require an extended right or left hepatectomy, with hepatic duct anastomosis to a loop of jejunum. There is some evidence to support routine removal of segment I. In a series of 66 patients reported by Nimura,[148] 55 cases of hilar carcinoma were resected. Of these 46 were thought to be curative resections, 45 including segment I, and tumour invasion of segment I was found histologically in 44. The three- and five-year survivals of 55% and 40% in these patients are exceptional, and offer support for caudate lobe resection as part of an attempt at curative surgery for advanced hilar cholangiocarcinoma.

Stenting
Several trials have now demonstrated that stenting and surgical bypass are equally effective in the relief of obstructive jaundice due to pancreatic cancer[154] and stenting is attended by a lower hospital mortality rate and

a shorter stay. However, for patients with this relatively favourable tumour and anticipated longer survival the rate of recurrent jaundice and cholangitis may be greater for those with an endoprosthesis than for those treated by surgical bypass. The development of large calibre (up to 1 cm) self-expanding metallic stents has produced a significant improvement, albeit at considerable expense.[155] Their principal application may therefore be in patients with primary malignancy of the bile ducts rather than adenocarcinoma of the head of the pancreas.

Percutaneous stenting The use of percutaneous drainage as a preliminary to operative treatment is addressed below. For patients unsuitable for resection, permanent percutaneous stenting may follow diagnostic and staging PTC.[156,157] Percutaneous placement of conventional stents may require a period of external drainage and dilatation of the track, but self-expanding metal stents can be placed in a single stage. Tumour ingrowth may be less of a problem with cholangiocarcinoma than with pancreatic or ampullary tumours because of their relatively low cellularity and dense stroma. Tumour 'overgrowth' above or below the stent may be more of a problem, but this can be overcome by placing the longest stent available. Occluded stents can be cleared by diathermy,[158] or further stents can be inserted through the obstructed stent (Fig. 7.12), or even from another segmental duct passed through the wall. Our own experience in 202 patients with malignant biliary strictures treated with Wallstent endoprosthesis over seven years showed a re-intervention rate of 12% compared with 22% in a retrospective series of 100 patients treated with plastic stents.[155]

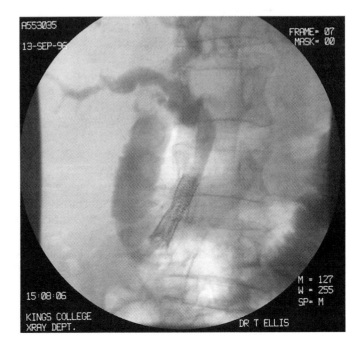

Figure 7.12 *A metallic stent was placed through a distal bile duct tumour in this elderly lady. After 2 years of symptom-free survival, she developed jaundice and cholangitis, and at ERCP the stent was cleared and a plastic stent placed through its lumen, giving rapid relief of symptoms.*

Endoscopic stenting Metallic stents can also be placed endoscopically (Fig. 7.12), combining the advantages of both techniques.[159] The techniques must not be looked upon as competitive, but complementary, and when intubation from below proves difficult or impossible, a combined procedure may be considered, using a percutaneous wire passed through the tumour from above. When endoscopic stenting is possible, it is usually regarded as a less-invasive procedure, and is the first choice for a route of access over percutaneous methods.

Adjuvant therapy

Radiotherapy There are as yet few studies which show any clear survival advantage. Lokich *et al.*[160] reviewed nine such studies, with a total number of only 124 patients. Larger numbers have been reported in the Japanese literature. In 122 patients treated with radiotherapy Nakama[161] reported a longer overall survival in patients who had a good local response, but no clear effect on survival in the group as a whole. Terblanche *et al.*[136] reported several long survivors after radiotherapy with transhepatic U-tubes, but not all had histologically proven tumours.

External beam radiotherapy (total doses used varying between 20 and 60 Gy), may cause radiation duodenitis and intractable gastrointestinal bleeding. To circumvent this problem brachytherapy has been given, using iridium 192, a beta emitter with only a few millimetres depth of penetration, which might slow local progression and delay the onset of biliary obstruction or stent overgrowth. The local dose of 30–50 Gy can be supplemented by another 30–45 Gy external beam irradiation. Delivery has mostly been transhepatic,[162,163] but can be achieved endoscopically via nasobiliary tubes.[164,165] The need for controlled studies has been stressed.[137] The author's experience in treating 39 patients with cholangiocarcinoma over 7 years with combinations of external beam and iridium-192 therapy showed that although treatment was generally well tolerated, no additional benefit could be demonstrated from the addition of the brachytherapy.[166] If radiotherapy is to be used postoperatively, metal clips may be placed to mark the area of the anastomosis after resection, or areas of known or suspected residual tumour.

Intraoperative radiotherapy has been reported from a few specialised centres. Busse *et al.*[167] treated 15 patients with advanced bile duct cancer over a five-year period, using 5–20 Gy, with postoperative radiotherapy also in 13. There was little morbidity and a low mortality, though again the effects on survival are undefined. One study of nine patients,[168] found no significant difference in mean survival or 1-year survival between those patients treated with intraoperative radiotherapy (16.8 months, 56%) and those treated by external beam irradiation with or without iridium-192 (11 months, 46%).

Chemotherapy Bile duct cancer has conventionally been regarded as chemoresistant. Oberfield and Rossi[169] reported a significant local response rate in 29% of 97 patients treated with 5-fluorouracil (5FU) and mitomycin C, alone or in combination with adriamycin (FAM). A report from UCLA[170] described significant response rates and possible survival improvement in seven patients receiving continuous 5FU, with intermittent leucovorin, mitomycin-C and dipyridamole. A number of the author's patients treated recently at the Royal Marsden Hospital, London, have also shown promising responses to continuous infusional 5FU with intermittent epirubicin and cisplatin (D. Cunningham, personal communication). Intra-arterial therapy produced a partial response rate of more than 50%, and a complete response in one of 11 patients in one series including both bile duct and gall bladder cancers, and suggested improved survival for both groups.[171] There remains, however, little evidence from controlled studies for the value of chemotherapy for tumours of the bile duct.

Finally, there is the intriguing but untested possibility of hormone manipulation in biliary cancer. Hudd et al.[172] showed retardation of tumour growth by cholecystokinin in a metastatic cholangiocarcinoma cell line in nude mice.

Liver transplantation

The literature is confused by the reporting of intrahepatic and extrahepatic cholangiocarcinomas as one group. Provided regional nodal metastases and other sites of extrahepatic tumour can be excluded, then total hepatectomy with transplantation may be possible for these patients. The Hanover group have investigated this extensively.[144] In nine patients found to have extrahepatic metastases after liver transplant, most developed tumour recurrence, and the longest survival was 27 months. However all of seven patients without apparent residual tumour appeared to be tumour-free at a follow-up at 21 months. The dilemma, therefore, remains that patients with well localised tumours are likely to survive transplantation and immunosuppression, but these are also the patients likely to be amenable to conventional local resection. Few of those patients whose tumours have transgressed the boundaries of local resectability will be suitable for transplantation. Current studies therefore remain opposed to transplantation for this indication.

Results

There remains no clear consensus as to the optimum methods of evaluation or as to treatment of these difficult cases. On the one hand, several authors are reporting higher resectability rates and more complex forms of resection, whereas, on the other hand, radiologists and endoscopists have made technical advances resulting in more expeditious treatment of patients and shorter hospital stay. Although philosophically it is reasonable to accept that the only prospects of cure are afforded by complete resection of the cancer, it is by no means certain that this is so, nor indeed that complete as opposed to almost complete resection followed by adjuvant therapy confers a significant survival advantage in the majority of cases.[173] Little[174] has reviewed this dichotomy of views. The one thing which stands out through all these reports is the need for a unified approach to assessment of quality of survival and palliation. Bismuth[123] defined the 'Comfort Index', the proportion of a patient's actual survival which is spent in good condition, effectively palliated, and demonstrated excellent results from a left-sided biliary–enteric anastomosis.

What survival results can actually be obtained? It is important to take account of the mortality of surgical treatment, which is not inconsiderable. Mortality is reasonably low for those not requiring hepatectomy, but has been reported as high as 70% for those in whom liver resection is required, though the most recent series[148] reported only four deaths in 51 patients undergoing liver resection, including in the majority of cases resection of the caudate lobe. Few authors quote five-year survival rates following radical treatment, and the reported mean survivals vary from nine months to 3.6 years and the median from 7 to 15 months. Among the best results are those from Nimura,[151] detailed below. Our own experience[173] in almost 200 patients treated over a ten-year period was that 22% of patients were suitable for resection. A total of 44 cases underwent resection. Three of these were carried out as emergency procedures because of liver necrosis or abscess formation due to previous treatment, and one patient who underwent local resection subsequently went on to liver transplantation. Thus there were 40 patients who underwent elective resection alone available for follow-up. Comparison with patients who underwent bypass or stenting showed a significant survival advantage for this (highly selected) resection group. The 40 patients who underwent resection were classified retrospectively into those with residual disease (either involved lymph nodes or tumour at the resection margins) and those without: 17 patients with known or suspected residual disease and 18 with potentially curative resection left hospital and were available for follow-up. All those with involved margins died within five years, whereas the actuarial five-year survival for those with clear margins approached 25%. Thus the likelihood of complete cure in the treatment group as a whole remains small, and it is important to concentrate the aims of surgery for cholangiocarcinoma on the relief of obstruction and prevention of cholangitis. Most patients not suitable for resection can be treated by internal drainage, 87% in the first five years of our series, and 97% in the second five years. This reflects both greater determination to achieve internal drainage and improvements in radiological technology.

Nimura et al.[151] described the management of 127 cases of hilar cholangiocarcinoma over 16 years; 110 were operated upon with 100 resections. All but nine patients had combined hepatic and hilar ductal resection, including the caudate lobe, with an overall hospital mortality following resection of 10%. Resection was thought to be 'curative' in 82/100, and in this group there was a 33-month median survival and a 31% 5-year actuarial survival. In the 'palliative' group the comparable figures were 18 month median and 14% 3-year survival, and no patient survived 4 years. The 'curative' group included 27 patients with portal vein resection and 12 with synchronous pancreatoduodenectomy en bloc (five with both), a formidable procedure: the 5-year survival for those with portal vein resection was only 5%, and for those without this manoeuvre it was 43%.

Recommendations

In the light of these findings we must stress the basic principles of treatment of hilar cholangiocarcinoma. The first of these is accurate diagnosis, followed by a full anatomical assessment of the tumour. Preoperative diagnosis may be aided by cytological examination. Long-term palliation depends on draining the maximum volume of functioning hepatic tissue possible, and if this includes tumour clearance, then that is the ideal. Stenting, especially with metallic stents, provides reliable palliation in most irresectable patients, and operative bypass is mostly now confined to patients who are explored but found to be irresectable, or in whom stenting has failed or been attended by severe recurrent cholangitis. Radiotherapy will probably occupy a declining role, and chemotherapy an increasing one. Finally, many patients in the past have died due to inadequate treatment of recurrent cholangitis, and such episodes must be treated vigorously. Stenting is well worthwhile for local recurrence and can give a useful period of prolonged palliation. Attention to these basic principles will give the best overall results for this difficult condition, even when curative resection is not possible.

Carcinoma of the gall bladder (GB)

This tumour represents only 2% of all cancers, but is the commonest site of cancer in the biliary tract.

Aetiology

Up to 70% of patients with GB cancer have gallstones, in contrast to some 13% for other biliary cancers.[109] The incidence of GB cancer is increased 14.7-fold 20 years after surgery for gastric ulcer.[114] Chronic inflammation due to typhoid appears to carry an increased risk. 'Porcelain' GB, with intramural calcification, is a premalignant condition. There is, however, little convincing evidence that benign polyps undergo malignant change. There are high risk ethnic groups, most notably South-West American Indians. The high incidence of the anomalous common bile duct and pancreatic duct junction has already been noted above.

Pathology

These are mostly mucus-secreting adenocarcinomas, though a few are squamous or adenosquamous. The staging and grading system adopted for these tumours is that of Nevin et al.[175] The grade is divided into I–III: well, moderately, or poorly differentiated. The Stages are I–V. Stage I tumours are confined to the mucosa; stage II tumours breach the muscularis mucosae; stage III tumours extend through the muscularis propria; stage IV additionally involves the cystic node; and stage V involves the liver or other organs, usually segments IV and V in the gallbladder bed. Nevin's score, a sum of stage and grade, directly affects survival: no patients in his series with a score of more than 6 survived 1 year.

Presentation

The peak age of incidence is 70–75 years. GB cancer may be silent for a long time, and the commonest diagnosis is made postoperatively in GBs removed for stone disease. This may be a particular problem in laparoscopic cholecystectomy, because of the risk of tumour implantation at the extraction port.

Symptomatic cancers may present with biliary obstruction, and preoperative investigation including ERCP, PTC and scanning may fail to make the distinction between cancer of the GB, Klatskin tumour and Mirizzi syndrome. Some patients with GB cancer present with acute cholecystitis or with empyema of the GB: in order not to miss such a diagnosis biopsy of the gall bladder is mandatory in patients treated by cholecystostomy.[176]

Investigation

Laboratory tests are non-specific. Plain abdominal radiograph is of limited value, but may show calcification suggestive of gallstones or gall bladder wall calcification ('porcelain gall bladder'). The preoperative diagnosis may be suggested by a mass on ultrasound, which has a reported sensitivity of 44%.[177] These findings may be confirmed by CT scanning. Direct cholangiography is usually required. Involvement of the duct of segment V by a GB mass is highly suggestive of cancer. Arteriography may show vascular involvement in advanced disease.

Management

Prophylactic cholecystectomy, except in cases of porcelain GB, is not indicated, as the risks outweigh the benefits. Treatment of the established tumour depends on staging, and on the mode of presentation. Once cancer of the gall bladder has invaded the hilar ducts and caused obstructive jaundice, it is rarely resectable for cure. When cancer of the gall bladder occurs as an incidental finding at open cholecystectomy the surgeon should if possible make a full assessment at the time of operation and decide whether a curative excision is reasonable. If a well-localised tumour is found, a wedge resection of the gall bladder bed or a formal excision of segments IV and V may be considered. Adson and Farnell[178] in the Mayo Clinic found only 12 patients of 112 whose tumours were resectable. Seven out of eight who had simple cholecystectomy were dead within 15 months, and the four who underwent radical excision had a longer survival. Shirai et al.[179] reoperated on 14/98 stage III cancers, and found residual tumour at re-resection in seven: however, only two of these seven survived 22 and 105 months. Evander and Ihse[180] demonstrated no survival advantage for radical resection in ten of 44 patients. Local invasion remains the overwhelming determinant of survival even after radical excision, and a significant number of patients with early (stage I) disease found incidentally will survive for many years.

In symptomatic (usually jaundiced) patients in whom the diagnosis is made or suspected preoperatively, very few will be resectable. These patients are best treated by stenting or by internal bypass, as described above. The round ligament or left duct approach may be valuable, because the anastomosis is at a safe distance from the tumour.

Adjuvant therapy

Some authors have reported useful responses and some long survival after external beam radiotherapy, but there are no controlled data. Conventionally regarded as chemoresistant, some GB cancers have shown significant responses to combination chemotherapy, similar to that used in bile duct tumours (see above).

Results

The factors influencing survival are described above: overall the five-year survival of patients with primary gall bladder cancer is usually less than 5%.

Functional disorders

Functional disorders causing pain have been difficult to define in the past, but improved understanding of the complex pressure relationships within the biliary tract (see above) has allowed a reasonable classification. Pain of 'biliary' origin in the absence of gallstones or other organic biliary disease may be attributed to gall bladder dyskinesia or sphincter of Oddi dysfunction (SOD). Administration of cholecystokinin to simulate biliary symptoms has a long history, but its specificity is very poor. This may be improved by quantitative scintigraphy, in which the gall bladder ejection fraction is measured in response to an infusion of cholecystokinin (CCK).[181] Toouli's group randomised patients with a gall bladder ejection fraction of less than 40% to cholecystectomy or follow-up: patients who had a cholecystectomy were cured of their symptoms and found to have histological changes of chronic cholecystitis. Most of the control patients continued to experience pain, and many later underwent cholecystectomy.

The second category (SOD) includes patients with organic stenosis (due to passage of small stones, to postoperative trauma or to an intrinsic stenosis of the sphincter) or sphincter of Oddi dyskinesia. Manometric studies may show retrograde propagation of phasic waves or an increased frequency of phasic contraction, or a paradoxical response in which the sphincter of Oddi contracts rather than relaxes to cholecystokinin. Elegant controlled follow-up studies have been conducted in which these patients were treated either by endoscopic sphincterotomy or manometry alone.[182] Most patients with raised sphincter of Oddi basal pressure became asymptomatic after sphincterotomy, whereas most controls continued to have symptoms.

Evaluation of these complex conditions remains difficult, but has now become more objective. Selection of patients for endoscopic sphincterotomy or for transduodenal sphincteroplasty and transampullary septectomy[183] can be based on rational criteria and futile procedures avoided. However, the investigations involved remain confined to specialist units.

Operative approaches

Preoperative preparation

Attention to nutrition is of great importance, both because of the general effects of the tumour and of obstructive jaundice and malabsorption. An assessment of weight loss should be made preoperatively, and there is an argument for instituting parenteral feeding in patients who have lost more than 10% of body weight. It has been suggested that a period of percutaneous transhepatic biliary drainage may allow more rapid improvement of nutrition by means intravenous feeding,[184] though this has been disputed.[185]

Renal function is extremely important. It has long been known that there is an increased tendency to acute renal failure in obstructive jaundice.[186] Intravenous fluids should be administered to all patients who are deeply jaundiced, especially if they are to be fasted overnight for operation. Mannitol diuresis is still sometimes used intraoperatively. Adminstration of bile salts to reduce the absorption of endotoxins, has been shown to be of value in this respect though not all preparations are equally efficacious.[187] A controlled trial of percutaneous transhepatic biliary drainage showed that rehydration alone produced as great an improvement in renal function as rehydration combined with biliary drainage.[188] Nakayama *et al*[189] claimed a significant reduction in mortality by using external biliary drainage. However, several controlled trials have been reported,[190–192] most of which showed no such improvement. Returning bile to the gastrointestinal tract may be better than relief of biliary obstruction by means of external drainage.[193] Internal drainage by means of endoscopic stenting may still be indicated for patients who are severely jaundiced, and particularly those suffering from acute cholangitis and some authors use this routinely.

Biliary resection and reconstruction – a general operative approach

Incisions and exploration

The bilateral subcostal ('rooftop') incision is widely used, giving wide access to the upper abdomen, and allows mobilisation of the liver. The use of a fixed retractor system (such as the Omnitract®) allows constant wide exposure.

After opening the abdomen the liver and supracolic compartment are inspected. The umbilical ligament is divided between ligatures and the falciform ligament is divided using the diathermy, to allow the placement of a retractor. If liver resection is to be performed this division is taken back to the level of the suprahepatic IVC. The liver is gently mobilised upwards. If there are dense adhesions following previous surgery it may be helpful to start from the right side, mobilising the colon and greater omentum from the undersurface of the liver. The duodenum is frequently adherent to the gall bladder bed or to the area of a biliary stricture, and this is gently retracted downwards and adhesions divided.

Principles

The ideal of biliary–enteric anastomosis is to secure drainage of all liver segments if possible, preferably by a wide mucosa-to-mucosa anastomosis to a well-defunctioned loop of jejunum. The observation that the left hepatic duct is invariably an extrahepatic structure, and can be accessed below segment IV of the liver, allows a useful approach to the hilar ducts, even in cases where there is dense stricture formation below this level.

Dissection of the hilar plate

A broad-bladed retractor is placed beneath segment IV and gently lifted, and adhesions freed until the region of the hilar plate is identified. When there are dense adhesions medially, it is best to work from the left side, commencing close to the umbilical fissure. The bridge connecting segments III and IV across the base of the fissure is of variable thickness, but contains no important structures, and can be divided safely. This allows the space beneath segment IV to be more readily opened, and dissection along the hilar plate commenced from left to right allowing the left hepatic duct to be gradually lowered. In cases where there is tumour involvement of the left duct this approach may have to be abandoned in favour of accessing the intrahepatic duct of segment III to the left of the umbilical ligament (see below).

The left hepatic duct can be identified if necessary by aspiration with a fine needle. Stay sutures are placed in the duct, the duct opened using a knife, and the opening extended with fine angled scissors. A length of 2–3 cm may be obtained by extending the opening in the left duct as far as the base of the umbilical fissure. Pursuing the opening towards the confluence will allow access to the right duct above the level of a high stricture (Bismuth type III). However, if there is complete separation of the right and left ducts (Bismuth type IV) then a separate approach to the right duct may have to be adopted. The lowering of the hilar plate can be continued across to the right side, though it is less easily defined here. In some difficult circumstances the duct of segment V may be accessed at the base of the gallbladder bed, and used for separate anastomosis.

In treating benign biliary strictures this wide opening in the hepatic duct may be adequate for anastomosis. It is, however, important to determine that all the segmental ducts are represented, and if there is doubt then cholangiography through separate ductal orifices may be helpful. This is most readily done using fluoroscopy, using a fine irrigating catheter with an occlusion balloon in each orifice in turn.

Preparation of Roux limb

This will not be described in detail. The limb of jejunum should be long enough to prevent reflux of liquids as far as the anastomosis. Reflux can be demonstrated along the full length of a 40 cm limb, and it is this author's practice to use a 70 cm length, brought up in a retrocolic position to the right of the middle colic vessels. Although an anastomosis can be performed to the very apex of the loop, if an access loop is to be used then a side-to-side anastomosis will be performed more distally to allow tension-free apposition to the peritoneum of the abdominal wall.

Anastomosis

Many variants have been described, but a safe, reliable and almost universally applicable technique is that described by Voyles and Blumgart.[194] Fine absorbable sutures are used, such as 4/0 PDS or Vicryl. The anterior row of sutures is placed first, starting from the apex of the left duct and working to the right, and placing the sutures from inside the duct to outside. Each suture is held (needles attached) in turn with a rubber-shod clamp, and kept in order. Once the upper row of sutures is in place then a jejunotomy is made, shorter than the apparent length required, to allow for the invariable stretching of the jejunotomy. The posterior row of sutures is then placed, again working from left to right, placing the needles from within the lumen of the gut to the serosa, and from outside to inside the posterior lip of the hepatic duct or ducts. Once again all the sutures are held in order and then the jejunum can be 'railroaded' down into position and all the stitches tied to complete the back row. If a trans-anastomotic tube is to be used (see below) this is best brought through the blind end of the Roux loop and led out through the jejunotomy before the back row is tied down. The tube is then placed into the selected hepatic duct, and may be sutured in place with a finer absorbable stitch, which will not resist removal of the tube in about a week's time. The held anterior row of sutures is now used to pick up the anterior wall of the jejunum, moving from right to left, and the sutures held in order again. When the final suture has been placed they are tied, moving from left to right, so that the knots are on the inside of the anastomosis, achieving a good mucosal apposition with a small amount of inversion. The anastomosis is now complete.

Access loop

Various techniques have been described for this.[195] Some authors use the technique selectively when a problem with the anastomosis is anticipated, but it has been the author's practice to use it almost universally. The purpose of the access loop is to allow radiological intervention avoiding a transhepatic route, and the ability of the radiologist to puncture the loop successfully is entirely dependent on the quality of the marking of the loop.[196] The author has evolved a simple method of doing this using a 2/0 stainless steel braided suture, which is placed around the end of the Roux loop using shallow seromuscular bites, encircling the point of exit of the trans-anastomotic tube. The tube is then brought out through the abdominal wall, and the end of the loop tacked to the peritoneum using four quadrant sutures of Vicryl. The position of the loop is important: it should lie away from the midline to avoid difficulties for the radiologist, and should be neither redundant nor under tension. This position must be carefully assessed before choosing the site for the hepaticojejunostomy.

Variants

The above technique is almost universally applicable, but a number of variants may be necessary. If there is complete separation of hepatic ducts which are to be used for anastomosis, a row of orifices can be treated as if there were a single duct, and the sutures placed and held in order in the same manner. Separate jejunotomies are made in appropriate positions for each duct, but again the posterior rows are placed in order from left to right and the anastomoses completed as described above. This is in practice much easier than attempting to complete each anastomosis separately, since access may become very difficult once the limb of jejunum is in place at the hilus.

If there are adjacent orifices of hepatic duct which can easily be apposed without tension then it is reasonable to do this with a few interrupted sutures, converting two ducts into one for the purpose of anastomosis. However, this should not be done if there is any degree of separation, or if extensive dissection is required between the ducts, because there is danger of damaging intervening intrahepatic vessels at this level.

The round ligament approach

This technique is useful when tumour obliterates the left hepatic duct. The approach is based on the fact that the duct of segment III runs in a relatively constant position to the left of the umbilical fissure, and can be accessed by dividing the liver just to the left of the falciform ligament. If this is done from the anterior surface of the liver then no significant portal vein branches should be encountered in front of the duct. Intraoperative ultrasound may be useful in locating the duct in difficult cases. The use of the cavitron ultrasonic surgical aspirator (CUSA) to divide the liver to the left of the falciform ligament may help to keep the field bloodless, which is important for identifying the duct. Once the duct is found an opening is made which can be extended proximally and distally, and often an anastomosis of 1 cm or longer can be achieved. The technique of anastomosis is as described above, except that if the liver is stiff and the duct deeply placed it may be difficult to get the side of the jejunal limb to lie comfortably in position for anastomosis. In this case the 'corner' of the jejunum (which has been divided with an intestinal stapling device) can be opened and will provide less of an obstacle in creating the anastomosis. This does not preclude the use of an access point, which can be achieved by attaching the side of the jejunal loop to an appropriate point on the peritoneum of the abdominal wall, marked as before.[196]

Postoperative management

The general management of the patient will not be detailed here, except to note that continued attention must be paid to fluid and electrolyte balance, to renal function and to the coagulation status. It is the author's practice to place a closed tube drain close to the anastomosis in every case. This drain can often be removed after 48 h, but if there is any bile leakage it should be left in place longer. If a trans-anastomotic tube has been placed then a cholangiogram can be performed at one week, and the anastomosis checked for any small residual leaks. This cholangiogram allows identification of all anastomosed ducts, which may be important for the future if problems of cholangitis should arise. The tube can usually be removed at seven days. The marked site of the access loop remains visible for future radiological access (Fig. 7.10).

Resections for bile duct cancer

The principles of the anastomosis following local resection, or after removal of the extrahepatic ducts combined with liver resection, are those described above. Local resection of a bile duct cancer is reasonable if it can be demonstrated that adequate ducts will be available for anastomosis after removing the hilar mass. This should be ascertained initially by dissection in the region of the hilar plate as described above or by intraoperative ultrasound. Once it appears likely that this can be achieved then there is nothing to lose by dividing the bile duct distally as low as possible, and gradually mobilising the duct and associated tumour off the underlying vessels. These tumours are often attended by a considerable thickening of lymphatic tissues and the peritoneum overlying the free edge of the lesser omentum may be quite stout. All of this tissue should be elevated en bloc, and the lymphatics surrounding the hepatic artery dissected forward with the specimen. It is at this point that invasion of the anterior surface of the portal vein may be identified for the first time, and a decision must then be made whether to continue with a palliative resection leaving if necessary a small rim of tumour on the portal vein, or whether dissection of part of the wall of the portal vein is feasible. Sometimes only part of the circumference of the vein needs to be removed, and this can be done using a curved vascular clamp. On other occasions it may be necessary to remove a segment of vein, which can be re-anastomosed end-to-end after Kocherisation of the duodenum to remove tension from the vein, or a short length of graft of jugular vein or artificial material inserted. It has already been noted above that the results of such resections and reconstructions are often poor and the justification for their performance is dubious. However, minor resection of the portal venous wall may well be justified and delay local recurrence.

Once the tumour can be lifted as far as the confluence, the dissection can be continued from below to above, or the left hepatic duct divided and the tumour removed from left to right. The value of frozen section of the resection margins at this stage is limited because of difficulties in identifying tumour. The techniques for combining resection of hilar tumours with major liver resection have been described in detail elsewhere, and will not be elaborated upon in this chapter.[124]

If postoperative radiotherapy is to be contemplated then metal clips may be used to mark areas of residual tumour or the area of the anastomosis. The use of an access loop is valuable for bile duct cancers, because local recurrence may require treatment by stenting, which can be readily performed through such an access loop.

References

1. Hadjis NS, Adam A, Gibson R *et al*. Non-operative approach to hilar cancer determined by the atrophy–hypertrophy complex. Am J Surg 1989; 157: 395–9.
2. Couinaud, Le Foie. Etudes anatomiques et chirurgicales. Paris: Masson, 1957.
3. Northover JMA, Terblanche J. Applied surgical anatomy of the biliary tree. In: Blumgart LH (ed.) Biliary tract. Edinburgh: Churchill Livingstone, 1982; vol. 5.
4. Beinart C, Efremedis S, Cohen B, Mitty HA. Obstruction without dilation. Importance in evaluating jaundice. JAMA 1981; 245 353–6.
5. McPherson GAD, Blenkharn JI, Nathanson B, Bowley NB, Benjamin IS, Blumgart LH. Significance of bacteria in external biliary drainage systems: a possible role for antisepsis. J Clin Surg 1982b; 1: 22–6.
6. Maki T. Pathogenesis of calcium bilirubinate gallstones: role of *E. coli* betaglucuronidase and coagulation by inorganic ions, polyelectrolytes and agitation. Ann Surg 1966; 164: 90–100.
7. Lipsett PA, Pitt HA. Cholangitis: non-toxic and toxic. In: Blumgart LH (ed.) Surgery of the liver and biliary tract, 2nd edn. London: Churchill Livingstone, 1992, vol 2, pp. 1081–9.
8. Sandblom P. Haemobilia. In: Blumgart LH (ed.) Surgery of the liver and biliary tract, 2nd edn. London: Churchill Livingstone, 1992, vol 2, pp. 1259–74.
9. McPherson GAD, Benjamin IS, Boobis AR, Blumgart LH. Antipyrine elimination in patients with obstructive jaundice: a predictor of outcome. Am J Surg 1985; 149: 140–3.
10. McPherson GAD, Benjamin IS, Hodgson HJF, Bowley NB, Allison DJ, Blumgart LH. Preoperative percutaneous transhepatic biliary drainage: the results of a controlled trial. Br J Surg 1984; 71: 371–5.
11. Howard ER. Surgery of liver disease in children. Oxford: Butterworth Heinemann, 1991.
12. Jenner RE, Howard ER. Unsaturated monohydroxy bile acids as a cause of idiopathic obstructive cholangiography. Lancet 1975; ii: 1073–4.
13. Kasai M, Suzuki S. A new operation for 'non-correctable' biliary atresia: hepatic portoenterostomy. Shujitsu 1959; 13: 733–9.
14. Mieli-Vergani G, Howard ER, Portmann B, Mowat AP. Late referral for biliary atresia – missed opportunities for effective surgery. Lancet 1989; i: 421–3.
15. Ohi R, Chiba T, Ohkochi N *et al*. The present status of surgical treatment for biliary atresia: reports of the questionnaire for the main institutions in Japan. In: Ohi R (ed.) Biliary

atresia. Professional Postgraduate Services, Tokyo, 1987; pp. 125–30.

16. Iwatsuki S. Liver transplantation for children with biliary atresia. In: Ohi R (ed.) Biliary atresia. Professional Postgraduate Services, Tokyo, 1987; pp. 315–19.

17. Howard ER, Driver M, McClement J, Mowat AP. Results of surgery in 88 consecutive cases of extrahepatic biliary atresia. J R Soc Med 1982; 75: 408–13.

18. Kato T, Hebiguchi T, Matsuda K, Yoshino H. Action of pancreatic juice on the bile duct: pathogenesis of congenital choledochal cyst. J Paediatr Surg 1981; 16: 146–51.

19. Alonso-Lej F, Rever WB Jr, Pessagno DJ. Congenital choledochal cysts, with a report of 2, and an analysis of 94 cases. Surg Gynecol Obstet 1959; 108: 1–30.

20. Ono J, Sakoda K, Akita H. Surgical aspects of cystic dilatation of the bile duct – an anomalous junction of the pancreatobiliary tract in adults. Ann Surg 1982; 195: 203–8.

21. Voyles CR, Smadja C, Shands C, Blumgart LH. Carcinoma in choledochal cysts – age-related incidence. Arch Surg 1983; 118: 986–8.

22. Davenport M, Howard ER. Spontaneous perforation of the bile duct in infancy. In: Howard ER (ed.) Surgery of liver disease in children. Oxford: Butterworth Heinemann, 1987, pp. 91–3.

23. Khuroo MS, Sarjar SA, Mahajan R. Hepatobiliary and pancreatic ascariasis in India. Lancet 1990; 335: 1503–6.

24. Fan ST, Wong J. Recurrent pyogenic cholangitis. In: Blumgart LH (ed.) Surgery of the liver and biliary tract. London: Churchill Livingstone, 2nd ed., 1994, pp. 1151–73.

25. Jan Y, Chen M, Wang C et al. Surgical treatment of hepatolithiasis: long-term results. Surgery 1996; 120: 509–14.

26. Ludwig J. Surgical pathology of the syndrome of primary sclerosing cholangitis. Am J Surg Pathol 1989; (Supplement 1): 43–9.

27. Chapman RW, Kelly PM, Heryet A, Jewell DP, Flemming KA. Expression of HLA-DR antigens on bile duct epithelium in primary sclerosing cholangitis. Gut 1988; 29: 422–7.

28. Gavaler JS, Delemos B, Belle SH et al. Ulcerative colitis disease activity as subjectively assessed by patient-completed questionnaires following orthotopic liver transplantation for sclerosing cholangitis. Dig Dis Sci 1991; 36: 321–8.

29. Marsh JW, Iwatsuki S, Makoka L et al. Orthotopic liver transplantation for primary sclerosing cholangitis. Ann Surg 1988; 207: 21–5.

30. Standfield NJ, Salisbury JR, Howard ER. Benign non-traumatic inflammatory strictures of the extrahepatic biliary system. Br J Surg 1989; 76: 849–52.

31. Stamatakis JD, Howard ER, Williams R. Benign inflammatory strictures of the common bile duct. Br J Surg 1979; 66: 257–8.

32. Hadjis NS, Collier NA, Blumgart LH. Malignant masquerade at the hilum of the liver. Br J Surg 1984; 72: 659–61.

33. Smadja C, Bowley NB, Benjamin IS, Blumgart LH. Idiopathic localised bile duct strictures: relationship to primary sclerosing cholangitis. Am J Surg 1983; 146: 404–8.

34. Blumgart LH. Benign biliary strictures. In: Blumgart LH (ed.) Surgery of the liver and biliary tract. Edinburgh: Churchill Livingstone, 1988, vol. 1, pp. 721–52.

35. Smith R. Injuries of the bile ducts. In: Smith LR, Sherlock S (eds) Surgery of the gallbladder and bile ducts. London: Butterworth, 1981, pp. 361–81.

36. Andren-Sandberg A, Alinder G, Bengmark S. Accidental lesions of the common bile duct at cholecystectomy: pre- and perioperative factors of importance. Ann Surg 1985; 201: 328–32.

37. Moossa AR, Easter DW, van Sonnenberg E et al. Laparoscopic injuries to the bile duct: a cause for concern. Ann Surg 1992; 215: 203–8.

38. Davidoff AM, Pappas TN, Murray AE et al. Mechanisms of major biliary injury during laparoscopic cholecystectomy. Ann Surg 1992; 215: 196–202.

39. Peters JH, Gibbons GD, Innes JT et al. Complications of laparoscopic cholecystectomy. Surgery 1991; 110: 769–78.

40. Meyers WC, Branum GD, Farouk M et al. A prospective analysis of 1518 laparoscopic cholecystectomies. N Engl J Med 1991; 324: 1073–8.

41. Way LW. Bile duct injury during laparoscopic cholecystectomy. Ann Surg 1992; 215: 195.

42. Cameron JL, Gadacz TR. Laparoscopic surgery. Ann Surg 1991; 213: 1–2.

43. Smith R. Injuries to the common bile duct during laparoscopic cholecystectomy (letter). Br Med J 1991; 303: 1475.

44. Deziel DJ, Millikan KW, Economou SG, Doolas A, Ko ST, Airan MC. Complications of laparoscopic cholecystectomy: a national survey of 4292 hospitals and an analysis of 77 604 cases. Am J Surg 1993; 165: 9–14.

45. Larson GM, Vitale GC, Casey J et al. Multipractice analysis of laparoscopic cholecystectomy in 1983 patients. Am J Surg 1992; 163: 221–6.

46. Kozarek R, Gannan R, Baerg R, Wagonfeld J, Ball T. Bile leak after laparoscopic cholecystectomy: diagnostic and therapeutic applications in endoscopic retrograde cholangiopancreatography. Arch Intern Med 1992; 152: 1040–3.

47. Fullarton GM, Bell G. Prospective audit of the introduction of laparoscopic cholecystectomy in the west of Scotland. West of Scotland Laparoscopic Cholecystectomy Audit Group. Gut 1984; 35: 1121–6.

48. Schol FP, Go PM, Gouma DJ. Risk factors for bile duct injury in laparoscopic cholecystectomy: analysis of 49 cases. Br J Surg 1995; 82: 565–6.

49. Richardson MC, Bell G, Fullarton M. Incidence and nature of bile duct injuries following laparoscopic cholecystectomy: an audit of 5913 cases. Br J Surg 1996; 83: 1356–60.

50. Bismuth H. Postoperative strictures of the bile duct. In: Blumgart LH (ed.) The biliary tract. Clinical surgery international. Edinburgh: Churchill Livingstone, 1982, vol 5, pp. 209–18.

51. Peters JH, Ellison C, Innes JT et al. Safety and efficacy of laparoscopic cholecystectomy: a prospective analysis of 100 initial patients. Ann Surg 1991; 213: 3–12.

52. Chapman WC, Halevy A, Blumgart LH, Benjamin IS. Postcholecystectomy bile duct strictures. Arch Surg 1995; 130: 597–604.

53. Scott-Coombes D, Thompson JN. Bile duct stones and laparoscopic cholecystectomy: selective intraoperative cholangiography is the best strategy. Br Med J 1991; 303: 1281–2.

54. Berci G, Sackier JM, Partlow MP. Routine or selected intraoperative cholangiography during laparoscopic cholecystectomy? Am J Surg 1991; 161: 355–60.

55. Fletcher DR. Biliary injury at laparoscopic cholecystectomy: recognition and prevention. Aust NZ J Surg 1993; 63: 673–7.

56. Csendes A, Diaz JC, Burdiles P, Maluenda F. Late results of immediate primary end to end repair in accidental section of the common bile duct. Surg Gynecol Obstet 1989; 168: 125–30.

57. Smith LR. Obstructions of the bile duct. Br J Surg 1979; 66: 69–79.

58. Wexler MJ, Smith R. Jejunal mucosal grafts: a sutureless technique for repair of high bile duct strictures. Am J Surg 1975; 129: 204–11.

59. Hepp J, Couinaud C. L'abord et l'utilisation du canal hepatique gauche dans les reparations de la voie biliare principle. Presse Med 1956; 64: 947–8.

60. Vogel SB, Howard RJ, Caridi J et al. Evaluation of percutaneous transhepatic balloon dilatation of benign biliary strictures in high-risk patients. Am J Surg 1985; 149: 73–9.

61. Mueller PR, van Sonnenberg E, Ferrucci JT et al. Biliary stricture dilatation: multicenter review of clinical management in 73 patients. Radiology 1986; 160: 17–22.

62. Coons HG. Self-expanding stainless steel biliary stents. Radiology 1989; 170: 979–83.

63. Pitt HA, Kaufman SL, Coleman J et al. Benign postoperative biliary strictures: operate or dilate? Ann Surg 1989; 210: 417–27.

64. Warren KW, McDonald WM. Facts and fiction regarding strictures of the extrahepatic bile ducts. Ann Surg 1964; 159: 996–1010.

65. Pitt HA, Miyamoto T, Parapatis SK et al. Factors influencing outcome in patients with postoperative biliary strictures. Am J Surg 1982; 144: 14–21.

66. Braasch JW, Bolton JS, Rossi RL. A technique of biliary tract reconstruction with complete follow-up in 44 consecutive cases. Ann Surg 1981; 194: 635–8.

67. Bismuth H, Franco D, Corlette MB et al. Long term results of Roux-en-y hepaticojejunostomy. Surg Gynecol Obstet 1978; 146: 161–7.

68. Moossa AR, Block GE, Skinner DB. Reconstruction of high biliary tract strictures employing transhepatic intubation. Surg Clin North Am 1976; 56: 73–81.

69. Beazley RM, Blumgart LH. Benign tumours and pseudotumors of the biliary tract. In: Blumgart LH (ed.) Surgery of the liver and biliary tract. Edinburgh: Churchill Livingstone, 1988; vol. 2, pp. 807–18.

70. Albores-Saavedra J, Henson DE, Sobin LH. The WHO histological classification of tumors of the gallbladder and extrahepatic bile ducts. A commentary on the second edition. Cancer 1992; 70: 410–14.

71. Yeung EC, McCarthy P, Gompertz RH, Benjamin IS, Gibson RN, Dawson P. The ultrasonographic appearances of hilar cholangiocarcinoma (Klatskin tumour). Br J Radiol 1988; 61: 991–5.

72. Cho C, Rullis I, Rogers LS. Bile duct adenomas as liver nodules. Arch Surg 1978; 113: 272–4.

73. Foulk WT. Congenital malformations of the intrahepatic biliary tree in the adult (Editorial). Gastroenterology 1970; 58: 253–6.

74. Kozuka S, Tsubone M, Hachisuka K. Evolution of carcinoma in the extrahepatic bile ducts. Cancer 1984; 54: 65–72.

75. Hubens G, Delvaux G, Willems G, Bourgain C, Kloppel G. Papillomatosis of the intra- and extrahepatic bile ducts with involvement of the pancreatic duct. Hepato-Gastroenterology 1991; 38: 413–18.

76. Mercadier M, Bodard M, Fingerhut A, Chigot J. Papillomatosis of the intrahepatic bile ducts. World J Surg 1984; 8: 30–5.

77. Gouma DJ, Mutum S, Benjamin IS, Blumgart LH. Intrahepatic biliary papillomatosis. Br J Surg 1984; 71: 72–4.

78. Hadjis NS, Slater RN, Blumgart LH. Mucobilia: an unusual cause of jaundice. Br J Surg 1987; 74: 48–9.

79. Caroli J. Disease of the intrahepatic biliary tree. Clin Gastroenterol 1973; 2: 147–61.

80. Caroli J, Soupault R, Champeau M, Eteve J, Hivet M. Papillomes et papillomatons de la voie biliaire principale. Rev Med Chir Malad Foie 1959; 34: 191–230.

81. Smith MJG. Multiple biliary papillomatosis. Cancer 1974; 34: 1316–20.

82. Cattel RB, Braasch JW, Kahn F. Polypoid epithelial tumors of the bile ducts. N Engl J Med 1962; 266: 57–61.

83. Newmann R, Livolsi V, Rosental N, Burrell M, Ball T. Adeno-carcinoma in biliary papillomatosis. Gastroenterology 1976; 70: 779–82.

84. Padfield C, Ansell I, Furness P. Mucinous biliary papillomatosis: a tumor in need of wider recognition. Histopathology 1988; 13: 687–94.

85. Rogers KE. Papillary cystadenoma of the common hepatic duct. Can Med Assoc J 1956; 55: 597–9.

86. Melnick PJ. Polycystic liver. Analysis of seventy cases. Arch Pathol 1955; 59: 162–72.

87. Ishak KG, Willis GW, Cummins SD, Bullock AA. Biliary cystadenoma and cystadenocarcinoma. A report of 14 cases and review of the literature. Cancer 1977; 38: 322–38.

88. Forrest ME, Cho KJ, Shields JJ, Wicks JD, Silver TM, McCormick TLK. Biliary cystadenomas: sonographic–angiographic–pathologic correlations. Am J Roentgenol 1980; 135: 723–7.

89. Wheeler DA, Edmondson HA. Cystadenoma with mesenchymal stroma (CMS) in the liver and bile ducts. A clinicopathologic study of 17 cases, 4 with malignant change. Cancer 1985; 56: 1434–45.

90. Korobkin M, Stephens DH, Lee JKT *et al.* Biliary cystadenoma and cystadenocarcinoma. CT and sonographic findings. Am J Roentgenol 1989; 53: 507–11.

91. Lewis WD, Jenkins RL, Rossi RL *et al.* Surgical treatment of biliary cystadenoma. A report of 15 cases. Arch Surg 1988; 123: 563–8.

92. Choi BI, Lim JH, Han MC *et al.* Biliary cystadenoma and cystadenocarcinoma: CT and sonographic findings. Radiology 1989; 17: 57–61.

93. Short WF, Nedwich A, Levy HA, Howord JM. Biliary cystadenoma. Arch Surg 1971; 102: 78–80.

94. Cahill CJ, Bailey ME, Smith MGM. Mucinous cystadenomas of the liver. Clin Oncol 1982; 8: 171–7.

95. Cheung YK, Chan FL, Leong LLY, Collins RJ, Cheung A. Biliary cystadenocarcinoma. Some unusual features. Clin Radiol 1991; 43: 183–5.

96. Frick MP, Feiberg SB. Biliary cystadenoma. Am J Roentgenol 1982; 139: 393–5.

97. Eisen RN, Kirby WM, O'Quinn JL. Granular cell tumor of the biliary tree – a report of two cases and a review of the literature. Am J Surg Pathol 1991; 15: 460–5.

98. Sobel HJ, Schwarz R, Marquet E. Light and electron microscope study of the origin of granular-cell myoblastoma. J Pathol 1973; 109: 101–11.

99. Seo S, Azzarelli B, Warner TF, Coheen MP, Senteney GE. Multiple visceral and cutaneous granular cell tumors. Ultrastructural and

immunocytochemical evidence of Schwann cell origin. Cancer 1984; 53: 2104–10.

100. Curry B, Gray N. Visceral neurofibromatosis. Br J Surg 1972; 59: 494–6.

101. Sarma DP, Rodriguez FH, Hoffman EO. Paraganglioma of the hepatic duct. J South Med Assoc 1980; 73: 1677–8.

102. Crile G Jr. The advantages of bypass operation over radical pancreatoduodenectomy in the treatment of pancreatic carcinoma. Surg Gynecol Obstet 1970; 130: 1049–53.

103. Traverso LW, Longmire WP. Preservation of the pylorus in pancreaticoduodenectomy. Ann Surg 1994; 192: 306–10.

104. Grace PA, Pitt HA, Tompkins RK *et al.* Decreased morbidity and mortality after pancreatoduodenectomy. Am J Surg 1986; 151: 141–9.

105. Braasch JW, Rossi RC, Wakins E Jr *et al.* Pyloric and gastric preserving pancreatic resection. Experience with 87 patients. Ann Surg 1986; 204: 411–18.

106. Monson JRT, Donahue JH, McEntee GP *et al.* Radical resection for carcinoma of the ampulla of Vater. Arch Surg 1991; 126: 353–7.

107. Altemeier WA, Gall EA, Zinninger MM, Hoxworth PI. Sclerosing carcinoma of the major intrahepatic bile ducts. Arch Surg 1957; 75: 450.

108. Blumgart LH, Benjamin IS. Cancer of the bile ducts. In: Blumgart LH (ed.) Surgery of the liver and biliary tract, 2nd edn. Edinburgh: Churchill Livingstone, 1994, pp. 967–95.

109. Renard P, Boutron MC, Faivre J *et al.* Biliary tract cancers in Cote d'Ore (France): incidence and natural history. J Epidemiol Community Health 1987; 41: 344–8.

110. Green A, Uttaravichien T, Bhudhisawasdi V *et al.* Cholangiocarcinoma in North East Thailand. A hospital-based study. Trop Geogr Med 1991; 43: 193–8.

111. Olsen JH, Dragsted L, Autrup H. Cancer risk and occupational exposure to aflatoxins in Denmark. Br J Cancer 1988; 58(3): 392–6.

112. Lanes SF, Cohen A, Rothman KJ, Dreyer NA, Soden KJ. Mortality of cellulose fibre production workers. Scand J Work Environ Health 1990; 16: 247–51.

113. Bond GG, McLaren EA, Sabel FL *et al.* Liver and biliary tract cancer among chemical workers. Am J Ind Med 1990; 18: 19–24.

114. Caygill C, Hill M, Kirkham J, Northfield TC. Increased risk of biliary tract cancer following gastric surgery. Br J Cancer 1988; 57: 434–6.

115. Suda K, Miyano T, Suzuki F *et al.* Clinicopathologic and experimental studies on cases of abnormal pancreato-choledocho-ductal junction. Acta Pathol Jpn 1987; 37: 1549–62.

116. Ohta T, Nagakawa T, Ueno K *et al.* Clinical experience of biliary tract carcinoma associated with anomalous union of the pancreatic ductal system. Jpn J Surg 1990; 20: 36–43.

117. Kato I, Kuroishi T, Tominaga S. Descriptive epidemiology of subsites of cancers of the liver, biliary tract and pancreas in Japan. Jpn J Clin Oncol 1989; 20: 232–7.

118. Weinbren K, Mutum SS. Pathological aspects of cholangiocarcinoma. J Pathol 1983; 139: 217–38.

119. Klatskin G. Adenocarcinoma of the hepatic duct at its bifurcation within the porta hepatis: an unusual tumour with distinctive clinical and pathological features. Am J Med 1965; 38: 241–56.

120. Davis RI, Sloan MJH, Hood JM, Maxwell P. Carcinoma of the extrahepatic biliary tract: a clinicopathological and immunohistochemical study. Histopathology 1988; 12: 623–31.

121. Bhuiya MR, Nimura Y, Kamiya J *et al.* Clinicopathologic studies on perineural invasion of bile duct carcinoma. Ann Surg 1992; 215: 344–9.

122. Adam A, Benjamin IS. The staging of cholangiocarcinoma. Clin Radiol 1992; 46: 299–303.

123. Bismuth H, Castaing D, Traynor O. Resection or palliation: priority of surgery in the treatment of hilar cancer. World J Surg 1988; 12: 37–47.

124. Blumgart LH, Benjamin IS. Liver resection for bile duct cancer. Surg Clin North Am 1989; 69: 323–37.

125. Blumgart LH, Hadjis NS, Benjamin IS, Beazley R. Surgical approaches to cholangiocarcinoma at confluence of hepatic ducts. Lancet 1984; i: 66–70.

126. Paganuzzi M, Onetto M, Marroni P *et al.* CA19-9 and CA50 in benign and malignant pancreatic and biliary disease. Cancer 1988; 61: 2100–8.

127. Halliday AW, Benjamin IS, Blumgart LH. Nutritional risk factors in major hepatobiliary surgery. J Parent Ent Nutr 1988; 12: 43–8.

128. Engels JT, Balfe DM, Lee JKT. Biliary carci-

noma: CT evaluation of extrahepatic spread. Radiology 1989; 172: 35–40.

129. Benjamin IS. Biliary tract obstruction. Surg Gastroenterol 1983; 2: 105–20.

130. Nimura Y, Shionoya S, Hayakawa N, Kamiya J, Kondo S, Yasui A. Value of percutaneous transhepatic cholangioscopy (PTCS). Surg Endosc 1988; 2: 213–19.

131. Desa LA, Akosa AB, Lazzara S, Domizio P, Krausz T, Benjamin IS. Cytodiagnosis in the management of extrahepatic biliary stricture. Gut 1991; 32: 1188–91.

132. Warshaw AI, Gu Z-Y, Wittenberg J et al. Preoperative staging and assessment of resectability of pancreatic cancer. Arch Surg 1990; 125: 230–3.

133. Warshaw AI, Tepper JE, Shipley WU. Laparoscopy in the staging and planning of therapy for pancreatic cancer. Am J Surg 1986; 151: 76–80.

134. Cuesta MA, Meijer S, Borgstein PJ et al. Laparoscopic ultrasonography for hepatobiliary and pancreatic malignancy. Br J Surg 1993; 80: 1571–4.

135. Garden OJ. Intraoperative and laparoscopic ultrasonography. Oxford: Blackwell Science, 1995.

136. Terblanche J, Saunders SJ, Louw JH. Prolonged palliation in carcinoma of the main hepatic duct junction. Surgery 1972; 71: 720–31.

137. Cameron JL. Proximal cholangiocarcinomas. Br J Surg 1988; 75: 1155–6.

138. Longmire WP, Sanford MC. Intrahepatic cholangiojejunostomy with partial hepatectomy for biliary obstruction. Surgery 1948; 128: 330–47.

139. Guthrie CM, Banting SW, Garden OJ, Carter DC. Segment III cholangiojejunostomy for palliation of malignant hilar obstruction. Br J Surg 1994; 81: 1639–41.

140. Pinson CW, Rossi RL. Extended right hepatic lobectomy, left hepatic lobectomy and skeletonization resection for proximal bile duct cancer. World J Surg 1988; 12: 52–9.

141. Longmire WP Jr, McArthur MS, Bastounis EA, Hiatt J. Carcinoma of the extrahepatic biliary tract. Ann Surg 1973; 178: 333–45.

142. Guthrie CM, Haddock G, de Beaux AC, Garden OJ, Carter DC. Changing trends in the management of extrahepatic cholangiocarcinoma. Br J Surg 1993; 80: 1434–9.

143. Baer HU, Stain SC, Dennison AR, Eggers B, Blumgart LH. Improvements in survival by aggressive resections of hilar cholangiocarcinoma. Ann Surg 1993; 27: 20–7.

144. Pichlmayr R, Burckhardt R, Lauchert W, Beckstein WO, Gubernatis G, Wagner E. Radical resection and liver grafting as the two main components of surgical strategy in the treatment of proximal bile duct cancer. World J Surg 1988; 12: 68–77.

145. Launois B, Lebeau G, Kiroff G, Oddi R, Campion JP. Survival after surgical resection of carcinoma in the upper third of the biliary tract. Dig Surg 1979; 7: 106–10.

146. Tsuzuki Y, Ogata Y, Iida S, Nakanishi I, Takenaka Y, Yoshii H. Carcinoma of the bifurcation of the hepatic ducts. Arch Surg 1983; 118: 1147–51.

147. Iwasaki Y, Okamura T, Ozaki A et al. Surgical treatment for carcinoma at the confluence of the major hepatic ducts. Surg Gynecol Obstet 1986; 162: 457–64.

148. Nimura Y, Hayakawa N, Kamiya J, Kondo S, Shiyonoya S. Hepatic segmentectomy with caudate lobe resection for bile duct carcinoma of the hepatic hilus. World J Surg 1990; 14: 535–44.

149. Mizumoto R, Kawarada Y, Suzuki H. Surgical treatment of hilar carcinoma of the bile duct. Surg Gynecol Obstet 1986; 162: 153–8.

150. Nagino M, Nimura Y, Hayakawa N, Kamiya J, Kondoh S, Shionoya S. Diagnostic value of computed tomography for the detection of invasion of the caudate bile duct branch in carcinoma of the hepatic hilum. Nippon-Geka-Gakkai-Zasshi 1988; 89: 889–97.

151. Nimura Y, Hayakawa N, Kamiya J. Hilar cholangiocarcinoma: the surgical therapy. In: Serio G, Huguet C, Williamson RCN (eds) Hepatobiliary and pancreatic tumours. Edinburgh: Graffham Press, 1994, pp. 116–22.

152. Voyles CR, Bowley NJ, Allison DJ, Benjamin IS, Blumgart LH. Carcinoma of the proximal extrahepatic biliary tree. Radiological assessment and therapeutic alternatives. Ann Surg 1983; 197: 188–93.

153. Watanapa P, Nargrove NS, Sirivatanauksorn Y. The potential role of intraoperative ultrasonography in the surgical treatment of hilar cholangiocarcinoma. Hepatobiliary Surg 1996; 9: 93–6.

154. Hatfield ARW. Palliation of malignant obstructive jaundice – surgery or stent? Gut 1990; 31: 1339–40.

155. Adam A, Chetty N, Roddie N et al. Self-expanding stainless steel endoprosthesis for treatment of malignant bile duct obstruction. Am J Roentgenol 1991; 156: 321–5.

156. Dooley JS. External bile drainage – the state of the art. J Hepatol 1985; 1: 681–6.

157. Casola G, O'Laoide R. Hilar cholangiocarcinoma: percutaneous approach. In: Serio G, Huguet C, Williamson RCN (eds) Hepatobiliary and pancreatic tumours. Edinburgh: Graffham Press, 1994, pp. 123–6.

158. Cremer M, Deviere J, Sugai B, Baize M. Expandable biliary metal stents for malignancies: endoscopic insertion and diathermic cleaning for tumor ingrowth. Gastrointest Endosc 1990; 36: 451–7.

159. Huibregtse K, Carr-Locke DL, Cremer M, and the European Wallstent Study Group. Biliary stent occlusion – a problem solved with self-expanding metal stents? Endoscopy 1992; 24: 391–4.

160. Lokich JJ, Kane RA, Harrison DA, McDermott WV. Biliary tract obstruction secondary to cancer: management guidelines and selected literature review. J Clin Oncol 1987; 5: 969–81.

161. Nakama M, Sugawara T, Ohgawara K. Radiotherapy of carcinoma of the biliary system. Nippon-Igaku-Hoshasen-Gakki-Zasshi, 1990; 50: 398–403.

162. Fletcher MS, Brinkley D, Dawson JL, Nunnerley H, Williams R. Treatment of hilar carcinoma by bile drainage combined with internal radiotherapy using ^{192}iridium wire. Br J Surg 1983; 70: 733–65.

163. Meyers WC, Scott Jones R. Internal radiation for bile duct cancer. World J Surg 1988; 12: 99–104.

164. Urban MS, Siegel JH, Pavlou W et al. Treatment of malignant biliary obstruction with a high-dose rate remote afterloading device using a 10 F nasobiliary tube. Gastrointest Endosc 1990; 36: 292–6.

165. Levitt MD, Laurence BH, Cameron F, Klemp PFB. Transpapillary iridium-192 wire in the treatment of malignant bile duct obstruction. Gut 1988; 29: 149–52.

166. Vallis KA, Benjamin IS, Munro AJ et al. External beam and intraluminal radiotherapy for locally advanced bile duct cancer: role and tolerability. Radiother Oncol 1996; (in press).

167. Busse PM, Stone MD, Sheldon TA et al. Intraoperative radiation therapy for biliary tract carcinoma: results of a 5-year experience. Surgery 1989; 105: 724–33.

168. Deziel DJ, Kiel KD, Kramer TS, Doolas A, Roseman DL. Intraoperative radiation therapy in biliary tract cancer. Am J Surg 1988; 54: 402–7.

169. Oberfield RA, Rossi RL. The role of chemotherapy in the treatment of bile duct cancer. World J Surg 1988; 12: 105–8.

170. Isacoff WH, Botnick L, Tompkins R, Jacobs AD, Reber H, Taylor O. Treatment of patients with advanced tumours of the bile ducts with continuous infusion of 5-FU in conjunction with calcium leucovorin mitomycin-C and dipyridamole. ASCO Proceedings March 1993; 12: 225.

171. Smith GW, Bukowski RM, Hewlett JS, Groppe CW. Hepatic artery infusion of 5-fluorouracil and mitomycin C in cholangiocarcinoma and gallbladder carcinoma. Cancer 1984; 54: 1513–16.

172. Hudd C, LaRegina MC, Devine JE et al. Response to exogenous cholecystokinin of six human gastrointestinal cancers xenografted in nude mice. Am J Surg 1989; 157: 386–94.

173. Gompertz RH, Benjamin IS, Blumgart LH. Resection for hilar cholangiocarcinoma: does clearance matter? Gut 1988; 29: A736–7.

174. Little JM. Editorial comment: Hilar biliary cancer – are we getting it right? Hepatobiliary Surg 1989; 1: 93–6.

175. Nevin JE, Moran TJ, Kay S, King R. Carcinoma of the gallbladder. Cancer 1976; 37: 141–8.

176. Thomas MG, Grace PA, Benjamin IS, Williamson RCN. Carcinoma of the gallbladder, acute cholecystitis and cholecystostomy. Eur J Gastroenterol Hepatol 1991; (in press).

177. Hederstrom E, Forsberg L. Ultrasonography in carcinoma of the gallbladder. Acta Radiol 1987; 28: 715–18.

178. Adson MA, Farnell MB. Hepatobiliary cancer – surgical considerations. Mayo Clin Proc 1981; 56: 686–99.

179. Shirai Y, Yoshida K, Tsukada K, Muto T. Inapparent carcinoma of the gallbladder. Ann Surg 1992; 215: 326–31.

180. Evander A, Ihse I. Evaluation of intended radical surgery in carcinoma of the gallbladder. Br J Surg 1981; 68: 158–60.

181. Yap L, McKenzie J, Wycherley A, Toouli J. Gallbladder ejection fraction for acalculous gallbladder pain. Gastroenterology 1991; 101: 786–93.

182. Geenen JE, Hogan WJ, Dodds WJ, Toouli J, Venu RP. The efficacy of endoscopic sphincterotomy in post-cholecystectomy patients with sphincter of Oddi dysfunction. N Engl J Med 1989; 320: 82–7.

183. Moody FG, Becker JM, Potts JR. Transduodenal sphincteroplasty and transampullary septectomy for post-cholecystectomy pain. Ann Surg 1983; 197: 627–36.

184. Foschi D, Cavagna G, Callioni F, Morandi E, Rovati V. Hyperalimentation of jaundiced patients on percutaneous biliary drainage. Br J Surg 1986; 73: 716–19.

185. Halliday AW, McPherson GAD, Benjamin IS, Blumgart LH. Does preoperative biliary drainage allow an improvement of nutritional status in the jaundiced patient? Dig Surg 1987; 4: 187–91.

186. Dawson JL. The incidence of postoperative renal failure in obstructive jaundice. Br J Surg 1965; 52: 663–5.

187. Thompson JN, Cohen J, McConnell JS. A randomized controlled trial of pre-operative oral ursodeoxycholic acid in obstructive jaundice. Br J Surg 1985; 72: 1027.

188. McPherson GAD, Benjamin IS, Blumgart LH. Improving renal function in obstructive jaundice without preoperative drainage. Lancet 1984; i: 511.

189. Nakayama T, Ikeda A, Okuda K. Percutaneous transhepatic drainage of the biliary tract. Gastroenterology 1978; 74: 554–9.

190. Hatfield ARW, Terblanche J, Fataar S et al. Pre-operative external biliary drainage in obstructive jaundice. Lancet 1982; ii: 896–9.

191. McPherson GAD, Benjamin IS, Hodgson HJF, Bowley NB, Allison DJ, Blumgart LH. Pre-operative percutaneous transhepatic biliary drainage: the results of a controlled trial. Br J Surg 1984; 71: 371–5.

192. Pitt HA, Gomes AS, Lois JF, Mann LL, Deutsch LS, Longmire WP. Does preoperative percutaneous biliary drainage reduce operative risk or increase hospital cost? Ann Surg 1985; 201: 9–16.

193. Diamond T, Dolan S, Thompson RLE, Rowlands BJ. Development and reversal of endotoxemia and endotoxin-related death in obstructive jaundice. Surgery 1990; 108: 370–5.

194. Voyles CR, Blumgart LH. A technique for construction of high biliary enteric anastomosis. Surg, Gynecol Obstet 1983; 154: 885–7.

195. Krige JE, Bornman PC, Harris-Jones EP et al. Modified hepaticojejunostomy for permanent biliary access. Br J Surg 1987; 74: 612–13.

196. Roddie ME, Benjamin IS. Transjejunal radiological intervention in hepatobiliary disease. Semin Intervent Radiol 1995; 12: 55–62.

8 Acute pancreatitis

David C. Carter

Definitions

Acute pancreatitis can be defined as an acute inflammatory condition which presents typically with abdominal pain, usually in association with raised levels of pancreatic enzymes in blood or urine. There is variable involvement of other regional tissues and/or remote organ systems, and there may be little correlation between clinical severity and morphological findings. Exocrine and endocrine function may be impaired for a variable time and to a variable extent. While acute pancreatitis can recur, it seldom progresses to chronic pancreatitis and a return to clinical, morphological and functional normality is usual if the primary cause is eliminated and complications do not supervene.

Mild acute pancreatitis is characterised by interstitial oedema, minimal organ dysfunction and uneventful recovery. The gland is swollen and pale and peripancreatic fat necrosis may be present.

Severe acute pancreatitis is associated with organ failure and/or local complications such as necrosis, pseudocyst and abscess. Clinically severe disease is usually associated with pancreatic and peripancreatic necrosis, although it is occasionally seen in patients with oedematous pancreatitis. Necrotising pancreatitis accounts for some 15% of attacks of acute pancreatitis. The necrosis can be diffuse or focal, and mortality doubles if it becomes infected. When necrosis is fully established, the organ may resemble oily mud in which necrotic tissue, fat and haemorrhage coalesce.

Acute fluid collections may be found in and around the pancreas. They develop early in the course of acute pancreatitis and do not have an enclosing wall of granulation tissue or fibrous tissue. **Acute pseudocysts** differ in that they take four or more weeks to form and have a wall of fibrous or granulation tissue.

Pancreatic abscess is a circumscribed collection of pus which lies in close proximity to the pancreas and which contains little or no pancreatic necrosis.

Terms such as haemorrhagic pancreatitis and phlegmon are confusing and are now obsolete.

Incidence of acute pancreatitis

Acute pancreatitis accounts for approximately 2% of hospital admissions because of abdominal pain and its incidence in the United Kingdom has risen over the past 25 years from 5–10 cases per million to over 20 cases per million. In Scotland, the incidence rose 11-fold in men and fourfold in women between 1961 and 1985, the increase being marked in young and middle-aged men and in elderly women.[1] Although this may reflect increasing awareness and improved diagnosis, the rising incidence in men in some European countries has been linked to a rising alcohol consumption and incidence of liver cirrhosis.[2] Gallstone disease probably accounts for the increased incidence of acute pancreatitis in women.

Aetiology of acute pancreatitis

As a useful generalisation, approximately one half of cases of acute pancreatitis in the United Kingdom are associated with gallstones and up to one-third with alcohol. The causes of acute pancreatitis in a recent series of patients admitted to Edinburgh Royal Infirmary is shown in Table 8.1.

Cholelithiasis

Some 5% of patients with gallstones will develop pancreatitis[3,4] and cholelithiasis is by far the commonest cause of acute pancreatitis in patients over 60 years of age. Pancreatitis is more likely to develop in patients who have multiple small stones, a wide cystic duct, a less acute angle then usual between bile duct and pancreatic duct and a long common channel between them, and in those who show a greater frequency of reflux into the pancreatic duct on operative cholangiography[5–8] (Fig. 8.1). The increased risk of pancreatitis in pregnancy is now attributed to the associated increase in the incidence of gallstones.

Table 8.1 *Aetiology, severity and mortality of acute pancreatitis in 279 cases admitted to the Royal Infirmary of Edinburgh, 1989–1993*

Aetiology	n	Severe disease	Mortality (%)
Gallstones	116	39 (34%)	4 (3%)
Alcohol	97	16 (16%)	1 (1%)
Idiopathic	41	12 (29%)	6 (15%)
Post-ERCP	11	4 (36%)	3 (27%)
Pancreatic cancer	5	1	0
Postoperative	3	3	1
Other	6	4	2
Total	279	79 (28%)	17 (6%)

Figure 8.1.
Operative cholangiogram taken during laparoscopic cholecystectomy in a patient who had previously presented with gallstone-associated pancreatitis. Note the 'common channel' and reflux of contrast material into the pancreatic duct.

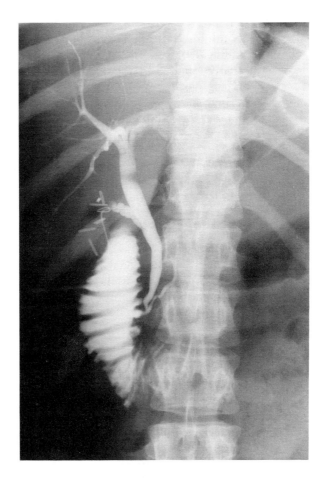

Alcohol

Alcohol is the major cause of acute pancreatitis in North American inner cities, but in UK centres it accounts for between 5% and 35% of cases. It is not understood why alcohol is more likely to cause acute pancreatitis in some individuals and not in others. The amount consumed may determine the severity of the first attack of acute pancreatitis but not of recurrent attacks.[2] It is also appreciated that 'acute alcoholic pancreatitis' can be an early stage of chronic pancreatitis.

Postoperative and post-ERCP pancreatitis

Direct trauma may cause pancreatitis after gastric, pancreatic or biliary surgery, particularly when there has been instrumentation or manipulation of the common bile duct and papilla of Vater. Pancreatitis may also occur after cardiac surgery involving cardiopulmonary bypass (see below).

Endoscopic retrograde cholangiopancreatography (ERCP) is the third commonest defined cause of pancreatitis in modern practice (Table 8.1). Clinical pancreatitis after ERCP varies from 0.7 to 12%[9] although as many as 50% of patients have hyperamylasaemia without clinical signs. Excessive manipulation, diathermy and high injection pressures (with acinarisation) are all risk factors, although non-ionic contrast media may have reduced some of the risks. Therapeutic manoeuvres generally increase risk but in skilled hands the incidence of pancreatitis after endoscopic sphincterotomy for bile duct stones can be less than 1%. Endoscopic sphincterotomy for sphincter of Oddi dysfunction carries a risk of about 3.5%.[10]

Local obstructive factors

Pancreatitis is occasionally caused by chronic duodenal or afferent loop obstruction, duodenal diverticula, duodenal and periampullary cysts, stenosis of the papilla of Vater, biliary ascariasis, and obstructing pancreatic and periampullary neoplasms.[11]

Pancreas divisum

Pancreas divisum is a congenital abnormality in which the dorsal and ventral pancreatic ducts fail to fuse. It has been postulated that pancreatitis arises because secretions from the larger dorsal pancreas have to pass through the small accessory papilla, and papillary stenosis may be a cofactor. However, pancreas divisum is present in about 6% of individuals and is probably an incidental finding in most patients with idiopathic pancreatitis.

Trauma

Pancreatitis may result from abdominal injury, and blunt trauma is recognised increasingly as a cause of pancreatitis in children.

Infections and infestations

Acute pancreatitis can be associated with viral (mumps, Coxsackie, hepatitis A, Ebstein–Barr and cytomegalic virus) and bacterial (*Campylobacter, Mycoplasma pneumoniae* and *Legionella*) infection, and with infestation by ascariasis and *Clonorchis sinensis*.

Drugs

Drugs associated with acute pancreatitis include thiazide diuretics, angiotensin converting enzyme (ACE) inhibitors, frusemide, sulphonamides, tetracycline, azathioprine and oestrogens. Drugs with a less certain association include corticosteroids, L-asparaginase, 6-mercaptopurine, chlorthalidone, methyldopa, ethacrynic acid, phenformin, procainamide, agents causing hypercalcaemia, and cytosine arabinoside.

Lipid abnormalities

Acute pancreatitis has a recognised association with types I, IV and V primary hyperlipoproteinaemia, and can occur in secondary hyperlipoproteinaemia.[12] Hyperlipidaemia in acute pancreatitis is usually characterised by high serum triglyceride and normal cholesterol levels.

It is uncertain whether hypertriglyceridaemia triggers pancreatitis in alcoholics. However, it is no commoner in patients with alcoholic pancreatitis than in alcoholics without pancreatitis, and plasma triglyceride levels do not explain individual susceptibility to either alcoholic or gallstone pancreatitis.[13] It may be that hypertriglyceridaemia is a result of pancreatic inflammation and pancreatic lipase could conceivably hydrolyse triglyceride with release of toxic fatty acids. A high fat intake, with or without alcohol, could precipitate pancreatitis through such a mechanism. Hypertriglyceridaemia is present in 50% of patients with necrotising pancreatitis[14] but is almost certainly pre-existing and not the result of pancreatic necrosis.

Ischaemia and cardiovascular disease

Hyperamylasaemia is present in about 25% of patients undergoing cardiac surgery, but only 1% of cases develop significant pancreatitis.[15] Factors implicated include hypotension and hypoperfusion, embolisation of cholesterol plaques, non-pulsatile perfusion, hypothermia and perioperative administration of calcium chloride.

Acute pancreatitis is a common finding in patients dying from rupture of an aortic aneurysm, and may be a consequence of prolonged hypotension. Other vascular diseases associated with acute pancreatitis include disseminated lupus erythematosus, polyarteritis nodosa and thrombotic thrombocytopenic purpura.

Hypercalcaemia

Pancreatitis due to hypercalcaemia was once diagnosed in up to 2% of cases of hyperparathyroidism. Earlier diagnosis of hyperparathyroidism now means that advanced malignancy has become the commonest cause of pancreatitis due to hypercalcaemia.

Miscellaneous causes

Acute pancreatitis can occur after scorpion stings, in fulminant hepatic failure and after organ transplantation. Post-transplantation pancreatitis is probably multifactorial with contributions from altered perfusion, drug therapy, infection and rejection. Pancreatitis in hypothermia and hypotensive states is probably due to impaired vascular perfusion and thrombosis.

Idiopathic pancreatitis

It is now appreciated that very small gallstones and biliary debris can cause pancreatitis,[16,17] and the proportion of cases without a defined aetiological cause has fallen. However, idiopathic pancreatitis still accounts for 30–40% of cases in the elderly and carries a high morbidity and mortality[18] (Table 8.1).

Pathogenesis of acute pancreatitis

Acute pancreatitis may involve events within the acinar cell and duct system, inflammation of the pancreas and peripancreatic tissues, and a systemic inflammatory response. The involvement of activated pancreatic proteases such as trypsin and phospholipase A has long been appreciated; more recently it has become apparent that oxygen-derived free radicals, inflammatory mediators (cytokines) and activated macrophages and polymorphonuclear leucocytes may also be important.

Activation of enzymes within the acinar cell[19]

Digestive enzymes and lysosomal hydrolases are normally both synthesised by ribosomes on the rough endoplasmic reticulum. They are then transported to the Golgi complex where secretory proteins accumulate in zymogen granules while lysosomal hydrolases are segregated in lysosomes. In experimental pancreatitis induced by a choline-deficient diet or caerulein, there is evidence that early co-localization and fusion of digestive and lysosomal enzymes causes activation of proteases in the resulting 'autophagic vacuoles'.[20,21] Zymogen granules normally discharge from the apical surface of the acinar cell, but disruption of this process may cause them to discharge from the basolateral surface into the intercellular space.[22] Entry of activated proteases into the tissues could then cause inflammation with activation of macrophages and polymorphonuclear leucocytes.

Despite the attractions of the concept of intracellular activation of proteases, the phenomenon has only been demonstrated in animal models and its role in human disease remains uncertain.

Reflux of duodenal juice and bile

The pancreas normally protects itself from its own proteolytic enzymes by synthesising them as proenzymes which are only activated in the duodenal lumen. Trypsinogen is cleaved by the duodenal brush border enzyme, enterokinase, releasing the active proteolytic enzyme, trypsin. Trypsin then triggers a cascade effect leading to activation of other pancreatic enzymes. Trypsinogen cleavage also releases trypsinogen activation peptides (TAPs), the concentration of which in urine and plasma reflects the severity of pancreatitis.[23,24] Other important enzymes include elastase (which with the locally released vasodilator, kallikrein, has a key role in local vascular changes) and phospholipase A (which may damage cell membranes and contribute to necrosis).

Other factors may help to avoid the pancreas becoming exposed to activated proteolytic enzymes. Inhibitors present in pancreatic tissue and juice can inactivate proteases, whereas reflux of activated enzymes from the duodenum is normally prevented by the secretion pressure in the pancreatic duct, the oblique course of the pancreatic duct through the duodenal wall, the high pressure within the sphincter of Oddi, and the valvular arrangement of mucosal folds at the termination of the pancreatic duct.

Compromise of these protective mechanisms may favour the development of pancreatitis. For example, reflux of duodenal contents would allow enterokinase to activate trypsin within the pancreatic duct, whereas continued secretion into a duct obstructed by an impacted gallstone could favour extravasation of enzymes. Activated proteases have been recovered from pancreatic tissues and juice in human pancreatitis, although available evidence suggests that pancreatic secretion, and in particular the response to cholecystokinin, is reduced soon after the onset of acute pancreatitis.[25] Refluxing bile salts could also cause inflammation by disrupting the pancreatic mucosal barrier[26,27] or liberating intracellular trypsin which could activate other zymogens.

Keynes[28] has argued that necrosis in pancreatitis is not caused by proteolytic autodigestion but by reflux of the lysolecithin formed from intraduodenal activation of phospholipase. Reflux of infected bile could also trigger the release of this cytotoxic agent, and there is a recognised clinical association between cholangitis and acute pancreatitis.[29]

Pathogenesis of gallstone pancreatitis

Opie[30] proposed that obstruction of the common pancreatobiliary channel by a gallstone allowed bile to reflux into the pancreatic duct, and so activate pancreatic enzymes. Some 80–90% of individuals possess a common channel, and reflux into the pancreatic duct is seen on operative cholangiography in up to two-thirds of patients who have had gallstone pancreatitis but in to less than 20% of patients with cholelithiasis who have not had pancreatitis.[5,7,31] Acute pancreatitis can be induced experimentally by closed-loop obstruction of the duodenum and prevented by prior ligation of the pancreatic duct,[32] findings which may be relevant to the pancreatitis which can follow Polya gastrectomy or chronic duodenal obstruction.

Despite these observations, it is still unclear whether duodenopancreatic or biliary-pancreatic reflux is responsible for triggering acute pancreatitis. Increasing pancreatic ductal pressure in itself can damage the mucosal barrier,[27,33] and ligation of the pancreatic duct of the oppossum produces necrotising pancreatitis which is just as severe as that caused by ligating the common pancreaticobiliary channel.[34] It is clear that duodenal or biliary reflux is not essential for the development of experimental pancreatitis.

Removal of the gallbladder cures patients with gallstone pancreatitis, probably because it removes the risk of further stones passing down the biliary tree to occlude the papilla of Vater. Most obstructing stones which cause pancreatitis pass on spontaneously within days,[35] but persisting impaction can lead to severe and complicated disease. It is also possible that the passage of a stone into the duodenum leaves a patulous orifice which permits duodenal content to reflux into the pancreatic duct.

Pathogenesis of alcoholic pancreatitis

Potential mechanisms whereby alcohol might cause pancreatitis include ductal obstruction by protein precipitates, acetaldehyde toxicity, increased pancreatic duct permeability, and hypertriglyceridaemia. Ethanol is metabolised to acetaldehyde in the liver (and perhaps in the pancreas) by alcohol dehydrogenase, and acetaldehyde induces pancreatitis when perfused into the isolated canine pancreas.[36] Acetaldehyde could also serve as a substrate for the generation of oxygen-free radicals. Less likely mechanisms include a direct toxic effect on the acinar cell, spasm of the sphincter of Oddi, promotion of sphincter incompetence and duodenal reflux, and pancreatic hypersecretion.

Role of ischaemia

Factors implicated in ischaemic pancreatitis include diffuse small vessel disease as in disseminated lupus, diminished perfusion as in shock, and thrombosis as in hypothermia. Altered blood flow and increased capillary permeability are factors in all forms of pancreatitis, and ultrastructural changes have been detected in the microvasculature within 30 minutes in experimental pancreatitis.[37] Ischaemia is a potent cause of necrosis. Alpha-adrenergic vasoconstrictors[38] and intravenous contrast agents[39] accentuate vascular damage in experimental pancreatitis, and could conceivably trigger necrosis or compound its development.

Clinical features

Abdominal pain is usually the predominant feature but the disease can be painless.[40] Nausea, vomiting and retching are often prominent. The attack is occasionally precipitated by a large meal and/or alcohol. The pain is usually epigastric but may radiate to the back or become generalised. It is usually constant and severe, and leaning forwards may afford some relief whereas vomiting and simple analgesics usually do not. Acute pancreatitis is easily confused with other causes of the acute abdomen, occasionally mimics myocardial infarction, pneumonia, pleurisy or uraemia, and must always be considered in patients who present with unexplained shock or anuria.

Abdominal tenderness and guarding are often less marked than might be expected from the severe pain and prostration. They may become generalised, and ileus can produce abdominal distension. Troublesome hiccoughs reflect irritation of the diaphragm. Low-grade pyrexia is common and jaundice can develop, particularly in those with obstructing gallstone pancreatitis. Shock may supervene, and confusion and toxicity sometimes produce 'pancreatic encephalopathy'. An abdominal mass is rarely palpable on admission but may develop, particularly if there are complications such as a pseudocyst. Bleeding into fascial planes produces discolouration around the umbilicus (Cullen's sign) or in the flanks (Grey–Turner's sign) in 1–3% of patients.[41] Neither sign is pathognomic of acute pancreatitis, but they denote severe although not necessarily fatal disease.[41] Subcutaneous fat necrosis occasionally produces small red tender nodules in the limbs.

In postoperative pancreatitis, pain, vomiting and abdominal tenderness are often masked by the original operation and diagnosis is difficult. Pancreatitis should be suspected in any patient who develops prolonged hypotension or jaundice within days of upper gastrointestinal, pancreatic or biliary surgery.

Investigations

Biochemical investigations

Serum and urinary amylase[42]

Only about 40% of the amylase activity in the serum normally originates from the pancreas, the rest being derived from other tissues, notably the salivary glands. Serum amylase activity is normally less than $300\,iu\,l^{-1}$ and most centres regard a level of greater than $1000\,iu\,l^{-1}$ as diagnostic. In acute pancreatitis, the rise in serum amylase activity is confined largely to pancreatic amylase. It is not proportional to disease severity, and pancreatic necrosis is sometimes associated with levels of less than $1000\,iu\,l^{-1}$. Amylase levels are highest during the first 25 hours and fall rapidly thereafter, unless there is recurrent pancreatitis, pseudocyst or abscess formation. The rapid fall in serum amylase activity may explain why some patients have normoamylasaemic pancreatitis by the time that they are admitted. In one recent study, admission serum amylase activity was diagnostic in 96% of patients with mild pancreatitis and in 87% of those with severe disease, whereas 48 hours later these values were 33% and 48% respectively.[43]

In general, alcoholic pancreatitis produces lower amylase levels than gallstone pancreatitis and as many as one-third of patients with ultrasonographic or CT scan evidence of acute alcoholic pancreatitis do not have hyperamylasaemia.[44] Some of these alcoholic patients may have subclinical chronic pancreatitis, and 20% have hyperlipidaemia which may help to explain the normality of their amylase levels. Patients with non-alcoholic forms of pancreatitis are less likely to have normoamylasaemia, but normoamylasaemic and hyperamylasaemic patients do not differ in terms of the severity or clinical course of their disease.[45]

Hyperamylasaemia can be found in conditions other than acute pancreatitis (Table 8.2). Isoenzyme determinations show that up to one-

Table 8.2 *Conditions associated with hyperamylasaemia*

Abdominal causes	Non-abdominal causes
Pancreatitis	Thoracic
Pancreatic cancer	Myocardial infarct
Biliary tract disease	Pulmonary embolism
Perforated peptic ulcer	Pneumonia
Acute perforated appendicitis	Metastatic lung cancer
Intestinal obstruction	Cardiopulmonary bypass
Mesenteric infarction	Salivary gland
Liver disease	Salivary trauma
Dissecting aortic aneurysm	Infection (mumps)
Ruptured ectopic pregnancy	Salivary duct obstruction
Prostatic disease	Irradiation
Ovarian neoplasm	Metabolic
	Diabetic ketoacidosis
Recent abdominal operation	Drugs
Afferent loop syndrome	Opiates
	Phenylbutazone
	Trauma
	Cerebral trauma
	Burns
	Renal disease
	Renal insufficiency
	Renal transplantation

third of patients with hyperamylasaemia do not have acute pancreatitis, and the circulating amylase in such cases is salivary amylase. Serum amylase activity rarely exceeds $1000\,\mathrm{iu}\,l^{-1}$ in the absence of pancreatitis, although in some such cases there may be degree of pancreatic inflammation; for example, after rupture of an aortic aneurysm or perforation of a duodenal ulcer.

Hyperamylasaemia is occasionally caused by impaired renal function, or more rarely because circulating amylase is bound to an abnormal immunoglobulin and forms a complex which is too large to be excreted. Macroamylasaemia should be suspected when there is hyperamylasaemia in association with low urinary amylase levels in a patient with normal renal function. Macroamylasaemia is found in up to 3% of cases of acute pancreatitis and more importantly, in 1–2% of the normal population. Uncertainty about whether pancreatitis is present is best resolved by measuring serum lipase activity.

Urinary amylase levels frequently remain elevated in acute pancreatitis after serum levels have returned to normal. Detection of urinary amylase and measurement of the amylase:creatinine clearance ratio has not proved useful in clinical practice,[42] but current interest surrounds a strip test for urinary trypsinogen-2.

Serum lipase

Serum lipase activity is one of the most reliable markers of acute pancreatitis, having a sensitivity and specificity of almost 90%.[46] Lipase activity remains elevated for longer than amylase activity, and does not increase when there is hyperamylasaemia in the absence of pancreatitis.[47] Serum lipase activity can now be measured rapidly and reliably and may yet be used more widely in clinical practice.

Radiology and other imaging procedures

Plain radiographs of the abdomen and chest radiograph

There are no radiological signs which are specific for acute pancreatitis but a chest radiograph and plain abdominal films should be obtained on admission.[48] Their principal value is to exclude other causes of the acute abdomen, notably gastrointestinal perforation and obstruction. Changes which may be seen in acute pancreatitis include the presence of a soft tissue mass, gas in the pancreatic bed, and soft tissue mottling due to fat necrosis. Gastrointestinal changes include dilatation of the stomach, duodenum, small and large intestine, and there may be a 'sentinel' loop of jejunum or a colon 'cut-off' sign in which gas is seen in the ascending and descending colon but not the transverse colon. Other relevant abnormalities are loss of psoas and renal outlines, radio-opaque gallstones, elevation of the diaphragm, gas in the biliary tract and evidence of ascites.

Chest radiography may reveal pleural effusion (usually left-sided), elevation of the diaphragm, widening of the mediastinum, basal atelectasis, lobar consolidation, pulmonary infarction and evidence of the adult respiratory distress syndrome. Chest radiographs are abnormal in one-third of patients with acute pancreatitis and in over 70% of those with severe pancreatitis, and left-sided pleural effusion is particularly common in patients with severe disease. It cannot be overemphasised that significant arterial hypoxia can be present or can develop in patients without marked changes on chest radiography.

Ultrasound scanning

Ultrasonography is a useful means of detecting gallstones and biliary obstruction and its introduction has virtually eliminated the need for cholecystography and cholescintigraphy.[48] Ultrasonography can be used to monitor the development of pseudocysts and abscesses, to establish the presence of pancreatitis in ill patients with normal or marginally increased amylase activity, and to guide needle insertion if infected necrosis is suspected. The investigation can be frustrated by gaseous distension or when tenderness prevents good skin contact.

Acute pancreatitis produces interstitial oedema which may alter the size and sonographic texture of the pancreas and blur its outlines. The swelling may be localised or diffuse. As oedema increases, the gland becomes less echogenic than normal and may be indistinguishable from the contiguous portal and splenic veins. In necrotising disease, echogenicity may increase as a consequence of necrosis, saponification and bleeding. Dilatation of the pancreatic duct is occasionally visible.

Computed tomography[48,49]

The morphological changes are similar to those seen on ultrasonography and include pancreatic enlargement, reduced attenuation or a mixed pattern, dilatation and irregularity of the pancreatic duct, loss of clarity of the gland margin with soft tissue oedema and abnormal peripancreatic fat planes, and pancreatic or peripancreatic fluid collections. The fat around the mesenteric artery is usually preserved, a helpful point in differentiating inflammatory from malignant disease.

The pancreas is a vascular organ and its density on CT scanning normally enhances following intravenous injections of contrast medium. Incremental dynamic bolus computed tomography is the best method of detecting the extent and severity of pancreatic and peripancreatic necrosis.[49–51] Oral contrast is also given to opacify the upper gastrointestinal tract whenever possible. Contraindications to intravenous contrast include a previous severe allergic reaction to iodinated media and severely restricted renal function in a patient not already on renal dialysis. Non-ionic contrast media such as iopamidol may carry less risk of renal and cardiovascular complications,[49] but both ionic and non-ionic contrast models can convert borderline ischaemia into irreversible necrosis in an experimental model.[39] The significance of these findings in human disease remains uncertain but dynamic CT scanning is best avoided early in the course of severe pancreatitis and should not be used routinely in all patients with acute pancreatitis.

The severity of inflammation on CT scanning can be graded. Stage A denotes a normal CT scan, stage B focal or diffuse pancreatic enlargement, stage C inflammatory change in the peripancreatic fat, stage D a single ill-defined fluid collection and phlegmon, and stage E two or more fluid collections or abscess. A 'CT score' (A = zero, E = 4) can then be added to a 'necrosis score' (no necrosis = zero, up to one-third = 2, up to one half = 4, more than half = 6) to give a CT Severity Index (CTSI) which shows strong correlation with morbidity and mortality.[52,53] Although such scoring systems may be valuable for research purposes, they are not used as a basis for clinical decision making.

Necrosis is a major determinant of morbidity and mortality. Virtually all patients without necrosis survive whereas mortality rates of 5%, 7% and 18%, respectively, have been reported in patients with focal necrosis, extended necrosis and subtotal/total necrosis.[54] Mortality rates are almost twice as high when necrosis becomes infected as it does in 40–70% of cases.[55–57] Fine needle aspiration under CT guidance can be used to detect infection[56] although it is sometimes obvious radiologically from the presence of gas in the pancreatic and peripancreatic tissues.

The soft tissues around the lesser sac and in front of the kidneys are commonly involved in pancreatitis. The changes are commoner on the left but may be bilateral. Fluid collections may develop in the pancreas, in the peritoneum and retroperitoneum, in the mediastinum and in the groin. Large peripancreatic collections may be indistinguishable from fat necrosis on CT scanning. Low CT attenuation (<15 Hounsfield units) is more often associated with fluid whereas high attenuation (>25 Hounsfield units) suggests fat necrosis. Other CT findings include vascular complications such as erosion of arteries with bleeding or pseudoaneurysm formation, venous thrombosis and formation of varices, biliary tract disease (gallstones, bile duct obstruction) and gastrointestinal complications (oedema, bleeding, obstruction, necrosis and fistula).

ERCP

ERCP is not used to establish the diagnosis of acute pancreatitis but is used in selected patients with gallstone pancreatitis to confirm the diagnosis and extract obstructing stones (see below).

Other investigations

There have been numerous attempts to define demographic, haematological and biochemical variables which can identify patients with severe pancreatitis and predict outcome. The multiple prognostic factor grading systems developed by Ranson[58] and Imrie[59] (Table 8.3) have proved the most reliable and popular systems in this regard. In addition, they have provided a basis for controlled clinical trials by defining patients with disease likely to be severe, and have allowed comparisons between centres.[60] In the 11 factor Ranson system (Table 8.4) mortality was 1% when up to two factors were positive; 16% with three or four positive; 40% with five or six positive; and 100% with seven or eight positive factors. With the modified Imrie system, 39% of 92 attacks classified as severe proved to be so (i.e. proved fatal, or were associated with the development of complications or need for operation) as opposed to 9% of the 313 attacks graded as mild.[59] As a rule of thumb, approximately one-in-four attacks are classified as severe using such systems and approximately one-in-four of those with severe disease will die. The drawback of these forms of assessment is that 1–2 days usually elapse before all of the information is available.

The volume and colour of free peritoneal fluid or the colour of return peritoneal lavage fluid has also been used to assess the severity of an attack of pancreatitis,[61] although this approach is now rarely employed.

Individual serum markers used to predict severity and identify high-risk patients include those reflecting release of active proteolytic enzymes (phospholipase A_2, ribonuclease), consumption of protease inhibitors (alpha-2 macroglobulin and alpha-1-antiprotease), complement activation or consumption and activation of inflammation and the acute phase response (granulocyte elastase, interleukin 6, C-reactive protein).[62,63] Although these markers have all thrown interesting light on the pathophysiology of acute pancreatitis, they have found limited clinical application with the possible exception of C-reactive protein levels.

Table 8.3 *Significant factors in predicting severity of acute pancreatitis*[59]

Factors	Episodes		
	n	Mild (%)	Severe (%)
Calcium (mmol l^{-1})			
<2.00	58	62	38
>2.00	305	91	9
Urea (mmol l^{-1})			
>16	13	31	69
<16	385	86	14
Lactic dehydrogenase (LDH) (u l^{-1})			
>600	70	67	33
<600	165	94	6
Glucose (mmol l^{-1})			
>10	29	48	52
<10	181	74	26
Arterial oxygen saturation (Pa_{O_2}) (mmHg)			
<60	114	75	25
>60	262	89	11
White blood cell count ($\times 10^9$ l^{-1})			
>15	130	73	27
<15	237	90	10
Albumin (g l^{-1})			
<32	28	64	36
>32	344	87	13
Age (years)			
>55	198	80	20
<55	207	88	12

As discussed earlier, extensive activation of trypsinogen in severe pancreatitis is reflected in increased urinary levels of trypsinogen activation peptides.[23] As yet, a TAP assay has not been available for routine use.

The APACHE-II score has also been used to assess and monitor patients with severe acute pancreatitis.[64]

Complications

Acute pancreatitis may give rise to local or generalized complications. In the first few days, hypovolaemic shock is the major threat to life; thereafter sepsis and multiple organ failure are the major dangers.

Hypovolaemic shock

Release of enzymes and vasoactive substances increases capillary permeability and produces oedema in and around the pancreas. Hypovolaemia is reflected in tachycardia, hypotension and decreased sys-

Table 8.4   *Basis of factor scoring systems to predict the severity of acute pancreatitis. In both systems, disease is classified as severe when three or more factors are present*

Ransom *et al.* (1974)[58]	Imrie *et al.* (1978)[79]
On admission	
Age >55 years	Age >55 years
White blood cell count 16 × 10^9 l^{-1}	White blood cell count >15 × 10^9 l^{-1}
Blood glucose >10 mmol l^{-1}	Blood glucose >10 mmol l^{-1} (no diabetic history)
Lactic dehydrogenase >700 u l^{-1}	Serum urea >16 mmol l^{-1} (no response to i.v. fluids)
Aspartate aminotransferase >250	Arterial oxygen saturation (Pao_2) <60 mmHg
Sigma Frankel units %	
Within 48 hours	
Blood urea nitrogen rise >5 mg %	Serum calcium <2.0 mmol l^{-1}
Arterial oxygen saturation (Pao_2) <60 mmHg	Serum albumin <32 g l^{-1}
Serum calcium <2.0 mmol l^{-1}	Lactic dehydrogenase >600 u l^{-1}
Haematocrit fall >10%	Aspartate aminotransferase/alanine aminotransferase
Base deficit >4 mmol l^{-1}	>100 u l^{-1}
Fluid sequestration >6 l	

temic vascular resistance,[65] hyperdynamic cardiovascular changes being significantly more marked in necrotising pancreatitis.[66] Bleeding into the pancreas, peritoneal cavity and fascial planes may compound the circulatory upset in necrotising pancreatitis. Less common complications include cardiac arrhythmias, myocardial infarction, pericarditis and pericardial effusion. Hypovolaemia, disseminated intravascular coagulation and intra-abdominal inflammation may predispose to thrombosis and cause infarction of the small intestine or colon.[67]

Respiratory failure

Respiratory failure makes a significant contribution to mortality in at least one-third of fatal cases. Asymptomatic hypoxaemia occurs in two-thirds of cases and a Pao_2 of less than 60 mmHg is used as a predictor of severity.[59] Patients developing the adult respiratory distress syndrome (ARDS) have tachypnoea and hypoxia results from impaired gaseous exchange and right-to-left shunting. Initially, there are no changes on the chest radiograph but pulmonary oedema may develop. Other factors which adversely affect pulmonary function include atelectasis due to abdominal pain, distension and elevation of the diaphragm, pneumonitis secondary to vomiting and aspiration, and pleural effusion caused by activated pancreatic enzymes. All of these complications take place against a background of the increased requirements for tissue oxygenation caused by intra-abdominal inflammation.

The histological features of ARDS have been well described.[68] In the first 7 days there is interstitial and intra-alveolar oedema, dilatation of lymphatics and capillaries with leucocyte adhesion. Fat droplets are occasionally seen in the pulmonary capillaries. Between days 3 and 7, hyaline microthrombi form within capillaries and there may be intra-alveolar bleeding. In the second week, hyaline membranes appear and pneumocytes proliferate. Thereafter, there is fibrous organisation of hyaline membranes and interstitial fibrosis.

At the time of admission to hospital, patients destined to develop ARDS often have little or no radiological change but they may already have high concentrations of interleukin-8 (IL-8) in bronchoalveolar lavage fluid.[69] Release of IL-8 by lung macrophages may be a major factor in pathogenesis of ARDS in that IL-8 may cause neutrophils to migrate into the alveoli, where they degranulate and release histotoxic products such as elastase and collagenase. Other mechanisms involved in ARDS include disseminated intravascular coagulation (which may be triggered by trypsin), phospholipase A-induced damage to membranes in the lung with increased pulmonary permeability, and fatty acid-induced damage to alveolar-capillary membranes (if high circulating levels of triglyceride are hydrolysed by pancreatic lipase). Complement may also cause acute pulmonary injury.

Hepatobiliary disorders

Mild jaundice occurs in about 15% of patients and can be due to impaired bilirubin clearance, biliary tract obstruction, or an increased bilirubin load from disseminated intravascular coagulation and intra-abdominal haemorrhage. More marked jaundice is usually obstructive and reflects compression of the bile duct by a gallstone, pancreatic oedema or pseudocyst. Cholecystitis can occur and portal hypertension due to thrombosis of the portal, splenic or hepatic vein is a rare but recognised complication.

Gastrointestinal complications

Ileus reflects the severity of the attack, lasting 2–3 days in mild cases, and for more protracted periods in more severe cases. Intestinal obstruction may be caused by mechanical compression of the duodenum by the inflamed pancreas, intramural haematoma, abscess or pseudocyst formation.[70] Infarction of the bowel may lead to necrosis, fistula or stricture formation.[67] The transverse colon and splenic flexure are at particular risk.

Plain radiographs of the abdomen will reveal ileus or obstruction, but barium meal and/or enema may be necessary to define such complications as fistula or stricture.

Severe pancreatitis can be complicated by haemorrhage into the gastrointestinal tract, pancreas, peritoneal cavity or retroperitoneum. Severe upper gastrointestinal bleeding occurs in approximately 2% of cases and is a major cause of fatal pancreatitis.[71] It may be due to gastric or duodenal erosions or ulceration, direct involvement of the wall of the duodenum by inflammation, or erosion of vessels with or without pseudoaneurysm formation. Bleeding into the pancreatic duct is uncommon.[72] Gastric or oesophageal varices can develop following portal or splenic vein thrombosis and may bleed, whereas bowel infarction can lead to rectal bleeding.

Gastrointestinal bleeding is an indication for urgent endoscopy. Contrast-enhanced dynamic computed tomography is an excellent method of detecting vascular complications such as pseudoaneurysm formation.[73] Selective arteriography is, and therapeutic embolization can occasionally be, useful in defining and controlling the sources of haemorrhage.[74]

Renal failure

Oliguria or anuria are common manifestations of hypovolaemia in severe pancreatitis. Hypovolaemia, hypoxaemia, sepsis, endotoxaemia and disseminated intravascular coagulation are all factors in the development of cortical or tubular necrosis.

Role of endotoxin in multiple organ failure

Endotoxin may have an important pathophysiological role in multiple organ failure.[75,76] It may translocate from the gut lumen if the gut mucosal barrier is impaired, and then passes through the portal venous system and hepatic reticuloendothelial system to produce bursts of systemic endotoxaemia. Endotoxaemia can induce complement and activate coagulation, generate vasoactive kinins, and stimulate mononuclear phagocytes to produce cytokines such as IL-1, IL-6, IL-8 and tumour necrosis factor (TNF). The bursts of systemic endotoxaemia may be difficult to detect without frequent blood sampling, but a fall in serum IgG antiendotoxin antibodies implies binding of endotoxin and its removal from the circulation, and signals a high risk of multiple organ failure.[77]

Metabolic abnormalities

At least one-third of pancreatitis patients have abnormal glucose tolerance in the first few days and transient hyperglycaemia and glycosuria are common in severe pancreatitis. If pancreatic resection is undertaken because of necrotising pancreatitis, up to 50% of patients will develop diabetes mellitus.[78]

The importance of hypocalcaemia is reflected in its inclusion in prognostic scoring systems.[58,79] Calcium is bound in 'calcium soaps' when fatty acids are liberated by the action of pancreatic lipase on body fat. This may account for some, but by no means all, of the fall in ionised calcium levels in the first 24 hours[80] but tetany is truly exceptional. Much of the subsequent hypocalcaemia reflects the reduction in serum albumin concentration and bound calcium.[81] Patients with hypocalcaemic severe pancreatitis have raised parathyroid hormone levels soon after hospitalisation; the levels return to normal within three or four days.[79] This supports the contention that there is indeed a reduction in ionised calcium levels and that parathyroid failure is not the cause of hypocalcaemia.

Skin and bone lesions

Subcutaneous fat necrosis can follow release of pancreatic lipase and produces raised red nodules on the limbs which are very similar to those of erythema nodosum.[82] Periarticular fat necrosis may produce polyarthritis and synovitis. Intramedullary fat necrosis occasionally causes painful osteolytic bone lesions and intramedullary calcification.

Psychosis and encephalopathy

These problems are not uncommon in severe pancreatitis. Contributory factors include hypoxia, hypovolaemia, metabolic abnormalities, alcohol withdrawal, sepsis, opiate administration and cerebral emboli.

Treatment of acute pancreatitis and its complications

Treatment of pain

Prompt treatment of pain is essential. Pethidine (75–100 mg given 4-hourly intravenously or by intravenous infusion) is usually preferred, despite the fact that most narcotic drugs produce some degree of spasm of the sphincter of Oddi.

Circulatory support

Hypotension, tachycardia and haemoconcentration reflect loss of fluid from the circulation. Treatment is commenced with intravenous isotonic saline but colloid solutions such as albumin are needed in shocked patients. Recent evidence suggests that isovolaemic dilution with dextran 60 may improve the pancreatic microcirculation and avoid necrosis.[83] Central venous pressure should be monitored, and the patient should be catheterized and urine output maintained as >30 ml h^{-1}. In patients with marked fluid shifts or associated cardiopulmonary disease, monitoring of pulmonary wedge arterial pressures with a Swan–Ganz catheter is of immense value.

Fluid and electrolyte balance, nutrition and metabolic support

Parenteral fluid and electrolytes are usually required for a day or two in mild pancreatitis, but may be needed for much longer in severe disease. Parenteral nutrition is initiated if oral intake has not been commenced after 3–5 days in patients with complicated disease. Treatment of hypocalcaemia is necessary only in the extremely rare event that it is symptomatic. When there is severe hypocalcaemia, serum magnesium should also be measured, and levels below $0.6\,\mathrm{mmol\,l^{-1}}$ ($1.5\,\mathrm{mg\,d^{-1}}$) are corrected by infusions of 10 ml of 50% magnesium sulphate dissolved in at least 200 ml of 5% dextrose. Persistent hyperglycaemia may require insulin therapy, particularly if ketosis develops.

Renal failure

The usual cause of low urine output is inadequate fluid replacement. If output remains below $30\,\mathrm{ml\,h^{-1}}$ despite apparently adequate intra-venous therapy, an attempt should be made to induce a diuresis, by giving 25–50 g of mannitol or 400 mg frusemide. If oliguria persists despite adequate volume replacement and dopamine infusion (2–$5\,\mu\mathrm{g}$ $\mathrm{kg^{-1}\,min^{-1}}$), a programme for acute renal failure must be instituted.

Respiratory support

Arterial blood gas concentrations should be measured on admission and as often as necessary in patients with severe disease. Oxygen is given if the patient is shocked or anoxic, and inability to maintain arterial oxygen tension above 8.0 kPa (60 mmHg) is an indication for endotracheal intubation and mechanically assisted ventilation with positive end-expiratory pressure.

Measures to suppress pancreatic inflammation[84]

Agents found to be beneficial in animal models have rarely been beneficial clinically, and most clinical trails have been weakened by inclusion of patients with mild disease and a lack of statistical power. The long list of agents without proven clinical value includes atropine, glucagon, cimetidine, calcitonin, aprotinin, corticosteroids, and soya bean trypsin inhibitor. The value of the protease inhibitor gabexate mesilate[85,86] and somatostatin and its analogues is at present uncertain but they cannot be recommended unequivocally for prophylaxis or treatment.[87] Earlier suggestions that fresh frozen plasma, which contains proteinase inhibitors, might be beneficial[88] have not been sustained.[89]

Gastric aspiration has been used traditionally in attempts to reduce pancreatic secretion but several studies have shown that it is of no significant benefit, at least in patients with mild disease. However, nasogastric aspiration may relieve persistent vomiting, and trials are still needed to assess whether it is beneficial in patients with severe pancreatitis. Oral feeding is normally withheld until pain and tenderness have resolved, although there is preliminary evidence that early naso-enteric tube feeding may reduce the incidence of endotoxaemia and septic complications.[90]

Antibiotics

It used to be held that prophylactic antibiotics do not prevent the septic complications of acute pancreatitis and may even promote infection with organisms which are particularly difficult to treat, such as *Candida albicans*. Nevertheless, many centres use prophylactic broad-spectrum antibiotics in gallstone pancreatitis with the intention of treating cholangitis, and some authorities advocate antibiotics for fulminant pancreatitis.[84]

Recent studies in rats have shown that early infection in necrotising pancreatitis can be reduced by gut decontamination (oral polymyxin, tobramycin, amphotericin) or by giving imipenem systemically.[91] Cefotaxime, which has a similar spectrum of activity to imipenem but which is not concentrated by the pancreas, was without effect. These findings suggest that the gut is the principal source of the bacteria which infect the pancreas in necrotizing pancreatitis, and that systemic antibiotics may be useful in clinical practice. The importance of the gut bacteria in pancreatitis has been emphasised by studies in cats showing that transmural spread of *E. coli* from gut to pancreas can be prevented by enclosing the colon in an impermeable bag.[92]

In a recent controlled trial in Holland, selective gut decontamination (norfloxacin, colistin, amphotericin) significantly reduced mortality (22% versus 35%) and need for laparotomy in severe acute pancreatitis.[93] Similarly, a small controlled Finnish study of acute necrotising pancreatitis has shown that intravenous cefuroxime significantly reduced infectious complications and mortality (one death as opposed to seven in control patients).[94] These findings with cefuroxime are inconsistent with the animal data discussed earlier and the Finnish paper has been criticised, not least because of the poor penetration of antibiotics such as cefuroxime into necrotic pancreatic tissue. Interestingly, imipenem failed to influence the mortality of necrotising pancreatitis in earlier clinical trials,[95] and questions have been raised about the suitability of both imipenem and cephalosporins given their poor penetration into pancreatic juice. If pancreatic juice penetration does reflect concentration in pancreatic tissue, then antibiotics such as clindamycin (34%) or oxfloxacin (84%) may have greater potential in necrotising pancreatitis. Further controlled studies are urgently required.

Other therapeutic agents

Although anticoagulation is contraindicated in acute pancreatitis, heparin (750–1000 units h^{-1} monitored by partial thromboplastin time) may reduce the danger of disseminated intravascular coagulation in patients with a rising platelet count and serum fibrinogen.[84]

Therapeutic peritoneal lavage

Therapeutic lavage is now seldom used. Despite encouragement from animal experiments and uncontrolled clinical studies, most randomised studies in severe disease have failed to show benefit in terms of mortality, complication rate or hospital stay. However, in one recent randomised study involving 29 patients with severe disease, lavage for 7 days halved the incidence of pancreatic sepsis (22% versus 40%) and improved mortality (0 versus 20%) when compared to lavage for 2 days.[96]

Surgical treatment

Surgery in gallstone pancreatitis

It is vitally important to identify patients in whom pancreatitis is due to gallstones, as eradication of their gallstones virtually eliminates the risk of further attacks. However, gaseous distension and ileus means that ultrasonography is less accurate than normal in the first few days of an attack of acute pancreatitis; the gall bladder is visualised in only 70–80% of cases and only about two-thirds of patients with gallstone pancreatitis have their gallstones detected at this stage.[97,98] Although ultrasonography at six weeks is more reliable, it still detects only about 90% of gallstones[99] and ERCP should be considered in all patients with 'idiopathic' pancreatitis and normal ultrasonography.

There has been controversy regarding the timing of biliary surgery in gallstone pancreatitis. The policy at one time was to allow the pancreatitis to settle, confirm the presence of gallstones, and readmit the patient 6–8 weeks later for definitive biliary surgery. Unfortunately pancreatitis did not always settle on conservative management and a large number of patients developed further attacks of pancreatitis or cholecystitis while awaiting biliary surgery.[100] Few surgeons adopted the alternative policy of immediate biliary surgery,[101] arguing that many of the gallstones responsible for acute pancreatitis impact only transiently at the lower end of the common bile duct, and that most will pass on spontaneously if surgery is deferred. More recent controlled evaluation has failed to show any benefit if cholecystectomy and bile duct exploration is undertaken within 48 h in patients with mild pancreatitis;[102] in patients with severe disease, biliary surgery within 48 hours had prohibitive morbidity (83%) and mortality (48%) when compared to the results of later surgery (18% and 11%, respectively).

It is now recommended that whenever possible, patients with gallstone pancreatitis should be allowed to settle and undergo cholecystectomy thereafter in the course of the same hospital admission.[100] Operative cholangiography or ERCP (see below) can be used to detect any stones which remain in the bile duct; if such stones are left in the biliary tree, the reported incidence of further attacks of pancreatitis approaches 92%.[103] Although this policy has proved safe and effective in patients who settle promptly, it still leaves the real problem posed by patients with severe disease who fail to settle on conservative treatment. Rather than subject the latter group to immediate surgery with all of its hazards,[102] ERCP can be used to confirm the presence of gallstones and allow their removal by endoscopic papillotomy.[104] Clinical and bio-

Table 8.5 *Factors of significance in distinguishing between episodes of acute pancreatitis due to gallstones and those associated with alcohol*[105]

Factor	Value	Percentage with gallstone
Alkaline phosphate (iu l^{-1})	<300	28*
	>300	86
Age (years)	<50	28*
	>50	82
Alanine aminotransferase (iu l^{-1})	<100	34*
	>100	89
Sex	M	31*
	F	82
Aspartate aminotransferase (iu l^{-1})	<100	38*
	>100	37
Amylase (u l^{-1})	<4000	41*
	>4000	73
Bilirubin (μmol l^{-1})	<25	45*
	>25	73

Chi-squared analysis: *$P < 0.001$.

chemical factors which suggest that gallstones are responsible for an attack of pancreatitis are age over 55, female sex, high alkaline phosphatase and aminotransferase levels, and a serum amylase activity of greater than 4000 iu l^{-1} [105] (Table 8.5). If ultrasonography is equivocal in a patient with severe acute pancreatitis, the fact that four or five of these factors are positive means that urgent ERCP should be considered. The objective in such cases is to outline the bile duct and care must be taken to avoid overfilling the pancreatic duct system and exacerbating the pancreatitis.

Neoptolemos et al.[104] randomised patients thought to have gallstone pancreatitis to receive conservative management or urgent ERCP (with sphincterotomy if stones were present). In patients with mild disease on Glasgow criteria, urgent ERCP conferred no benefit whereas morbidity was significantly lower in the group of patients with severe disease who underwent urgent ERCP (Table 8.6). None of the patients with mild disease died in this study, but there were fewer deaths in patients with severe disease who received urgent ERCP as opposed to conservative management (although the difference was not statistically significant). In a similar study from Hong Kong, early ERCP (with sphincterotomy if stones were present) reduced the incidence of biliary sepsis but did not affect the mortality or the risk of developing local and systemic complications.[106]

Thus, it appears that early ERCP is unnecessary in patients with mild pancreatitis and should be avoided if at all possible in patients who do not have gallstones. Although the available results are encouraging, some believe that the severity of an attack of pancreatitis (and the risk of

Table 8.6 *Controlled trial of urgent ERCP (with or without endoscopic sphincterotomy, ± ES) and conventional treatment in patients with acute gallstone pancreatitis*[104]

	Group A (ERCP ± ES within 72 h)	Group B (conventional treatment)
Mild acute pancreatitis[a] (n)	34	34
With complications	4 (12%)	4 (12%)
Deaths	0	0
Severe acute pancreatitis (n)	25	28
With complications	6 (24%)	17 (61%)
Deaths	1	5

[a] Severity assessed by Glasgow criteria.[59]

necrosis) is determined early and that the amount of activated enzyme may be a more important factor than persisting impaction of a gallstone at the ampulla of Vater.[102] If there is indeed a 'window of opportunity' during which an attack of pancreatitis can be aborted by endoscopic sphincterotomy and stone extraction, the window is likely to be short and may well have passed by the time the patient reaches hospital. On the other hand, necrotising pancreatitis caused by obstruction of the biliopancreatic duct system by a balloon catheter in the opossum is less severe if the catheter is removed at 1 or 3 days as opposed to 5 days,[107] lending support to the practice of early endoscopic removal of obstructing stones in gallstone pancreatitis. It is our practice to undertake ERCP in all patients with severe pancreatitis which is not settling and where gallstones cannot be excluded by other means. Indeed, there is some evidence that leaving patients with an impacted stone is particularly dangerous.

If obstructing stones are found and removed at ERCP, the fact that sphincterotomy has been performed may in itself offer some protection against further attacks of pancreatitis. However, unless the patient is unfit for biliary surgery, most surgeons would still advocate early cholecystectomy, an operation which can be carried out laparoscopically where feasible. The potential importance of 'biliary sludge' as a cause of acute pancreatitis has been highlighted recently. Of 31 patients with idiopathic pancreatitis, 23 (74%) had microscopic evidence of sludge (i.e. calcium bilirubinate crystals or cholesterol monohydrate crystals) in duodenal aspirates. Pancreatitis recurred in only one of the 10 patients undergoing cholecystectomy or endoscopic papillotomy, as opposed to 8 of the 11 patients having no treatment.[17]

Surgery for necrotising pancreatitis
The development of extensive pancreatic necrosis remains a major cause of death in patients with severe pancreatitis. Although the risk of

complications and death can be predicted by clinical and biochemical grading systems[58,59] or examination of lavage fluid,[61] it may still be difficult to identify individuals who are developing severe necrosis which requires surgical intervention. Multisystem failure is an important marker of fulminant disease, and a rising pulse rate, serum creatinine, fever and white cell count in conjunction with difficulty in maintaining arterial blood pressure and PaO_2 are ominous signs.[108] In some patients it is apparent from the outset that multisystem failure is present and worsening, whereas others 'fail to thrive' or improve temporarily before beginning to deteriorate. As discussed earlier, serum markers which have been advocated for the early detection of pancreatic necrosis include raised levels of ribonuclease,[109] fibrinogen,[110] alpha-1-antitrypsin,[111] lactic dehydrogenase and C-reactive protein[112] and a falling level of alpha-2-macroglobulin.[111] Depletion of alpha-2-macroglobulin reflects its consumption during inactivation of circulating proteases and has a sensitivity of 85% in the detection of necrosis.[112] The acute phase protein, C-reactive protein (CRP), is a non-specific index of injury, inflammation, sepsis and ischaemia. The level used to signify a high probability of necrosis varies from centre to centre, but levels greater than 100 mg l^{-1} had a sensitivity of 95% in detecting necrosis in the Ulm series.[112] This is not to say that an elevated CRP level is an indication for surgery, rather that it may be an early indicator of the need for CT scanning to define the presence and extent of necrosis, and determine whether infection is present. Nonetheless, CRP is normally the serum marker most commonly used in clinical practice to monitor the progress of the individual patient.

As indicated earlier, incremental dynamic bolus computed tomography is the best method of detecting pancreatic and peripancreatic necrosis, defining its severity, and planning surgical intervention,[49–51] whereas percutaneous fine-needle aspiration under computed tomography guidance may be used to detect infection.[54] It must be emphasised that radiological appearances are not the sole determinant of the need for surgery, and that the clinical condition of the patient is also important. However, extensive necrosis and in particular, the presence of infected necrosis, are strong indications for surgery. Operation is usually undertaken through a bilateral subcostal incision with the lesser sac being opened widely, although some recommend a direct approach to the retroperitoneum through a left lateral subcostal incision.[113] Dead and liquefied pancreas is removed and dead retroperitoneal tissue is debrided thoroughly. Blunt (finger dissection) necrosectomy is used and it is now clear that formal pancreatic resection carries unacceptable morbidity and mortality (Table 8.7)[114–117] in addition to removing viable pancreas unnecessarily and incurring a high risk of insulin-dependent diabetes.[78] Fortunately, the head of the pancreas usually remains viable but the transverse colon may be affected by necrosis and may have to be resected, with creation of a temporary colostomy. Thorough intraoperative peritoneal lavage is mandatory and the pancreatic bed must be adequately drained. Opinions vary as to whether copious irrigation of

Table 8.7 *Effect of surgical treatment on the mortality of pancreatic necrosis and infection in surgical series reviewed by d'Egidio and Schein*[116]

	n	**% mortality**
Resection/necrosectomy + drainage	516	38 (32)[a]
Necrosectomy + lavage	216	23
Resection/necrosectomy + open management	188	24

[a]Resections excluded.

the lesser sac is advisable,[54,118] or whether the abdominal wound should be packed and left open to facilitate re-exploration, an approach sometimes called 'laparostomy'.[119,120] A recent review has concluded that necrosectomy followed by local lavage or open management with planned re-exploration offer better survival prospects than 'conventional' management by resection or necrosectomy followed only by drainage.[116] Open management may carry a higher risk of complications such as colonic necrosis, fistula formation and bleeding, but it is clear that specialist units can achieve acceptable results with open management or the lavage method provided that the initial debridement is thorough and re-exploration is undertaken promptly if sepsis persists or recurs. Regardless of the method used, a gastrostomy tube inserted at the time of surgery can avoid the need for prolonged nasogastric intubation in patients liable to protracted duodenal ileus. Insertion of a feeding jejunostomy is also advisable in that enteral nutrition is often practicable and total parenteral nutrition can be avoided. It has been postulated that enteral feeding also reduces the absorption of bacteria and their toxins from the gut by strengthening the intestinal mucosal barrier.[121]

Treatment of complications

Pseudocyst formation

Acute pseudocysts probably arise because of loss of pancreatic duct integrity and leakage of pancreatic juice and enzymes. The development of a pseudocyst should be suspected if signs of inflammation continue beyond one week or recur, if a mass develops, or if there is persisting or recurrent hyperamylasaemia. The diagnosis can be confirmed by ultrasonography or CT scanning, although CT scanning should be used selectively so as to avoid excessive doses of radiation. Given that the majority of acute pseudocysts will resolve spontaneously, they should be managed conservatively in the first instance.[122] Persistence of a pseudocyst for more than 4–6 weeks, particularly when the collection has a diameter of more than 5 cm, means that spontaneous resolution is unlikely (Fig. 8.2). Such 'mature pseudocysts' should not be allowed to persist as continuing enzymatic activity within the collection can erode major blood vessels leading to life-threatening haemorrhage. The

Figure 8.2. *CT scan undertaken five weeks after admission in a patient with severe pancreatitis. Note the large pseudocyst extending along the length of the pancreas behind the stomach.*

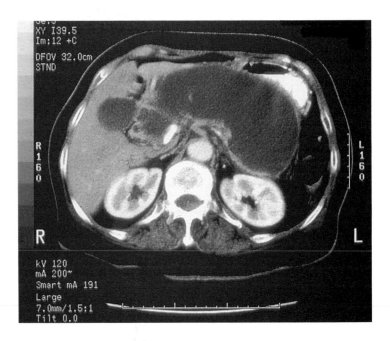

pseudocyst may also compress the common bile duct leading to obstructive jaundice and can impair gastric emptying.

The conventional open surgical treatment of a mature pancreatic pseudocyst is to drain the collection into the stomach, a Roux loop of jejunum, or more rarely, the duodenum. Dependent drainage is desirable and a sample of the pseudocyst wall is sent routinely for histological examination to exclude the presence of an epithelial lining and confirm that the collection was inflammatory rather than neoplastic. The gallbladder is removed at the same operation in patients with gallstone pancreatitis. Alternatives to open internal drainage now include percutaneous external drainage under radiological control and endoscopic internal drainage into the stomach or duodenum if the collection bulges into the gut lumen. External drainage has the disadvantage that it may introduce infection and leave the patient with an external fistula, whereas endoscopic drainage requires careful patient selection and skill if complications such as bleeding are to be avoided. In a series reporting the results of operative treatment of pancreatic pseudocysts, mortality rates of up to 12% have been observed with recurrence rates of 5–20%.[123] Internal drainage has had a lower complication rate (30%) and mortality rate (5%) than external drainage. More recently, internal drainage has been achieved by laparoscopic means but the role of this form of minimal access procedure in management is yet to be established.

Pancreatic abscess

Some 1–4% of patients with acute pancreatitis go on to develop an abscess following liquefaction of infected necrotic areas or secondary infection of a pancreatic pseudocyst. Abscess should not be confused with infected necrosis, the latter being defined as a diffuse bacterial inflammation of pancreatic and peripancreatic tissue without significant pus formation.[124] Infected necrosis usually becomes evident in the first week or two of an attack of acute pancreatitis whereas abscesses usually become manifest after 4–5 weeks, often after the acute pancreatitis appears to have subsided. About 85% of all pancreatic infections involve Gram-negative bacteria (particularly *E. coli*), but Gram-positive organisms are found in 10–55% of cases, and *Candida* infection has also been reported.[125]

Some four weeks after the onset of the attack of acute pancreatitis the patient's condition deteriorates, with recurrence of abdominal pain, anorexia, nausea, weight loss, fever and abdominal tenderness. A mass may be palpable. Cardiorespiratory and renal insufficiency are common (although not as common as in patients with infected necrosis) and the patient looks unwell. Leucocytosis is usual, but hyperamylasaemia, hypocalcaemia, hyperglycaemia and disturbed liver function are seldom present.[124]

Abscess formation can be inferred from organ distortion or displacement on a plain radiograph or barium meal, but CT scanning is the investigation of choice (Fig. 8.3). Survival increases dramatically with surgical drainage, and early computed tomography is imperative whenever abscess formation is suspected.[126,127] The demonstration of gas in the pancreas or peripancreatic tissues (usually due to gas-forming organisms) is a key diagnostic feature. However, gas is seen in only 30–50% of proven abscesses and in some it is related to a fistula, a

Figure 8.3. *CT scan undertaken three weeks after an attack of acute pancreatitis in a patient with persisting abdominal pain and fever. Note the 5 × 10 cm collection which contains gas and is situated behind the stomach.*

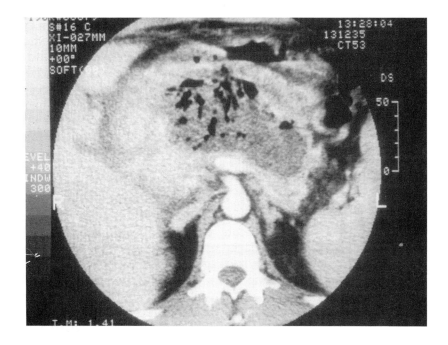

complication which should be excluded in doubtful cases by contrast radiology of the gastrointestinal tract. When gas is not present in an abscess the appearances are indistinguishable from those of a non-infected pancreatic mass or pseudocyst, and bacteriological culture following fine-needle aspiration can be invaluable. Abscesses are multiple in up to one-third of cases and may occur at distant sites. Computed tomography is a valuable aid in planning surgical drainage and in some cases, percutaneous aspiration.

Mortality rates following the conventional treatment of debridement and sump drainage of pancreatic abscess have commonly ranged from 30 to 50%.[128] The recent fall in the mortality of pancreatic abscess to 5–22% reflects early diagnosis by computed tomography and more aggressive surgical intervention with extensive drainage and debridement.[124,127,128] Warshaw and Jin[127] counsel against open packing or continuing local peritoneal lavage, although others regard these as valuable innovations.[128,129] It is essential to provide adequate nutrition after surgery and a feeding jejunostomy established at the time of surgery may be helpful. After drainage, recurrent abscess formation, haemorrhage from the abscess cavity and fistula are common and potentially lethal complications,[130] and the importance of eradicating further septic collections cannot be overemphasised. Recurrent abscess may require further surgical treatment, although CT-guided percutaneous drainage may be considered. Bleeding is second only to sepsis as a cause of death in patients with pancreatic abscess and may demand re-exploration, further debridement and packing for its control. Pancreatic fistulas usually close spontaneously but enteric fistulas are more troublesome and may require further surgery if conservative management fails.

Haemorrhage

Acute pancreatitis is complicated by life-threatening haemorrhage in about 2% of cases. Bleeding may occur into the gastrointestinal tract, pancreas, retroperitoneum, peritoneal cavity or pancreatic duct, and traditionally carried a mortality rate of 50–80%. Improved overall care in conjunction with improved diagnosis and management has reduced the number of patients who succumb from haemorrhage. In our own recent review of 279 patients with acute pancreatitis, significant bleeding was only encountered in four patients undergoing early necrosectomy, although it contributed to the demise in three of these patients.[131]

Gastritis, duodenitis, erosions and peptic ulceration

Haemorrhage from superficial mucosal erosions was once common in severe acute pancreatitis, particularly when complicated by sepsis. Prophylactic use of H_2 receptor antagonists, antacids or mucosal protectants such as sucralfate, appears to have reduced the incidence of bleeding from erosions and peptic ulceration. The onset of major upper gastrointestinal haemorrhage is an indication for endoscopy, and bleeding from defined ulcers is arrested by injection of adrenaline or sclerosants whenever possible. Bleeding from erosions and mucosal inflammation hardly ever responds to endoscopic measures, and surgery may have to be considered as a last resort.

Left-sided portal hypertension and variceal haemorrhage

The increasing use of CT scanning has revealed that splenic vein thrombosis is a not infrequent complication of pancreatitis and autopsy series suggest that approximately 15% of patients dying with acute pancreatitis will have such thrombosis.[132] The signs include failure of the splenic vein to outline with contrast, splenomegaly, and the development of collaterals around the greater curvature of the stomach. The subsequent left-sided or segmental portal hypertension may produce troublesome gastric and even colonic varices. Although variceal haemorrhage has been reported in 30–70% of patients with long-standing splenic vein thrombosis, variceal haemorrhage is unusual during an episode of acute pancreatitis. In patients coming to laparotomy for any reason, the development of splenic vein thrombosis is suggested by dilatation of the gastroepiploic vein in the absence of liver cirrhosis. If bleeding occurs as a consequence of splenic vein thrombosis, it almost always emanates from gastric varices, and splenectomy rather than portasystemic shunting is indicated.

Vascular complications of acute pancreatitis

Potentially lethal vascular necrosis may develop when arteries in or around the pancreas are bathed in activated proteolytic enzymes and the products of pancreatic suppuration. Segmental vascular thrombosis or pseudoaneurysm formation may follow, the vessel most commonly affected being the splenic artery. The gastroduodenal, pancreaticoduodenal, gastric and hepatic arteries may also be involved in descending order of frequency. Pseudoaneurysm formation is revealed by selective arteriography or by detecting the leakage of intravenous contrast on computed tomography (Fig. 8.4).

Fatal haemorrhage from direct intraperitoneal rupture can occur but rupture into the gastrointestinal tract is more common and is typically preceded by episodes of 'herald bleeding'. Bleeding into a pre-existing pseudocyst is often associated with the sudden development of a painful pulsatile abdominal mass, often associated with a bruit. Blood loss can be prodigious, and in the rare complication of 'hemosuccus pancreaticus', the pseudoaneurysm ruptures into the pancreatic duct system and blood is then lost into the gastrointestinal tract after passing through the papilla of Vater.

Conservative treatment of major bleeding in pancreatitis carries a mortality which may be as high as 90%. Surgical management used to carry mortality rates of up to 50%, and this led to the employment of angiographic embolisation in the first instance. Our own approach is to perform diagnostic angiography if time permits and embolise the offending artery with autologous clot, sponge pledgets or coils if the source of bleeding is located. Even if embolisation succeeds, there is a high incidence of recurrent haemorrhage from continued erosion of the

Figure 8.4.
(a) Contrast enhanced CT scan demonstrating a mass in the region of the head of the pancreas. Note the pooling of contrast (of the same density as that in the aorta) within this pseudoaneurysm.

(a)

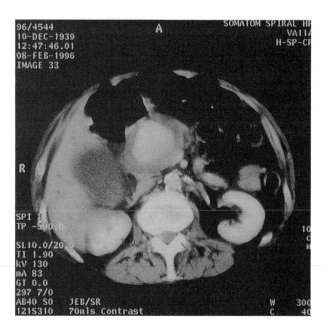

(b) Selective superior mesenteric angiogram demonstrating the pseudoaneurysm involving the gastroduodenal artery.

(b)

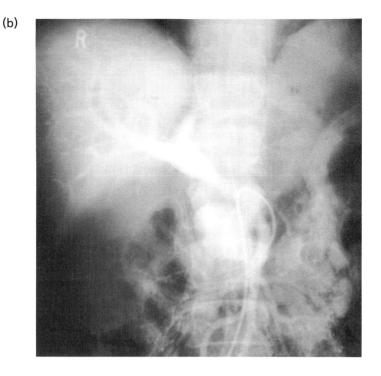

affected vessels, and planned surgical intervention is usually advisable. When surgery has to be undertaken without prior angiographic or CT localisation of the source of bleeding, the following policy is recommended. If blood is seen within the stomach, a longitudinal pylorotomy is used to search for duodenal, gastric or variceal haemorrhage. 'Hemosuccus pancreaticus' is excluded by inspecting the papilla of Vater. If haemorrhage is coming from a pseudocyst or a pseudoaneurysm which has eroded into the gastrointestinal tract, the vessel responsible can often be defined from the location of the inflammatory mass. Pulsation in the wall of a 'pseudocyst' will declare its true nature, and needle aspiration is always advisable before the wall of a pseudocyst is incised. Masses within the head of the pancreas usually involve the gastroduodenal or pancreaticoduodenal arteries, whereas those in the body and tail of pancreas involve the splenic artery. A bleeding vessel is controlled initially by compression followed by suture ligation if local conditions permit. In some cases where the splenic artery has eroded into a pseudocyst, control can be obtained by under-running the artery on either side of the point of rupture. Distal vascular lesions can be managed definitively by distal pancreatectomy and splenectomy, but proximal pancreatic resection is a formidable undertaking in sick patients and is avoided if possible.

Course and prognosis of acute pancreatitis

The mortality rate associated with acute pancreatitis has been of the order of 10–15% and has not changed substantially in 20 years.[133] However, there is some evidence that the situation may be improving. For example, in Scotland mortality rates fell from 17.8% in 1961 to 5.8% in 1985[1] whereas in Finland mortality rates fell from 5.9% in 1970 to 2.6% in 1989. Encouraging though these trends may be, it should be borne in mind that in as many as 40% of fatal cases, the diagnosis of acute pancreatitis is not made in life[134] and that the lethality of the disease may still be significantly underestimated.

Oedematous pancreatitis nearly always runs a benign course and patients admitted with mild disease on prognostic factor grading have a mortality of 0–3% whereas those with predicted severe disease have a mortality of 25–30%.[135] Necrotising pancreatitis develops in 5–15% of cases and has a particularly poor prognosis with reported mortality rates which average some 20–30%.[116] Patients who survive a first attack have a low mortality in subsequent attacks. In general, alcohol-associated pancreatitis has a lower mortality than gallstone pancreatitis[133] (Table 8.3), which in turn has a lower mortality than idiopathic and postoperative pancreatitis.[18,133] The elderly are at particular risk and mortality rates for those over 60 years of age in Bristol were 28% as opposed to 9% in younger patients,[136] whereas in Hong Kong, mortality rates rose from 6% in those under 50 years to 21% in older patients.[137] Obese patients appear to be at particular risk of developing severe necrotising pancreatitis and respiratory complications.[138,139] One large autopsy study involving 405 patients found that 20.5% of deaths occurred in the first 24 hours and 60% died within the first week. Pulmonary oedema and congestion were the prominent findings in deaths during the first week whereas sepsis was the major cause of death thereafter.[132] In a more recent multicentre audit involving 57 deaths, 32% of patients died within the first week, 12% in the second, 19% in the third and 37% died thereafter.[133]

References

1. Wilson C, Imrie CW. Changing patterns of incidence and mortality from acute pancreatitis in Scotland, 1961–1985. Br J Surg 1990; 77: 731–4.
2. Jaakkola M, Sillanaukee P, Lof K, Koivula T, Nordback I. Amount of alcohol is an important determinant of the severity of acute alcoholic pancreatitis. Surgery 1994; 115: 31–8.
3. Ranson JHC. The timing of biliary surgery in acute pancreatitis. Ann Surg 1979; 189: 654–63.
4. Moreau JA, Zinsmeister AR, Melton IJ, Di Magno EP. Gallstone pancreatitis and the effect of cholecystectomy. Mayo Clin Proc 1988; 63: 466–73.
5. Kelly TR. Gallstone pancreatitis. Local predisposing factors. Ann Surg 1984; 200: 479–84.
6. Armstrong CP, Taylor TV. The biliary tract in patients with acute gallstone pancreatitis. Br J Surg 1985; 72: 551–6.
7. Armstrong CP, Taylor TV. Pancreatic duct reflux and acute gallstone pancreatitis. Ann Surg 1986; 204: 59–64.
8. Jones BA, Salsberg BB, Bohnen JMA, Mehta MH. Common pancreatobiliary channels and their relationship to gallstone size in gallstone pancreatitis. Ann Surg 1987; 205: 123–5.
9. Roszler M, Campbell W. Post-ERCP pancreatitis: association with urographic visualization during ERCP. Radiology 1985; 157: 595.
10. Sherman S, Ruffolo TA, Hawes RH, Lehman GA. Complications of endoscopic sphincterotomy. Gastroenterology 1991; 101: 1068–75.
11. Warshaw AL. Obstructive pancreatitis: acute and chronic pancreatitis due to ductal obstruction by causes other than gallstones. In: Carter DC, Warshaw AL (eds) Clinical Surgery International 16. Edinburgh: Churchill Livingstone 1989, pp. 71–89.
12. Toskes PP. Is there a relationship between hypertriglyceridemia and development of alcohol- or gallstone-induced pancreatitis? Gastroenterology 1994; 106: 810–12.
13. Haber PS, Wilson JS, Apte MV, Hall W, Goumas K, Pirola RC. Lipid intolerance does not account for susceptibility to alcoholic and gallstone pancreatitis. Gastroenterology 1994; 106: 742–8.
14. Dominguez-Munoz JE, Malfertheiner P, Ditschuneit HH, Blanco-Chavez J, Uhl W, Buchler M, Ditschuneit H. Hyperlipidaemia in acute pancreatitis. Relationship with etiology, onset and severity of the disease. Int J Pancreatol 1991; 10: 261–7.
15. Fernandez-del Castillo C, Harringer W, Warshaw AL et al. Risk factors for pancreatic cellular injury after cardiopulmonary bypass. N Engl J Med 1991; 325: 382–7.
16. Neoptolemos JP, Davidson BR, Winder AF, Vallance D. Role of duodenal bile crystal analysis in the investigation of 'idiopathic' pancreatitis. Br J Surg 1988; 75: 450–3.
17. Lee SP, Nicholls JF, Park HZ. Biliary sludge as a cause of acute pancreatitis. N Engl J Med 1992; 326: 589–93.
18. Browder W, Patterson MD, Thompson JL, Walters DN. Acute pancreatitis of unknown etiology in the elderly. Ann Surg 1993; 217: 469–75.
19. Steer ML, Meldolesi J, Figarella C. Pancreatitis. The role of lysosomes. Dig Dis Sci 1984; 29: 934–8.
20. Adler G, Rohr G, Kern H. Alteration of membrane fusion as a cause of acute pancreatitis in the rat. Dig Dis Sci 1982; 27: 993–1002.
21. Bettinger JR, Grendell JH. Intracellular events in the pathogenesis of acute pancreatitis. Pancreas 1991; 6: S2–S6.
22. Adler G, Hahn C, Kern H, Rao K. Cerulein-induced pancreatitis in rats: increased lysosomal enzyme activity and autophagocytosis. Digestion 1985; 32: 10–14.

23. Gudgeon AM, Health DI, Hurley P, Jehanli A *et al*. Trypsinogen activation peptide assay in the early prediction of severity of acute pancreatitis. Lancet 1990; 335: 4–8.

24. Schmidt J, Fernandez-del Castillo C, Rattner DW *et al*. Trypsinogen-activation peptides in experimental rat pancreatitis: prognostic implications and histopathologic correlates. Gastroenterology 1992; 103: 1009–16.

25. Niederau C, Niederau M, Luthen R, Strohmeyer G, Ferrell LD, Grendell JH. Pancreatic exocrine secretion in acute experimental pancreatitis. Gastroenterology 1990; 99: 1120–7.

26. Farmer RC, Tweedie J, Maslin S, Reber HA, Adler G, Kern H. Effects of bile salts on permeability and morphology of main pancreatic duct in cats. Dig Dis Sci 1984; 29: 740–51.

27. Simpson CJ, Toner PC, Carr KE, Anderson JD, Carter DC. Effect of bile salt perfusion and intraduct pressure on ionic flux and mucosal ultrastructure in the pancreatic duct of cats. Virchows Arch Cell Pathol 1984; 42: 327–42.

28. Keynes M. Heretical thoughts on the pathogenesis of acute pancreatitis. Gut 1988; 29: 1413–23.

29. Neoptolemos JP, Carr-Locke DL, Leese T, James D. Acute cholangitis in association with acute pancreatitis; incidence, clinical features and outcome in relation to ERCP and endoscopic sphincterotomy. Br J Surg 1987; 74: 1103–6.

30. Opie EL. The etiology of acute hemorrhagic pancreatitis. Bull Johns Hopkins Hosp 1901; 12: 182–8.

31. Kelly TR. Gallstone pancreatitis; pathophysiology. Surgery 1976; 80: 488–92.

32. Pfeffer RB, Stasior O, Hinton JW. The clinical picture of sequential development of acute hemorrhagic pancreatitis in the dog. Surg Forum 1957; 8: 248–51.

33. Harvey MH, Wedgwood KR, Austin JA, Reber HA. Pancreatic duct pressure, duct permeability and acute pancreatitis. Br J Surg 1989; 76: 859–62.

34. Lerch MM, Saluja AK, Runzi M, Dawra R, Saluja M, Steer ML. Pancreatic duct obstruction triggers acute necrotizing pancreatitis in the opossum. Gastroenterology 1993; 104: 853–61.

35. Acosta JL, Rossi R, Ledesma CL. The usefulness of stool screening for diagnosing cholelithiasis in acute pancreatitis. A description of the technique. Am J Dig Dis 1977; 22: 168–74.

36. Nordback IH, Macgowan S, Potter JI, Cameron JL. The role of acetaldehyde in the pathogenesis of acute alcoholic pancreatitis. Ann Surg 1991; 214: 671–8.

37. Kelly DM, McEntee GP, Delaney C, McGeeney KF, Fitzpatrick JM. Temporal relationship of acinar and microvascular changes in caerulein-induced pancreatitis. Br J Surg 1993; 80: 1174–8.

38. Klar E, Rattner DW, Compton C, Stanford G, Chernow B, Warshaw AL. Adverse effect of therapeutic vasoconstrictors in experimental acute pancreatitis. Ann Surg 1991; 214: 168–74.

39. Foitzik T, Bassi DG, Schmidt J *et al*. Intravenous contrast medium accentuates the severity of acute necrotizing pancreatitis in the rat. Gastroenterology 1994; 106: 207–14.

40. Lankisch PG, Schirren CA, Kunze E. Undetected fatal acute pancreatitis: why is the disease so frequently overlooked. Am J Gastroenterol 1991; 86: 322–6.

41. Dickson AP, Imrie CW. The incidence and prognosis of body wall ecchymosis in acute pancreatitis. Surg Gynecol Obstet 1984; 159: 343–7.

42. Clavien P-A, Burgan S, Moossa AR. Serum enzymes and other laboratory tests in acute pancreatitis. Br J Surg 1989; 76: 1234–43.

43. Winslet M, Hall C, Londin NJM, Neoptolemos JP. Relation of diagnostic serum amylase levels to aetiology and severity of acute pancreatitis. Gut 1992; 33: 982–6.

44. Spechler SJ, Dalton JW, Robbins AH *et al*. Prevalence of normal serum amylase levels in patients with acute alcoholic pancreatitis. Dig Dis Sci 1983; 28: 865–9.

45. Clavien P-A, Robert J, Meyer P. Acute pancreatitis and normo-amylasaemia. Ann Surg 1989; 210: 614–20.

46. Ventrucci M, Pezilli R, Gullo L, Plate L, Sprovieri G, Barbara L. Role of serum pancreatic enzyme assays in diagnosis of pancreatic disease. Dig Dis Sci 1989; 34: 39–45.

47. Kolars JC, Ellis CJ, Levitt MD. Comparison of serum amylase pancreatic isoamylase and lipase in patients with hyperamylasaemia. Dig Dis Sci 1984; 29: 289–93.

48. Freeny PC. Pre-operative diagnosis of pancreatic disease. In: Trede M, Carter DC (eds)

Surgery of the pancreas. Edinburgh: Churchill Livingstone, 1993, pp. 51–86.

49. Larvin M, Chalmers AG, McMahon MJ. Dynamic contrast enhanced computed tomography: a precise technique for identifying and localising pancreatic necrosis. Br Med J 1990; 300: 1425–8.

50. London NJM, Leese T, Lavelle JM et al. Rapid-bolus contrast-enhanced dynamic computed tomography in acute pancreatitis: a prospective study. Br J Surg 1991; 78: 1452–6.

51. Freeny PC. Incremental dynamic bolus computed tomography of acute pancreatitis. Int J Pancreatol 1993; 13: 147–58.

52. Balthazar EJ. CT diagnosis and staging of acute pancreatitis. Radiol Clin North Am 1989; 27: 19–37.

53. Balthazar EJ, Robinson DL, Megibow AJ, Ranson JHC. Acute pancreatitis: value of CT in establishing prognosis. Radiology 1990; 174: 331–6.

54. Beger HG, Buchler M, Bittner R, Block S, Nevalainen T, Roscher R. Necrosectomy and postoperative local lavage in necrotizing pancreatitis. Br J Surg 1988; 75: 207–12.

55. Beger HG, Bittner R, Block S, Buchler M. Bacterial contamination of pancreatic necrosis. A prospective clinical study. Gastroenterology 1986; 91: 433–8.

56. Gerzof SG, Banks PA, Robbins AH et al. Early diagnosis of pancreatic infection by computed tomography-guided aspiration. Gastroenterology 1987; 93: 1315–20.

57. Rattner DW, Legemate DA, Meuller PR, Warshaw AL. Early surgical debridement of pancreatic necrosis is beneficial irrespective of infection. Am J Surg 1992; 163: 105–10.

58. Ranson JH, Rifkind KM, Roses DF, Fink SD, Eng K, Spencer J. Prognostic signs and the role of operative management in acute pancreatitis. Surg Gynecol Obstet 1974; 139: 69–81.

59. Blamey SL, Imrie CW, O'Neill J, Gilmour WH, Carter DC. Prognostic factors in acute pancreatitis. Gut 1984; 25: 1340–6.

60. Williamson RCN. Early assessment of severity in acute pancreatitis. Gut 1984; 25: 1331–9.

61. Corfield AP, Williamson RCN, McMahon MJ et al. Prediction of severity in acute pancreatitis: prospective comparison of three prognostic indices. Lancet 1984; ii: 403–7.

62. Viedma JA, Perez-Mateo M, Agullo J, Dominguez JE, Carballo F. Inflammatory response in the early prediction of severity in acute pancreatitis. Gut 1994; 35: 822–7.

63. Wilson C, Heath DI, Shenkin A, Imrie CW. C-reactive protein, antiproteases and complement factors as objective markers of severity in acute pancreatitis. Br J Surg 1989; 76: 177–81.

64. Larvin M, McMahon MJ. Apache-II score for assessment and monitoring of acute pancreatitis. Lancet 1989; ii: 201–5.

65. Bradley EL, Hall JR, Lutz J, Hamner L, Lattouf O. Hemodynamic consequence of severe pancreatitis. Ann Surg 1983; 198: 130–3.

66. Beger HG, Bittner R, Buchler M, Hess W, Schmitz JE. Hemodynamic data patterns in patients with acute pancreatitis. Gastroenterology 1986; 90: 74–9.

67. Aldridge MC, Francis ND, Glazer G, Dudley HAF. Colonic complications of severe acute pancreatitis. Br J Surg 1989; 76: 362–7.

68. Lankisch PG, Rahlf G, Koop H. Pulmonary complications in fatal acute hemorrhagic pancreatitis. Dig Dis Sci 1983; 28: 111–16.

69. Donnelly SC, Strieter RM, Kunkel SL et al. Interleukin-8 and development of adult respiratory distress syndrome in at-risk patient groups. Lancet 1993; 341: 643–7.

70. Bradley EL, Clements JL. Idiopathic duodenal obstruction. An unappreciated complication of pancreatitis. Ann Surg 1981; 193: 638–46.

71. Stroud WH, Cullom JW, Anderson MC. Hemorrhagic complications of severe pancreatitis. Surgery 1981; 90: 657–63.

72. Brown RA, Immelman EJ, Harries-Jones EP. Pancreatic duct haemorrhage. Br J Surg 1985; 72: 223–4.

73. Freeny PC, Lawson L (eds) Radiology of the pancreas. New York: Springer-Verlag, 1982.

74. Steckman ML, Dooley MC, Jaques PF, Powell DW. Major gastrointestinal hemorrhage from peripancreatic blood vessels in pancreatitis. Treatment by embotherapy. Dig Dis Sci 1984; 29: 486–97.

75. Foulis AK, Murray WR, Galloway D. Endotoxaemia and complement activation in acute pancreatitis in man. Gut 1982; 23: 656–61.

76. Kivilaakso E, Valtnen VV, Malkamaki M et al., Endotoxaemia and acute pancreatitis: correlation between the severity of the disease and the antienterobacterial common antigen antibody titre. Gut 1984; 25: 1065–70.

77. Windsor JA, Fearon KCH, Ross JA et al. Role of serum endotoxin and antiendotoxin core antibody levels in predicting the development of multiple organ failure in acute pancreatitis. Br J Surg 1993; 80: 1042–6.

78. Eriksson J, Doepel M, Widen E et al. Pancreatic surgery, not pancreatitis, is the primary cause of diabetes after acute fulminant pancreatitis. Gut 1992; 33: 843–7.

79. Imrie CW, Beastall GH, Allam BF, O'Neill J, Benjamin IS, McKay AJ. Parathyroid hormone and calcium homeostasis in acute pancreatitis. Br J Surg 1978; 65: 717–20.

80. Croton RS, Warren RA, Stott A, Roberts NB. Ionized calcium in acute pancreatitis and its relationship with total calcium and serum lipase. Br J Surg 1981; 68: 241–4.

81. Allam BF, Imrie CW. Serum ionized calcium in acute pancreatitis. Br J Surg 1977; 64: 665–8.

82. Higgins E, Ive FA. Subcutaneous fat necrosis in pancreatic disease. Br J Surg 1990; 77: 532–3.

83. Klar E, Foitzik T, Buhr H, Messmer K, Herfarth C. Isovolemic hemodilution with dextran 60 as treatment of pancreatic ischemia in acute pancreatitis. Clinical practicability of an experimental concept. Ann Surg 1993; 217: 369–74.

84. Ranson JHC. Non-operative management of acute pancreatitis. In: Trede M, Carter DC (eds) Surgery of the pancreas. Edinburgh: Churchill Livingstone, 1993, pp. 209–19.

85. Pederzzoli P, Cavallini G, Falconi M, Bassi C. Gabexate mesilate vs aprotinin in human acute pancreatitis. Int J Pancreatol 1993; 14: 117–24.

86. Buchler M, Malfertheiner P, Uhl W et al. Gabexate mesilate in human acute pancreatitis. Gastroenterology 1993; 104: 1165–70.

87. McKay CJ, Imrie CW, Baxter JN. Somatostatin and somatostatin analogues – are they indicated in the management of acute pancreatitis? Gut 1993; 34: 1622–6.

88. Cuschieri A, Wood RAB, Cumming JRG, Meehan SE, Mackie CR. Treatment of acute pancreatitis with fresh frozen plasma. Br J Surg 1983; 70: 710–12.

89. Leese T, Holliday M, Heath D, Hall AW, Bell PFR. Multicentre trial of low volume fresh frozen plasma therapy in acute pancreatitis. Br J Surg 1987; 74: 906–11.

90. Windsor ACJ, Li A, Guthrie A et al. Feeding the gut in acute pancreatitis: a randomised clinical trial of enteral vs parenteral nutrition. Br J Surg 1996; 77: 731–4.

91. Foitzik T, Fernandez-del Castillo C, Ferraro MJ, Mithofer K, Rattner DW, Warshaw AL. Pathogenesis and prevention of early pancreatic infection in experimental acute necrotizing pancreatitis. Ann Surg 1995; 222: 179–85.

92. Widdison AL, Karanja ND, Reber HA. Routes of spread of pathogens into the pancreas in a feline model of acute pancreatitis. Gut 1994; 36: 1306–10.

93. Luiten E, Hop W, Lange J, Bruining H. Controlled clinical trial of selective decontamination for the treatment of severe acute pancreatitis. Ann Surg 1995; 222: 57–65.

94. Sainio V, Kemppainen E, Puolakkainen P et al. Early antibiotic treatment in acute necrotising pancreatitis. Lancet 1995; 346: 663–7.

95. Pederzzoli P, Bassi C, Vesentini Sea. A randomized multicenter clinical trial of antibiotic prophylaxis of septic complications in acute necrotizing pancreatitis with imipenem. Surg Gynecol Obstet 1993; 176: 480–3.

96. Ranson JHC. The role of surgery in the management of acute pancreatitis. Ann Surg 1990; 211: 382–93.

97. McKay AJ, Imrie CW, O'Neill J, Duncan JG. Is an early ultrasound scan of value in acute pancreatitis? Br J Surg 1982; 69: 369–72.

98. Neoptolemos JP, Hall AW, Finlay DF, Berry JM, Carr-Locke DL, Fossard DP. The urgent diagnosis of gallstones in acute pancreatitis: a prospective study of three methods. Br J Surg 1984; 71: 230–3.

99. Goodman AJ, Neoptolemos JP, Carr-Locke DL, Finlay DB, Fossard DP. Detection of gallstones after acute pancreatitis. Gut 1985; 26: 125–32.

100. Osborne DH, Imrie CW, Carter DC. Biliary surgery in the same admission for gallstone associated acute pancreatitis. Br J Surg 1981; 68: 758–61.

101. Acosta JM, Rossi R, Galli OMR, Pellegrini CA, Skinner DB. Early surgery for acute gallstone pancreatitis: evaluation of a systematic approach. Surgery 1978; 83: 367–80.

102. Kelly TR, Wagner DS. Gallstone pancreatitis: a prospective randomized trial of the timing of surgery. Surgery 1988; 104: 600–5.

103. Kelly TR, Swaney PE. Gallstone pancreatitis: the second time around. Surgery 1982; 92: 571–5.

104. Neoptolemos JP, Carr-Locke DL, London NJM, Bailey IA, James D, Fossard DP. Controlled trial of urgent endoscopic retrograde cholangiopancreatography and endoscopic sphincterotomy versus conservative treatment in patients with acute pancreatitis due to gallstones. Lancet 1988; ii: 979–83.

105. Blamey SL, Osborne DH, Gilmour WH, O'Neill J, Carter DC, Imrie CW. The early identification of patients with gallstone pancreatitis using clinical and biochemical factors only. Ann Surg 1983; 198: 574–8.

106. Fan S-T, Lai ECS, Mok FPT, Lo C-M, Zheng S-S, Wong J. Early treatment of acute biliary pancreatitis by endoscopic papillotomy. N Engl J Med 1993; 328: 228–32.

107. Runzi M, Saluja A, Lerch MM, Dawra R, Nishino H, Steer ML. Early ductal decompression prevents the progression of biliary pancreatitis: an experimental study in the opossum. Gastroenterology 1993; 105: 157–64.

108. Aldridge MC, Ornstein M, Glazer G, Dudley HAF. Pancreatic resection for severe acute pancreatitis. Br J Surg 1985; 72: 796–800.

109. Warshaw AL, Lee H-L. Serum ribonuclease elevations and pancreatic necrosis in acute pancreatitis. Surgery 1979; 86: 227–32.

110. Berry AR, Taylor TV, Davies GC. Diagnostic tests and prognostic indicators in acute pancreatitis. J R Coll Surg Edinb 1982; 27: 345–52.

111. McMahon MJ, Bowen M, Mayer AD, Cooper EH. Relationship of alpha-macroglobulin and other antiproteases to the clinical features of acute pancreatitis. Am J Surg 1984; 147: 164–70.

112. Buchler M, Malfertheiner P, Beger HG. Correlation of imaging procedures, biochemical parameters, and clinical stage in acute pancreatitis. In: Malfertheiner P, Ditschuneit H (eds) Diagnostic procedures in pancreatic disease. Heidelberg: Springer-Verlag, 1986; pp. 123–9.

113. Fagniez PL, Rotman N, Kracht M. Direct retroperitoneal approach to necrosis in severe acute pancreatitis. Br J Surg 1989; 76: 264–7.

114. Kivilaakso E, Lempinen M, Makelainen A, Nikki P, Schroder T. Pancreatic resection versus peritoneal lavation for acute fulminant pancreatitis. A randomized prospective study. Ann Surg 1984; 199: 426–31.

115. Wilson C, McArdle CS, Carter DC, Imrie CW. Surgical treatment of acute necrotizing pancreatitis. Br J Surg 1988; 75: 1119–23.

116. D'Egidio A, Schein M. Surgical strategies in the treatment of pancreatic necrosis and infection. Br J Surg 1991; 78: 133–7.

117. Kiviniemi H, Makela J, Kairaluoma M. Acute fulminant pancreatitis: debridement or formal resection of the pancreas. HPB Surg 1993; 6: 255–63.

118. Larvin M, Chalmers AG, Robinson PJ, McMahon MJ. Debridement and closed cavity irrigation for the treatment of pancreatic necrosis. Br J Surg 1989; 78: 465–71.

119. Bradley EL. Management of infected pancreatic necrosis by open drainage. Ann Surg 1987; 206: 542–50.

120. Mughal MM, Bancewicz J, Irving MH. The surgical management of pancreatic abscess. Ann R Coll Surg Engl 1987; 69: 64–70.

121. Wilmore DW, Smith RJ, O'Dwyer ST et al. The gut: a central organ after surgical stress. Surgery 1988; 104: 917–24.

122. Bradley E III, Gonzalez AC, Clements LJ. Acute pancreatic pseudocysts: incidence and implications. Ann Surg 1976; 184: 734–7.

123. Yeo CJ, Bastidas JA, Lynch-Nyhas A et al. The natural history of pancreatic pseudocysts documented by computed tomography. Surg Gynecol Obstet 1990; 170: 411–17.

124. Bittner R, Block S, Buchler M, Beger HG. Pancreatic abscess and infected pancreatic necrosis. Different local septic complications in acute pancreatitis. Dig Dis Sci 1987; 32: 1082–7.

125. Beger HG. Management of pancreatic necrosis and pancreatic abscess. In Carter DC, Warshaw AL (eds) Pancreatitis. Clinical surgery international. 16. Edinburgh: Churchill Livingstone, 1989, pp. 107–19.

126. Ranson JHC, Balthazar E, Caccavale R, Cooper M. Computed tomography and the prediction of pancreatic abscess in acute pancreatitis. Ann Surg 1985; 201: 656–63.

127. Warshaw AL, Jin G. Improved survival in 45 patients with pancreatic abscess. Ann Surg 1985; 202: 408–15.

128. Bradley EL, Fulenwider JT. Open treatment of pancreatic abscess. Surg Gynecol Obstet 1984; 159: 509–13.
129. Van Vyve EL, Reynaert MS, Lengele BG, Pringot JT, Otte JB, Kestens PJ. Retroperitoneal laparostomy; a surgical treatment of pancreatic abscesses after an acute necrotizing pancreatitis. Surgery 1992; 111: 369–75.
130. Warshaw AL, Moncure AC, Rattner DW. Gastrocutaneous fistulas associated with pancreatic abscesses. An aggressive entity. Ann Surg 1989; 210: 603–7.
131. de Beaux AC, Palmer KR, Carter DC. Factors influencing morbidity and mortality in acute pancreatitis: an analysis of 279 cases. Gut 1995; 37: 121–6.
132. Renner IG, Savage WT, Pantoja JL, Renner VJ. Death due to acute pancreatitis: a retrospective analysis of 405 cases. Dig Dis Sci 1985; 30: 1005–18.
133. Mann DV, Hershman MJ, Hittinger R, Glazer G. Multicentre audit of death from acute pancreatitis. Br J Surg 1994; 81: 890–3.
134. Wilson C, Imrie CW, Carter DC. Fatal acute pancreatitis. Gut 1988; 29: 782–8.
135. Mayer AD, McMahon MJ, Corfield AP et al. Controlled clinical trial of peritoneal lavage for the treatment of severe acute pancreatitis. N Engl J Med 1985; 312: 399–404.
136. Corfield AP, Cooper MJ, Williamson RCN. Acute pancreatitis: a lethal disease of increasing incidence. Gut 1985; 26: 724–9.
137. Fan ST, Choi TK, Lai CS, Wong J. Influence of age on the mortality from acute pancreatitis. Br J Surg 1988; 75: 463–6.
138. Porter KA, Banks PA. Obesity as a predictor of severity in acute pancreatitis. Int J Pancreatol 1991; 10: 247–52.
139. Funnell IC, Bornman PC, Weakly SP, Terblanche J, Marks IN. Obesity: an important prognostic factor in acute pancreatitis. Br J Surg 1993; 80: 484–6.

9 Chronic pancreatitis

David C. Carter
O. James Garden

Incidence Chronic pancreatitis may be complicated by recurrent attacks of acute pancreatitis but it may escape detection in life. Recent data suggest that its incidence is increasing. A prospective Danish study noted an incidence of 8.2 per million with a prevalence of 27.4 cases per million,[1] figures which are in keeping with retrospective studies in Europe and North America. In England and Wales, the number of patients discharged from hospital with a diagnosis of chronic pancreatitis increased fourfold in men and twofold in women between two comparable five-year periods in the 1960s and 1980s. There has been a close correlation between alcohol consumption per head of the population and the number of patients discharged from hospital with a diagnosis of chronic pancreatitis six years later[2] (Fig. 9.1).

Figure 9.1 *Changes in annual alcohol consumption (litres per head of population), hospital discharges for chronic pancreatitis per million of population, and total number of deaths from chronic pancreatitis in England and Wales 1960–1988.* Reproduced from ref. 2 with permission of the publishers.

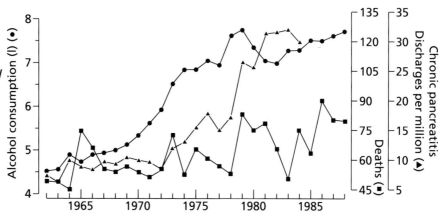

Aetiology

Alcohol

Alcohol is recognised as the prime aetiological factor in chronic pancreatitis, accounting for 60–70% of cases of chronic pancreatitis in the Western world. Due to their larger consumption of alcohol, men are more commonly affected than women. In contrast to research in patients with liver disease, no precise level of daily alcohol consumption has been demonstrated above which chronic pancreatitis is more likely to develop. Individual sensitivity to the toxic effects of alcohol must vary greatly since not all alcoholics develop clinical pancreatitis, although distinct morphological changes in the pancreas have been recorded at autopsy in 19–58% of cases.[3,4] In patients with alcohol-associated chronic pancreatitis, the average daily intake of pure alcohol generally exceeds 60–80 g, although, as in liver disease, women may have a lower threshold. The interval between the commencement of regular alcohol consumption and the clinical manifestations of chronic pancreatitis averages only 12 years in women and 18 years in men.[5] Tobacco has been identified as an additional risk factor[6] but it is difficult to separate its role from that of alcohol.

Nutritional factors

It has been suggested that the development of alcoholic pancreatitis may be associated with an increased diet comprising protein and fat. However, several studies have implicated a higher than normal, normal or lower than normal intake of calories, fat and protein, and an insufficient intake of the trace elements zinc and selenium.[7]

Tropical pancreatitis

There seems to be a definite link between nutrition and the development of tropical pancreatitis, a disease in which alcohol has no role. This particular form of pancreatitis is noted for the calcific changes in the pancreas and is reported in a number of countries situated within 15 degrees of the equator. Its main clinical features include abdominal pain, pancreatic calcification, diabetes mellitus, steatorrhoea related to exocrine insufficiency and early death.[8,9] Protein calorie malnutrition or childhood kwashiorkor was thought to be the main aetiological factor, but malnutrition is more likely to be the result of the disease. The fact that the disease is not seen in areas where protein energy malnutrition is prevalent, has further raised doubts as to whether malnutrition is truly an initiating factor in the pathogenesis of tropical pancreatitis. Pancreatic atrophy and insufficiency can be caused by juvenile kwashiorkor but is usually reversible. Epidemiological studies have implicated toxic cyanogenetic glycosides in cassava (*Manihot esculenta*), agents which could theoretically cause pancreatic injury by interfering with the action of free radical scavengers such as superoxide dismutase. A cassava-rich diet may also be deficient in methionine and trace elements such as zinc and selenium, leading to impaired detoxification of cyanogens and increased production of free radicals.

Obstructive pancreatitis

A form of chronic pancreatitis has been described which is thought to be secondary to ductal obstruction. Common causes would include congenital or acquired strictures, pancreatitis, neoplasia or trauma. Obstructive pancreatitis differs from alcoholic pancreatitis in that the epithelium of the obstructed ducts is usually preserved and the obstructive pancreas shows uniform chronic inflammatory changes rather than the patchy involvement which characterises alcoholic chronic pancreatitis. Intraductal protein plugs are not commonly found and progression to calcification and stone formation is not common.

Pancreas divisum, in which the dorsal and ventral pancreatic ducts fail to fuse, is the commonest congenital abnormality of the pancreas. Autopsy and ERCP studies have shown a prevalence affecting up to 7% of the population.[7] It is thought that pancreatitis may develop due to the impaired passage of juice through the small minor papillae from the larger dorsal pancreas. Although pressures are invariably abnormally high in the dorsal pancreas in pancreas divisum;[10] the condition is thought to represent a potential cause of recurrent acute pancreatitis rather than chronic pancreatitis.[11]

Hypercalcaemia

Hypercalcaemia associated with hyperparathyroidism and chronic renal failure can give rise to both acute and chronic pancreatitis. Given that hyperparathyroidism is diagnosed early on the basis of routine blood testing, this accounts for less then 2% of cases of chronic pancreatitis.

Hereditary chronic pancreatitis

This rare disease is inherited through a autosomal dominant gene of incomplete penetrance and does not normally become manifest until the age of 5 to 15 years. The diagnosis should be suspected if several members of a family develop chronic pancreatitis without obvious reason. Associated conditions include hyperlipidaemia and aminoaciduria.[12] Although hyperlipidaemia on its own can be associated with acute pancreatitis, there is no evidence that it is involved in the pathogenesis of chronic pancreatitis. Hereditary chronic pancreatitis may increase the risk of developing pancreatic cancer, the risk being reported to be as high as 25% in some families.

Biliary tract disease

Although gallstone disease is the most frequent cause of acute pancreatitis in many industrialised countries, it is not clear whether patients experiencing recurrent episodes of acute pancreatitis due to biliary disease proceed to the development of chronic pancreatitis. As many as one-half of patients with gallstones have an abnormal pancreatogram and one in six have changes resembling those of chronic pancreatitis.[13] However, the significance of these abnormal findings is uncertain and it is felt that choledocholithiasis is therefore an exceptional cause of chronic pancreatitis. It should be noted, however, that chronic pancreatitis not infrequently causes biliary stasis and the formation of stones in the common bile duct.

Idiopathic chronic pancreatitis

In up to 40% of patients, no obvious aetiological factor is identified. Idiopathic chronic pancreatitis has an equal sex distribution, and in the absence of a defined aetiology, many of these patients are often wrongly labelled as having alcohol-associated disease. Juvenile idiopathic chronic pancreatitis has a median age of onset of 20 years and pursues a painful clinical course.

Late-onset idiopathic chronic pancreatitis is more common in men, often pursues a painless clinical course but is associated with weight loss, exocrine and endocrine insufficiency and pancreatic calcification.[14] Pancreatic atrophy, functional impairment and morphological change (including calcification) is an accepted form of ageing, and it remains unclear whether late-onset chronic pancreatitis represents an exaggeration of this process.

Other factors

Rare causes of chronic pancreatitis include cystic fibrosis and previous abdominal radiotherapy.[15]

Pathogenesis The precise mechanism by which alcohol induces chronic pancreatitis remains uncertain.

One theory suggests that the initial step is a primary effect of alcohol on pancreatic exocrine secretion. Chronic alcohol uptake decreases pancreatic bicarbonate and water secretion and results in an increase in protein secretion. The increased viscosity of the pancreatic juice, activation of enzyme and a reduction in the amount of substances which keep protein soluble may contribute to the formation of protein plugs and their calcification. It is thought that a 14 000-dalton pancreatic stone protein called lithostatine is the major component of the organic matrix of the resulting stones. There is *in vitro* evidence which suggests that this substance prevents the nucleation and growth of calcium carbonate crystals.[16] Its concentration in the pancreatic juice of patients with chronic pancreatitis has been reported to be decreased, particulary in those patients with marked calcification in the gland.[16–18] There is evidence that eosinophilic protein precipitates have been found in the pancreatic secretions before histological damage to acinar and ductal cells is evident. Levels of messenger RNA encoding for lithostatine are lower in the juice of patients with chronic calcific pancreatitis than in controls, regardless of the aetiology of the disease.[19,20] There is not universal support for this particular theory and some investigators have been able to identify differences in lithostatine concentrations in groups of patients with chronic pancreatitis, pancreatic neoplasia and non-pancreatic disease.[21] Other factors may favour calcification of protein in the pancreatic ductules. In alcohol chronic pancreatitis, the pancreatic juice may be more viscous due to increased protein secretion, increased secretion of calcium by acinar cells and a decreased concentration of citrate in pancreatic juice.[22,23]

A second theory has been proposed which suggests that acinar cell damage may be primarily due to ductular obstruction by protein precipitates secondary to fatty degeneration of pancreatic cells. There may be associated loss of zymogen content and periacinar fibrosis.[24–26] It has also been suggested that alcohol may lead to the production of toxic metabolites of lipid metabolism within pancreatic cells, thereby precipitating the development of chronic pancreatitis.[27]

A third hypothesis has implicated impaired hepatic detoxification which may generate toxic free radicals and reactive intermediates which are excreted in bile and reflux into the pancreatic duct system.[28] The process may be initiated by the induction of hepatic mixed function oxidases by alcohol. This theory offers an explanation for the varied genetic susceptibility to alcohol whilst stressing the potential importance of toxic factors in the pathogenesis of chronic pancreatitis.

Pathology

The morphological changes in chronic pancreatitis are extremely variable and range from minimal morphological and histological change to dense fibrosis with destruction of gland architecture.[29] Oedema, acute inflammation and necrosis are often superimposed on chronic inflammatory change with marked fibrosis, loss of acinar cells, and ultimate loss of endocrine cells. The duct system shows variable dilatation and stricture formation with protein plugs and calcification (Fig. 9.2). Perineurial disintegration and eosinophilic infiltration are typical features and are associated with an increase in mean nerve diameter. These changes may account for pain being the predominant feature of chronic pancreatitis.[30]

Abnormally large amounts of serotonin and calcitonin gene-related peptide are present and may be related to altered pain thresholds.[29] Extension of the inflammatory process into neighbouring organs can produce common bile duct obstruction, splenic vein thrombosis, segmental portal hypertension and duodenal stenosis.

It may be difficult to exclude the presence of carcinoma and the two conditions may co-exist. Recent evidence suggests that some 4% of patients develop malignancy within 20 years of the onset of chronic pancreatitis.[31]

Figure 9.2 *Factors implicated in the calcification of chronic pancreatitis.*

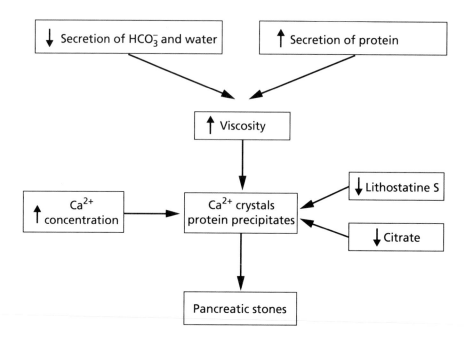

Clinical features Pain is the principal presenting feature of chronic pancreatitis and is generally felt centrally in the epigastric region or subcostally with radiation to the back or shoulder tip. The pain is typically constant, severe and dull. Some patients say pain is eased by leaning forward or to one side. Some patients indicate that they avoid lying supine or even resort to kneeling on hands and knees to obtain relief. Some patients note that the pain is exacerbated by meals or the ingestion of certain foods such as those high in fat. In others, bouts of pain are associated with drinking alcohol. Application of a hot water bottle or a hot bath may ease the pain. The pain is often intermittent and may last for considerable periods of time, although some patients are rarely free of pain. Many patients may require high doses of opiates by the time of presentation, and fear of addiction is a recurring anxiety in management. Loss of sleep, time off work and the need for admission to hospital are useful pointers to severity and it is important to establish whether the pain does significantly impair the patient's quality of life. Assessment of pain can be difficult in these patients, some of whom remain addicted to alcohol and have manipulative personalities. Steatorrhoea is not an invariable feature of chronic pancreatitis, but the patient should be carefully questioned regarding the passage of pale bulky or oily stools which may be offensive in smell and difficult to flush away. Some patients are socially incapacitated because of this symptom. There is some evidence that functional impairment and calcification is associated with relief from pain[32] but this is not generally accepted and the concept that chronic pancreatitis eventually 'burns itself out' has been overemphasised. It is unusual for diabetes mellitus to declare itself at an early stage and it usually only develops once overt exocrine insufficiency has occurred. There may be a transition from diet control to the use of oral hypoglycaemic agents and ultimately to the use of insulin. Patients with diabetes mellitus and chronic pancreatitis are exposed to the same risks of complications such as diabetic neuropathy and vascular disease.

Endocrine and exocrine insufficiency may contribute to the weight loss often observed in these patients, although anorexia, nausea and vomiting may be a contributing factor. Duodenal obstruction due to inflammation in the head of the pancreas is uncommon. The development of jaundice suggests biliary tract obstruction by inflammation, fibrosis or cyst formation. Haemorrhage from gastro-oesophageal varices may arise as a consequence of splenic vein thrombosis, and major bleeding can follow involvement of the major pancreatic vessels by the inflammatory process.

Examination may be unrewarding and there are no specific features of chronic pancreatic disease. Evidence of weight loss and malnutrition may be present and mottled burn marks (erythema *ab igne*) may be associated with the use of heat pads or hot water bottles. The patient should be examined for evidence of jaundice, palpable abdominal mass and splenomegaly which may indicate splenic vein thrombosis. Stigmata of chronic liver disease are unusual in patients with known alcohol-associated pancreatitis. Rupture of the pancreatic duct or pseudocyst may present with pancreatic ascites or a pleural effusion.

Investigations

Biochemical and haematological investigation

In chronic pancreatitis, serum amylase levels are usually normal and may be only slightly elevated. Liver function tests may demonstrate a cholestatic pattern with elevation of serum alkaline phosphatase and/or gamma glutamyl transpeptidase levels if there is associated biliary tract obstruction or continuing ethanol abuse. The presence of leucopenia and thrombocytopenia suggests that splenic vein thrombosis may have resulted in hypersplenism and the prothrombin time should be assessed in patients with cholestasis. A random blood glucose level should be measured to exclude diabetes mellitus.

Tests of pancreatic exocrine function (Table 9.1)[33]

Few centres use pancreatic function tests routinely in diagnosis, which is generally made based on the history and imaging of the pancreas. Function tests may be helpful when chronic pancreatitis is suspected and the imaging studies are normal or show minimal change, but none of the available tests is sufficiently sensitive to exclude chronic pancreatitis when negative. The established direct tests involve measuring the concentrations of bicarbonate and enzymes in duodenal juice after stimulating the pancreas by a meal (Lundh test) or by exogenous secretin with or without cholecystokinin or caerulein (secretin–pancreozymin

Table 9.1 *Pancreatic exocrine function tests*[33]

Direct pancreatic function tests
   Secretin–pancreozymin test
   Lundh test
Indirect pancreatic function tests
   Measurement of enzymes
      Serum pancreatic isoamylase
      Serum immunoreactive trypsin
      Faecal trypsin
      Faecal chymotrypsin
   Measurement of enzyme actions
      NBT-PABA (bentiromide) test
      Pancreolauryl test
      Faecal fat analysis

test). These tests are, however, time consuming, invasive and expensive. In addition, they are difficult to standardise and are therefore now used in very few centres. Indirect tests measure digestive capacity, since they are easier to standardise, non-invasive and more commonly undertaken. These include measurement of enzymes, including pancreatic isoamylase, immunoreactive trypsin, faecal trypsin and faecal chymotrypsin. Pancreatic function can also be assessed by measurement of enzyme actions and these include NBT-PABA (Bentiromide) test, pancreolauryl test and faecal fat analysis. Function tests are a non-specific means of diagnosing exocrine insufficiency and cannot differentiate between chronic pancreatitis and pancreatic cancer.

Imaging studies

Plain abdominal radiography may demonstrate the presence of calcification within the pancreas but this finding is non-specific and its presence does not exclude pancreatic cancer. Ultrasonography may demonstrate pancreatic calcification, although it is normally employed to assess the presence of pancreatic enlargement, duct dilatation, cysts or pseudocysts. The demonstration of splenomegaly or biliary dilatation may indicate splenic vein thrombosis and/or biliary tract obstruction. Computed tomography has a high sensitivity and specificity for the diagnosis of chronic pancreatitis and is the best method of detecting calcification (Fig. 9.3). It should be seen as complementary to ultrasonography in its ability to detect chronic pancreatitis and pancreatic cancer, which, if suspected, can be confirmed by either ultrasound or CT guided fine needle aspiration or biopsy. Endoscopic retrograde cholangiopancreatography (ERCP) is the most effective method of detecting chronic pancreatitis and differentiating it from pancreatic cancer. In practice, ERCP is used to complement ultrasonography or CT scanning. When all

Figure 9.3 *CT scan of a patient with chronic pancreatitis showing extensive calcification in tail of the pancreas.*

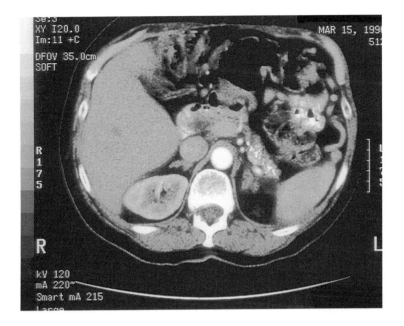

three investigations are combined a sensitivity of 95–97% and specificity of 100% are obtained for the diagnosis of both chronic pancreatitis and pancreatic cancer.[34] Ductal changes are classified as mild (normal main duct and three or more abnormal side branches), moderate (abnormal main duct with more than three abnormal side branches) or severe (as in moderate disease but with additional features such as a large cavity, filling defect and severe duct dilatation or irregularity) (Fig. 9.4). These

Figure 9.4 *Endoscopic retrograde pancreatogram in a patient with chronic pancreatitis showing irregular areas of narrowing and gross dilatation of the pancreatic duct system.*

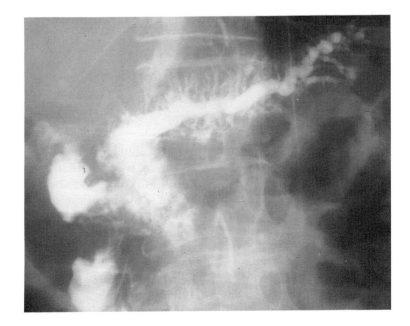

morphological changes do not parallel the degree of functional impairment.

Angiography is used only to locate a source of bleeding and may be required to evaluate portal and splenic thrombosis, although dynamic computed tomography and Doppler ultrasonography may similarly display vascular abnormalities. Barium studies may be used if duodenal stenosis or colonic obstruction is suspected. Endoscopic ultrasonography and magnetic resonance imaging are emerging as investigations which may be of value in the future. If cancer is suspected, brush cytology at ERCP and fine needle aspiration cytology may be of value. In practice, it may be extremely difficult to exclude a diagnosis of cancer in patients presenting with symptoms and signs suggestive of chronic pancreatitis and the diagnosis may only be made following pathological examination of the resected portion of pancreas.[35]

Management

In the majority of patients diagnosed as having chronic pancreatitis, symptoms can be managed conservatively for long periods, and in some cases indefinitely. No surgical procedure can reverse the loss of endocrine and exocrine function. Nonetheless, medical treatment often fails to control pain and prevent the development of complications, so that the majority of patients will come to surgical intervention.

Conservative management

Irrespective of whether the patient has surgery, it is well established that abstinence from alcohol is crucial in determining the long-term outcome. Patients will require considerable support, which may include counselling, self-help groups, and, where necessary, psychiatric support. The clinician will need to develop a strong rapport with the patient. Some patients will attempt to conceal continuing alcohol abuse, and others, in whom there may be doubt regarding the contribution of alcohol to their symptoms, may show considerable resentment to the stigma of an alcohol-related disease.

There is some debate about whether alcohol withdrawal leads to pain relief and arrests functional deterioration.[36] In chronic alcoholic pancreatitis, serial ERCP studies have shown progression of ductal changes despite reduction in alcohol consumption or complete abstinence.[37]

Acute exacerbations of chronic inflammation may produce episodes of severe abdominal pain often necessitating admission to hospital. The surgeon should resist the temptation to abandon conservative treatment in favour of operation in the face of such acute exacerbations. In the majority of cases, symptoms can be brought under control by gut rest and the institution of intravenous nutritional support.

Non-opioid analgesics such as aspirin and paracetamol are more effective in the relief of muscular skeletal pain than in the treatment of visceral pain. Opioid drugs such as dihydrocodeine (DF118) and codeine (30 mg every 6 h) are suitable for patients with mild to moderate pain but often give rise to constipation, nausea and dizziness. Sublingual buprenorphine (200–400 μg every 6–8 h) can be used for more severe pain and has less risk of dependence than morphine. Withdrawal symptoms, including pain, may arise in patients dependent on other opioids because of its opioid agonist and antagonist properties. Diconal and/or pethidine are alternatives for those with severe pain, but the slow release morphine preparation (MST Continus) (starting dose 10–20 mg twice daily) is often the best option for long-term relief. Non-steroidal analgesics may be of value in the short term, but these may increase the risk of gastrointestinal haemorrhage. Alternative therapies such as percutaneous coeliac plexus blockade have proved disappointing, and the early experience with thoracoscopic splanchnicectomy is not encouraging.

Patients are often advised to avoid fat-rich diets and large meals, as these may give rise to pain. Avoidance of high fat, high protein diet should restrict cholecystokinin release and physiological stimulation of the pancreas. Elemental diets, although theoretically beneficial, are no longer employed routinely. There has been considerable debate as to whether luminal proteases reduce pancreatic exocrine secretion by a negative feedback mechanism and whether oral enzyme supplements reduce pancreatic pain in addition to combating steatorrhoea.[38,39] All of the currently available pancreatic enzyme supplements consist of crude extracts of porcine pancreas, known in many countries as Pancreatin. The enzymes are rapidly and irreversibly inactivated below pH5 but more recently enteric-coated microspheres have been developed in which hundreds of individually coated microspheres are contained in a gelatine capsule. Supplements such as Creon and Pancrease have a high lipase content and are taken with meals in doses of some 10–15 capsules a day. An H_2 receptor antagonist such as cimetidine is usually prescribed but if steatorrhoea is still troublesome, fat intake may have to be restricted or replaced by medium chain triglycerides. Malnutrition, weight loss and muscle-wasting are common in chronic pancreatitis. Vitamin deficiency is common and supplements may require to be prescribed, especially in alcoholics.

Diabetic control may be difficult for patients on oral hypoglycaemic drugs or insulin, particularly if food intake is variable. Lack of endogenous glucagon contributes to a greater sensitivity to insulin and risk of hypoglycaemia. However, diabetic ketoacidosis is uncommon in the patient with chronic pancreatitis, since there is usually sufficient insulin secretion to prevent the release of fatty acids from adipose tissue and their subsequent metabolism to ketone bodies in the liver.

Indications for surgery[40]

It should, again, be emphasised that surgical intervention will not reverse the progressive loss of endocrine and exocrine pancreatic function. Equally, the surgeon should not be pressurised into offering surgery to the symptomatic patient until a thorough evaluation and

Table 9.2 *Indications for surgery in chronic pancreatitis*

Intractable pain
Pancreatic duct stenosis
Cysts and pseudocysts
Biliary tract obstruction
Splenic vein thrombosis with gastric/oesophageal varices
Portal vein compression/mesenteric vein thrombosis
Pancreatic ascites/pleural effusion
Duodenal stenosis
Colonic stricture
Suspicion of pancreatic carcinoma

assessment of the pancreatic disease has been undertaken. The principal objectives of patients undergoing surgery include the improvement of intractable pain, to exclude the suspicion of carcinoma and to bypass or remove the complications of the disease. Table 9.2 lists the principal indications for operation.

Biliary obstruction

Obstruction of the biliary tree occurs in 30–65% of patients[41,42] but is seldom complete and is rarely the sole indication for surgery. The stenosis involves the retropancreatic portion of the common bile duct but is usually the tapering-type rather than the abrupt cut-off seen in malignant obstruction. Obstruction can be caused by oedema, a cyst or pseudocyst but is seldom complete and is rarely the sole indication for surgery. About 20% of patients with asymptomatic common duct stenosis on ERCP have raised alkaline phosphatase levels.[43] In such patients, deterioration of liver function is exceptional but if biliary obstruction is symptomatic, relief should be sought before hepatic sequelae result. Endoscopic insertion of a stent is indicated only as a temporary measure, since prolonged disease would require repeated change of stent. If biliary obstruction is the only complication of chronic pancreatitis, some form of bilioenteric bypass is indicated. There has been a move away from choledochotomy, since this anastomosis depends on a well-dilated duct for longer-term patency, a condition which seldom applies in chronic pancreatitis. Although satisfactory results with cholecystojejunostomy have been reported, hepaticojejunostomy utilising a long Roux-en-Y loop is preferred by most surgeons since this will avoid the risk of reflux of enteric contents into the biliary tree.[43] Although isolated biliary obstruction is rare, it is interesting that pain is often improved with the jaundice following bypass in some patients.

Intestinal obstruction

Some degree of duodenal obstruction is commonly found in chronic pancreatitis during endoscopy or in upper gastrointestinal radiology and should be distinguished from stenosis related to peptic ulceration. If isolated duodenal obstruction occurs, this is best managed by gastro-jejunostomy combined with some form of vagotomy to avoid peptic ulceration. A colonic stricture may mimic carcinoma but once this diagnosis has been excluded by colonoscopy, expectant conservative treatment should be pursued. Surgical intervention for this complication is exceptional.

Pseudocyst

True cystic dilatation of the pancreatic duct as well as pseudocysts outside the confines of the pancreas complicate chronic pancreatitis in some 25% of patients. Pseudocysts of less than 6 cm in diameter can be observed for a period of up to six weeks since a spontaneous resolution may occur but, for larger collections, simple observation carries the risk of complication that is greater than that of elective surgery.[44] Although percutaneous drainage is feasible and has often been attempted prior to referral, recurrence occurs in almost 70% of cases. Endoscopic transgastric cyst drainage by means of a stent may be undertaken but this assumes an adherence between the stomach and cyst wall which may not be present in up to 60% of cases.[44] It is used in selected cases where a collection with a relatively thin wall bulges into the gut lumen.[45] After puncture with a diathermy needle-knife a pigtail stent is inserted over a guidewire or the site of puncture can be extended using a conventional papillotome. Complications (bleeding, pancreatitis and abscess) are reported in 5–15% of cases but are rarely fatal.

There has been little support for non-surgical drainage, since there is a risk of draining an unrecognised neoplastic cyst. Open biopsy of the cyst wall is an integral part of every operation on pseudocysts. Often treatment is indicated for all pseudocysts of more than 6 cm in diameter which show no sign of resolution within a six-week observation period. Drainage will be achieved by anastomosing the stomach, duodenum or a Roux-en-Y limb of jejunum at the lowest point of the cyst wall and this latter method has been most popular in Europe. For cysts situated near the tail of the pancreas, resection is often considered. It should be borne in mind, however, that biliary or pancreatic duct obstruction causing intractable pain may require additional drainage procedures or even resection.

Pancreatic ascites and pleural effusion are ominous complications of both chronic and acute pancreatitis. These result from rupture of a pseudocyst, cyst or pancreatic duct and complicate about 1% of cases. The ascites is often wrongly attributed to liver disease in a patient with a history of alcohol abuse, but paracentesis reveals a high amylase content and protein levels which exceed $30 \, g \, l^{-1}$. Similarly, sampling of the pleural effusion reveals fluid with a high amylase content. Such patients are generally malnourished and treatment consists of paracentesis, pleural aspiration, intravenous nutritional support and administration of somatostatin (octreotide 50–200 µg twice daily by subcutaneous injection) to minimise pancreatic secretion. The treatment should be continued for several weeks and ERCP should be undertaken to accurately localise the site of the leak. This examination will generally identify an associated pancreatic duct obstruction which will require either to be managed by resection or surgical drainage into a Roux-en-Y limb of jejunum.[46] Pleural effusions will settle once the abdominal cause has been eradicated. Untreated pancreatic ascites carries a mortality of up to 30% and it is therefore unwise to persist with conservative treatment for more than two to three weeks.

Portal hypertension

Some involvement of the portal venous system is encountered in 10% of patients presenting with chronic pancreatitis. Involvement ranges from compression to frank occlusion with thrombosis. Splenic vein thrombosis causing segmental portal hypertension is the commonest manifestation and the resulting splenomegaly produces hypersplenism and the formation of gastric and oesophageal varices. Thrombosis confined to the splenic vein is best dealt with by distal pancreatectomy and splenectomy before bleeding occurs. Portal or superior mesenteric venous thrombosis resulting in portal hypertension and cavernous transformation of the peripancreatic veins is considered to be a contraindication to any procedure in the pancreas itself. Changes in the peripancreatic arteries are rarely seen in chronic pancreatitis and preoperative angiography but may include pseudoaneurysm formation. Bleeding may occur directly into the pancreatic duct, peritoneum or retroperitoneum but haemorrhage more commonly occurs into a pseudocyst and this may be fatal. A site of bleeding may be demonstrated by leakage of contrast on dynamic CT scanning and can be confirmed by emergency angiography prior to resection of the affected part of the pancreas. Angiography may allow embolisation and occlusion of the bleeding vessel but this should only be considered as a temporary manoeuvre.

Surgical options in management

Surgical drainage procedures may best arrest or slow the rate of decline of loss of pancreatic exocrine and endocrine function but will not reverse this process.[47] Resection almost invariably leads to further deterioration (partial pancreatectomy) or complete loss of function (total pancreatectomy). The selection of the patient is as important as the selection of the operative procedure and the decision to undertake surgery should only be made when a full and thorough evaluation of the patient has been made. The patient must understand the risks of intervention and be aware that pain may not be relieved. Operative mortality for pancreatic drainage procedures should be negligible and be less than 5% for resection. In general, all forms of pancreatic surgery offer complete or substantial pain relief in up to 70% of cases when patients are assessed at five years.[48]

Drainage procedures in chronic pancreatitis are based on the concept that ductal obstruction leads to distention and in turn pain. Since many patients with chronic pancreatitis do not have pancreatic duct dilatation, it is clear that other factors must contribute. Increased pancreatic ductal pressure has been recorded at operation and endoscopically.[49,50] A number of studies have cast doubt on the relationship between pain and chronic pancreatitis and pancreatic duct size and pressure. Similarly, although stenosis of the pancreatic duct system is a frequent finding in chronic pancreatitis, disordered biliary motility is unlikely to have a significant role in the pathogenesis of chronic pancreatitis. Calculi may also contribute to duct obstruction and a number of studies have reported pain relief in the short term in patients having a stone removed by transduodenal or endoscopic sphincterotomy but it remains to be seen whether endoscopic intervention will rival surgical drainage procedures in the long-term relief of pain.

Pancreaticojejunostomy

Although Cattel first described the use of a Roux limb of jejunum to bypass the obstructed pancreatic duct in a patient with pancreatic cancer,[51] it was Duval who popularised retrograde drainage of the pancreas into a Roux limb or jejunum following amputation of the tip of the pancreatic tail and splenectomy.[52] It was soon recognised that this procedure did not lend itself to providing adequate drainage of a pancreatic duct with multiple strictures and Peustow and Gillesby[53] extended the Duval procedure by unroofing the main pancreatic duct from the tail to the right of the portal and superior mesenteric veins. In this procedure, the tip of the gland was still amputated prior to implanting the body and tail of the pancreas into the open end of the Roux limb. This latter procedure was further modified by Partington and Rochelle[54] so as to preserve the spleen. A side-to-side pancreaticojejunal anastomosis is fashioned between the open pancreas and a Roux limb of jejunum. It was stressed in the original description that mucosa to mucosa anastomosis should be avoided to avoid occlusion of the side branches of the main pancreatic duct. It is this latter operation of side-to-side pancreaticojejunostomy which forms the basis of the modern operation (Fig. 9.5).

It is generally accepted that the operation should only be performed in patients with pancreatic ducts larger than 7–8 mm in diameter, although others have challenged this restriction.[55] The duct should be opened to within 1–2 cm of the hilus of the spleen and extended to the head of the gland and if possible in the uncinate process as well. Intraoperative ultrasonography may be used to locate the duct and it

Figure 9.5
Longitudinal pancreatico- jejunostomy. The pancreatic duct system is opened as widely as possible and anastomosed to a Roux loop of jejunum. Intestinal continuity is restored by an end-to-side jejunojejunal anastomosis. The same Roux loop can also be used to drain cystic collections or an obstructed bile duct, and to bypass an obstructed duodenum.

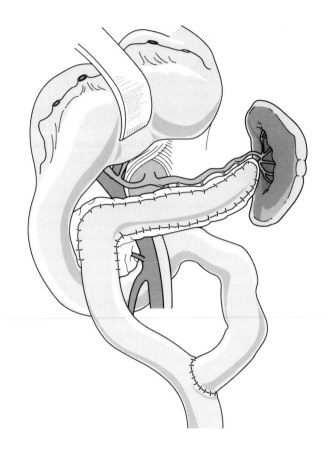

may be valuable to undertake a tru-cut biopsy of the liver at the time of surgery to assess hepatic damage. Although there is an argument against mucosa-to-mucosa apposition, it is our practice to use one layer of interrupted sutures and to pick up the mucosa of the pancreatic duct if the gland overlying the anterior aspect of the duct is thin. It is important to orientate the Roux limb so that its blind end is placed towards the tail of the pancreas allowing the possibility of using the same limb for anastomosis to the biliary system. Pseudocysts can also be drained into the same Roux limb without any increase in morbidity or mortality.

It has been argued by some[56] that if the head of the pancreas is more than 3 cm thick, it is unlikely to be drained adequately by a standard longitudinal pancreaticojejunostomy. Frey has therefore modified the longitudinal pancreaticojejunostomy to include partial excision of the head of the gland, removing cysts or other areas of necrosis and scarring. A 4–5 mm rim of pancreatic tissue is left between the superior mesenteric vein and the core incision. A similar sliver of pancreatic tissue is preserved along the inner aspect of the duodenum and retroperitoneally. Once this core out process is complete, all of the open pancreas is anastomosed to a Roux limb. Further modifications to this procedure have also been described, although it remains to be seen whether long-term results are improved by these modifications.[42]

Pancreaticogastrostomy has been advocated by some as a better form of drainage procedure than pancreaticojejunostomy, although this has generally been restricted to patients in whom the pancreatic duct was strictured at only one or two sites.[57] Surgical sphincterotomy and sphincteroplasty have similarly been attempted although most surgeons have moved away from this form of intervention. Although good short-term results are reported, 30% of patients relapsed within 36 months of follow-up.[58]

Pancreatic resection

Chronic pancreatitis generally affects the entire gland and the desire to remove all of the diseased pancreas has to be balanced against the problems posed by producing brittle insulin dependent diabetes and total loss of exocrine function which follow total pancreatectomy. A minority of patients have disease confined to the body and tail of the gland and can be dealt with effectively by distal pancreatectomy and in terms of pain relief, the results of distal pancreatectomy are said to be comparable to those of pancreaticojejunostomy and pancreaticoduodenectomy.[59] In a review of published series between 1972 and 1988, the operative mortality for distal pancreatectomy (4.1%) compared favourably with operative mortality rates of 5.2% and 9.6% for pancreaticoduodenectomy and total pancreatectomy, respectively. The risk of developing diabetes mellitus postoperatively is increased the more extensive the pancreatic resection. Less than 80% distal pancreatectomy is associated with a 19% incidence of clinical diabetes mellitus whereas this rises to approximately 60% for an 80–95% distal pancreatectomy. Up to 38% of patients will be troubled clinically by steatorrhoea on late follow-up. Although preservation of the pancreas is therefore desirable, distal pancreatectomy would be indicated where disease appears to be localised mainly in the body and tail of the gland and/or when there is concern regarding the presence of an underlying malignancy in a patient with an associated pseudocyst.

In chronic pancreatitis, the Whipple operation removes the head of the gland but conserves function in the remaining pancreas and improves its drainage. The conventional Whipple operation removes the duodenum, gallbladder and common bile duct, and antrum of the stomach in addition to the head of the pancreas (Fig. 9.6). Modern variants include pylorus-preserving pancreaticoduodenectomy and duodenum-preserving pancreaticoduodenectomy.[60] Preservation of the stomach and pylorus was thought to maintain normal gastric function of storage and mixing and digestion of fat and proteins, thereby minimising the incidence of dumping and affluent loop syndrome. Bile reflux would be reduced and the incidence of duodenal ulceration would be minimal. Concerns have been expressed regarding the duodenum-preserving

Figure 9.6
*Reconstruction
following resection of
the distal stomach,
duodenum and head
of pancreas by the
Whipple operation.
The hepaticojejunal (1),
pancreaticojejunal (2)
and gastrojejunal (3)
anastomoses are
shown. The side-to-
side jejunojejunostomy
is performed by some
surgeons.*

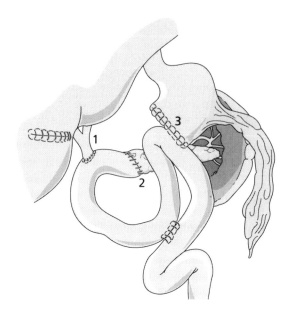

resection since prolonged gastric outlet obstruction and duodenal stricturing have been reported (Table 9.3).

A Whipples resection is often thought of as a relatively easy procedure because the residual pancreas is usually suitable for pancreaticojejunal anastomosis. However, the resection may be complicated by associated splenic vein obstruction and the fibrotic inflammatory reaction associated with chronic pancreatitis often destroys the natural planes of

Table 9.3 *Comparison of standard Whipple procedure with pylorus-preserving partial pancreaticoduodenectomy for chronic pancreatitis*[61]

	Standard	Pylorus-preserving
Number of cases[a]	15/18	19/20
Mean follow-up (years)	8.2	2.8
% Operative mortality	7	0
% Major postoperative complication	7	37
Gastric suction postoperatively (mean days)	4.5*	7*
% Pain improved	78	85
Number of significant jejunal ulcers	0	4
Number of stools per day	4*	2*
% Diabetes postoperatively[b]	47	26
Increase in body weight postoperatively, number of patients	9*	19*

[a] Numerator denotes patients having partial pancreaticoduodenectomy; denominator also indicates patients undergoing total pancreatectomy.
[b] Patients who had total pancreatectomy have been omitted.
* Statistically significant difference.

dissection rendering dissection in the area of the head and neck of the pancreas extremely difficult. Apart from the risk of complications common to all major abdominal procedures, the Whipples resection may be specifically associated with anastomotic leakage and the long-term sequelae of this extensive multivisceral resection. Operative mortality should be less than 5% although in most large series is close to 1%.[61] Good to excellent results are reported in up to 90% of patients although the postoperative incidence of diabetes is in excess of 50% with late mortality rates of 20% reported by some.[61] Gastric emptying can be a source of complication following surgery and does appear more marked following pylorus-preserving partial pancreaticoduodenectomy.[62]

Total pancreatectomy represents the final ablation of pancreatic tissue in an attempt to cure symptoms (Fig. 9.7). Patients must be selected with extreme care if they are to manage the ensuing brittle diabetes mellitus.[63] Similarly, rehabilitation of the patient undergoing total pancreatectomy may be made difficult if they come to the surgical procedure suffering from severe malnutrition and having symptoms which have not responded well to previous surgical intervention. In a review[64] of 324 patients 31 (9.6%) died usually related to haemorrhage or sepsis. The morbidity of the operation is high with as many as 40% of cases developing complications in the postoperative period.[65] Those patients who developed septic complications tend to develop multiple complications and infection of the pancreatic bed is difficult to eradicate. These admissions are rare but readmissions are frequent due to the metabolic effects of the operation. Some 15–30% of patients continue to experience significant discomfort or pain and patients who continue to drink alcohol have worse results than those who abstain.

Prognosis

Chronic pancreatitis has a mortality rate which approaches 50% over 20–25 years.[48,66] Up to 20% of patients die of complications of the disease whereas the remainder succumb to problems associated with alcohol abuse, tobacco smoking, malnutrition, infection, diabetes mellitus, insulin overdose and suicide. These patients are at greater risk of death from malignancy than the general population and are at particular risk of dying from carcinoma of the pancreas.

It is difficult to interpret the results of surgical procedures for chronic pancreatitis since case selection and type of operative procedure often differs. The results will be worse for patients who cannot abstain from alcohol and for those who become dependent on opiate analgesics. Pancreaticojejunostomy carries a lower operative mortality and morbidity than operations involving resection of the pancreas (Table 9.4). Satisfactory control of pain is achieved in up to 75% of patients undergoing pancreatic surgery for chronic pancreatitis. It is widely accepted that the prospects for pain relief are good if the pancreatic duct is dilated and pancreaticojejunostomy therefore offers the best prospects for such patients. Some 20% of patients will, however, require further surgical intervention in the long term for recurrent symptoms.

Figure 9.7 *The extent of resection (a) and the method of reconstruction (b) after total pancreatectomy.*

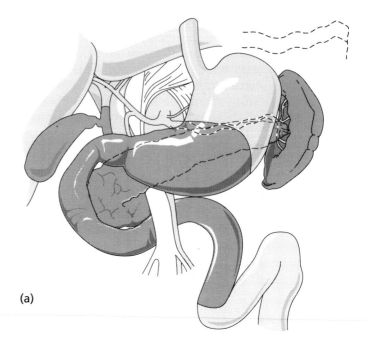

(a)

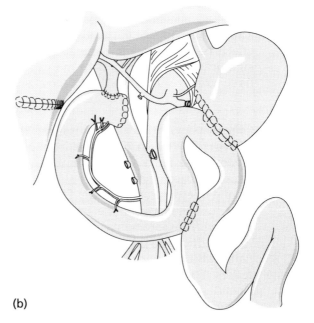

(b)

Failure to abstain from alcohol will inevitably reduce the chance of effecting satisfactory relief of pain and will reduce long-term survival.[67] Although it has been argued that extensive pancreatic calcification is indicative of marked exocrine dysfunction and this may lead to spontaneous diminution in pain,[32] pancreatic drainage in such patients does

Table 9.4 *Outcome following pancreaticojejunostomy and resection for chronic pancreatitis*[69]

	Pancreaticojejunostomy	Distal pancreatectomy	Pancreatico-duodenectomy
No. of patients	228	102	278
Operative mortality (%)	4.3	8.2	5.3
Late mortality (%)	399	36	30
Insulin dependent diabetes			
preoperative (%)	26	11	28
postoperative (%)	50	62	64

not appear to have produced better results in such patients.[68] In patients treated surgically, the long-term results depend more on the drinking habits of the patient than the type of surgery performed.

References

1. Copenhagen Pancreatitis Study. An interim report from a prospective epidemiological multicenter study. Scand J Gastroenterol 1981; 16: 305–12.
2. Johnson CD, Hosking S. National statistics for diet, alcohol consumption and chronic pancreatitis in England and Wales, 1960–1988. Gut 1991; 32: 1401–5.
3. Pitchuomi CS, Sonneshein M, Candido FM, Panchacharam P, Cooperman JM. Nutrition in the pathogenesis of alcoholic pancreatitis. Am J Clin Nutr 1980; 33: 631–6.
4. Renner IG, Savage WT, Pantoja JL, Renner VJ. Death due to acute pancreatitis: a retrospective analysis of 405 autopsy cases. Dig Dis Sci 1985; 30: 1005–18.
5. Durbec JP, Sarles H. Multicenter survey of the etiology of pancreatic diseases. Relationship between the relative risk of developing chronic pancreatitis and alcohol, protein, and lipid consumption. Digestion 1978; 18: 337–50.
6. Bourliere M, Barhtet M, Berthezene P, Durbec JP, Sarles H. Is tobacco a risk factor for chronic pancreatitis and alcoholic cirrhosis? Gut 1991; 32: 1392–5.
7. Muller MK, Singer MV. Aetiology and pathogenesis of chronic pancreatitis. In Trede M, Carter DC (eds) Surgery of the pancreas. Edinburgh: Churchill Livingstone, 1993.
8. Nwokolo C, Oli J. Pathogenesis of juvenile tropical pancreatitis syndrome. Lancet 1980; i: 456–9.
9. GeeVarghese PJ. Calcific pancreatitis. Causes and mechanisms in the tropics compared with those of the subtropics. St Joseph's Trivandrum. Varghese, Bombay, 1986.
10. Staritz M, Meyer-zum-Buschenfelde KH. Elevated pressure in the dorsal part of the pancreas divisum: the cause of chronic pancreatitis? Pancreas 1988; 3: 108–10.
11. Bernard JP, Sahel K, Giovanni M, Sarles H. Pancreas divisum is a probable cause of acute pancreatitis: a report of 137 cases. Pancreas 1990; 5: 248–54.
12. Dalton-Clarke HJ, Lewis MH, Levi AJ, Blumgart LH. Familial chronic calcific pancreatitis: a family study. Br J Surg 1985; 72: 307–8.
13. Misra SP, Dwivedi M. Do gallstones cause chronic pancreatitis? Int J Pancreatol 1991; 10: 97–102.
14. Layer P, Holtmann G. Pancreatic enzymes in chronic pancreatitis. Int J Pancreatol 1994; 15: 1–11.
15. Levy P, Menzelxhiu A, Palliot B *et al*. Abdominal radiotherapy is a cause for chronic pancreatitis. Gastroenterology 1993; 105: 905–9.
16. Sarles H, Bernard JP, Gullo L. Pathogenesis of chronic pancreatitis. Gut 1990; 31: 629–32.

17. Multinger I, Sarles H, Lombardo D, De Caro A. Pancreatic stone protein. II. Implication in stone formation during the course of chronic calcifying pancreatitis. Gastroenterology 1985; 89: 387–91.

18. Mariani A, Mezzi G, Malesci. Purification and assay of secretory lithostatine in human pancreatic juice by fast protein liquid chromatography. Gut 1995; 36: 622–9.

19. Giorgi D, Bernard JP, De Caro A et al. Pancreatic stone protein. I. Evidence that it is encoded by a pancreatic messenger ribonucleic acid. Gastroenterology 1985; 89: 381–6.

20. Giorgi D, Bernard JPO, Ranquir S, Iovanna J, Sarles H, Dagorn JC. Secretory pancreatic stone protein messenger RNA. Nucleotide sequence and expression in chronic calcifying pancreatitis. J Clin Invest 1989; 84: 100–6.

21. Schmiegel W, Buchert M, Kalthoft H et al. Immunochemical characterization and quantitative distribution of pancreatic stone protein in sera and pancreatic secretion in pancreatic disorders. Gastroenterology 1990; 99: 1421–30.

22. Lohse J, Schmid D, Sarles H. Pancreatic citrate and protein secretion of alcoholic dogs in response to graded doses of caerulein. Pflugers Arch 1983; 397: 141–3.

23. Lohse J, Pfeiffer A. Duodenal total and ionised calcium secretion in normal subjects, chronic alcoholics, and patients with various stages of chronic alcoholic pancreatitis. Gut 1984; 25: 874–80.

24. Noronha M, Bordalo O, Dreiling DA. Alcohol and the pancreas. II. Pancreatic morphology of advanced alcoholic pancreatitis. Am J Gastroenterol 1981; 76: 120–4.

25. Noronha M, Bapista A, Bordalo O. Sequential aspects of pathology in chronic alcoholic disease of the pancreas. In: Gyr KE, Singer MV, Sarles H (eds) Pancreatitis – concepts and classification. Excerpta Medica, International Congress Series No. 642, Amsterdam: Elsevier, 1984.

26. Bordalo O, Bapista A, Dreiling D, Noronha M. Early pathomorphological pancreatic changes in chronic alcoholism. In: Gyr KE, Singer MV, Sarles H (eds) Pancreatitis – concepts and classification. Excerpta Medica, International Congress Series No. 642, Amsterdam: Elsevier, 1984.

27. Apte M, Wilson JS, Korsten MA, McCaughan GW, Haber PS, Pirola RC. Effects of ethanol and protein deficiency on pancreatic digestive and lysosomal enzymes. Gut 1995; 36: 287–93.

28. Braganza JM. Pancreatic disease: a casualty of hepatic 'detoxification'. Lancet 1983; ii: 1000–3.

29. Walsh TN, Rode J, Theis BA, Russell RCG. Minimal change chronic pancreatitis. Gut 1992; 33: 1566–71.

30. Bockman D, Buchler M, Malfertheiner P, Beger HG. Analysis of nerves in chronic pancreatitis. Gastroenterology 1988; 94: 1459–69.

31. Lowenfels AB, Maisonneuve P, Cavallini G et al. Pancreatitis and the risk of pancreatic cancer. N Engl J Med 1993; 328: 1433–7.

32. Amman RW, Akovbiantz A, Largadier F, Schueler G. Course and outcome of chronic pancreatitis. Longitudinal study of a mixed medical-surgical series of 245 patients. Gastroenterology 1984; 86: 820–8.

33. Lankisch PG. Function tests in the diagnosis of chronic pancreatitis. Int J Pancreatol 1993; 14: 9–20.

34. Niederau C, Grendell JH. Diagnosis of chronic pancreatitis. Gastroenterology 1985; 88: 1973–5.

35. Carter DC. Cancer of the head of pancreas or chronic pancreatitis? A diagnostic dilemma. Surgery 1992; 111: 602–3.

36. Banks PA. Medical strategy in chronic pancreatitis. In: Carter DC, Warshaw AL (eds) Pancreatitis. Edinburgh: Churchill Livingstone, 1989, pp. 133–47.

37. Nagata A, Homma T, Tamai K et al. A study of chronic pancreatitis by serial endoscopic pancreatography. Gastroenterology 1981; 81: 884–91.

38. Layer P, Yamamoto H, Kalthoff L, Clain JE, Bakken LJ, DiMagno EP. The different courses of early- and late-onset idiopathic and alcoholic chronic pancreatitis. Gastroenterology 1994; 107: 1481–7.

39. Larvin MM, McMahon MJ, Puntis MCA, Thomas WEG. Marked placebo responses in chronic pancreatitis: final results of a controlled trial of Creon therapy. Br J Surg 1992; 79: 457 (abstract).

40. Trede M, Carter DC. Preoperative assessment and indication for operation in chronic pancreatitis. In Trede M, Carter DC (eds) Surgery of the pancreas. Edinburgh: Churchill Livingstone, 1993.

41. Wilson D, Auld CD, Schlinkert R *et al*. Hepatobiliary complications in chronic pancreatitis. Gut 1989; 30: 520–7.

42. Beger HG, Buchler M. Duodenum-preserving resection of the head of the pancreas in chronic pancreatitis with an inflammatory mass in the head. World J Surg 1990; 14: 83–7.

43. Bornman PC, Kalvaria I, Girdwood AH, Marks IN. Clinical relevance of cholestatis syndrome in chronic pancreatitis: the Cape Town experience. In: Beger HG, Buchler M, Ditschuneit H, Malfertheiner P (eds) Chronic pancreatitis. Berlin: Springer-Verlag, 1990, pp. 256–9.

44. Bradley EL, 3rd. Pseudocysts in chronic pancreatitis: development and clinical implications. In: Beger HG, Buchler M, Ditschuneit H, Malfertheiner P (eds) Chronic pancreatitis. Berlin: Springer-Verlag, 1990, pp. 260–8.

45. Maydeo A, Grimm H, Soehendra N. Endoscopic interventional techniques in chronic pancreatitis. In: Trede M, Carter DC (eds) Surgery of the pancreas. Edinburgh: Churchill Livingstone, 1993.

46. Bradley EL, Allen KA. Complications of acute pancreatitis and their management. In: Trede M, Carter DC (eds) Surgery of the pancreas. Edinburgh: Churchill Livingstone, 1993.

47. Nealon WH, Thompson JC. Progressive loss of pancreatic function in chronic pancreatitis is delayed by main pancreatic duct decompression. Ann Surg 1993; 217: 458–68.

48. Horn J. Late results of surgical treatment for chronic pancreatitis. In: Trede M, Carter DC (eds) Surgery of the pancreas. Edinburgh: Churchill Livingstone, 1993.

49. Bradley EL. Pancreatic duct pressure and chronic pancreatitis. Am J Surg 1982; 144: 313–16.

50. Novis BH, Bornman PC, Girdwood AW, Marks IN. Endoscopic manometry of the pancreatic duct and sphincterozone in patients with chronic pancreatitis. Dig Dis Sci 1985; 30: 225–8.

51. Cattel RB. Anastomosis of the duct of Wirsung: its use in palliative operations for cancer of the head of the pancreas. Surg Clin North Am 1947; 27: 636–42.

52. Duval NK. Total pancreaticojejunostomy for chronic pancreatitis. Ann Surg 1954; 140: 775–85.

53. Peustow CB, Gillesby WJ. Retrograde surgical drainage of the pancreas for chronic relapsing pancreatitis. Arch Surg 1958; 76: 898–907.

54. Partington PF, Rochelle REL. Modified Peustow procedure for retrograde drainage of the pancreatic duct. Ann Surg 1960; 152: 1037–43.

55. Delcore R, Rodriguez FJ, Thomas JH, Forster J, Hermreck AS. The role of pancreaticojejunostomy in patients without dilated pancreatic ducts. Am J Surg 1994; 168: 598–601.

56. Frey CF, Smith GJ. Description and rationale for a new operation for chronic pancreatitis. Pancreas 1987; 2: 701–5.

57. Pain JA, Knight MJ. Pancreaticogastrostomy: the preferred operation for pain relief in chronic pancreatitis. Br J Surg 1988; 75: 220–2.

58. Grimm H, Meyer W-H, Nam VC, Soehendra N. New modalities for treating chronic pancreatitis. Endoscopy 1989; 21: 70–4.

59. Frey CF. Distal pancreatectomy in chronic pancreatitis. In: Trede M, Carter DC (eds) Surgery of the pancreas. Edinburgh: Churchill Livingstone, 1992, pp. 321–8.

60. Beger HG, Imaizumi T. Duodenum-preserving head resection in chronic pancreatitis. J Hepatobil Pancreat Surg 1995; 2: 13–18.

61. Gall FP, Gebhardt C, Meister R, Zirngibl H, Schneider MU. Severe chronic cephalic pancreatitis: use of partial duodenopancreatectomy with occlusion of the pancreatic duct in 289 patients. World J Surg 1989; 13: 809–17.

62. Morel P, Mathey P, Corboud H, Huber O, Egeli RA, Rohner A. Pylorus-preserving duodenopancreatectomy: longterm complications in comparison with a Whipple procedure. World J Surg 1990; 14: 642–7.

63. Cooper MJ, Williamson RCN, Benjamin IS *et al*. Total pancreatectomy for chronic pancreatitis. Br J Surg 1987; 74: 912–15.

64. Frey CF, Suzuki M, Isaji S, Znu Y. Pancreatic resection for chronic pancreatitis. Surg Clin North Am 1989; 69: 499–528.

65. Trede M, Schwall G. The complications of pancreatectomy. Ann Surg 1988; 207: 39–47.

66. Steer ML, Waxman I, Freedman S. Chronic pancreatitis. N Engl J Med 1995; 332: 1482–90.

67. Prince RA, Greenlee HB. Pancreatic duct drainage in 100 patients with chronic pancreatitis. Ann Surg 1981; 194: 313–18.

68. Homberg TJ, Isaacsson T, Ihse I. Long-term results in pancreaticojejunostomy in chronic pancreatitis. Surg Gynecol Obstet 1985; 160: 339–46.

69. Eckhauser FE, Strodel WE, Krol JA, Harper M, Turcotte JG. Near-total pancreatectomy for chronic pancreatitis. Surgery 1984; 96: 599–607.

10 Pancreatic neoplasia

James N. Crinnion
Robin C. N. Williamson

Introduction

Pancreatic neoplasms comprise a spectrum of exocrine and endocrine tumours, most of which are malignant. This chapter focuses on the management of pancreatic ductal adenocarcinoma or 'pancreatic cancer' but will incorporate a discussion of other periampullary tumours.

Over 6000 people die from pancreatic cancer in the United Kingdom each year, and it is the sixth leading cause of cancer-related death.[1] Surgical resection offers the only hope of long-term survival, but the aggressive nature of the disease together with its late presentation results in an extremely poor overall prognosis. Only 10% of affected patients are alive 12 months after diagnosis, and the overall five-year survival is less than 3%.[2,3] Recent progress in the diagnosis and staging of pancreatic cancer means that only those with a realistic hope of cure need undergo laparotomy. Nonetheless, although radiological and endoscopic techniques provide useful alternatives for palliating patients with unresectable disease, there is still a role for surgical bypass in selected patients.

The differential diagnosis of periampullary cancer includes tumours of the head of pancreas, ampulla, distal third of bile duct and duodenum. Pancreatic cancer is by far the commonest type, accounting for over 80% of such tumours. Although the four types of periampullary cancer differ in their prognosis, they have a similar clinical presentation and the preferred method of treatment is surgical resection. Furthermore, the intraoperative appearance may not allow a clear distinction between the different types, and the exact origin of the tumour often remains in doubt until it has been excised and examined histologically. In this chapter we have concentrated on describing the assessment, special investigation and treatment of patients with adenocarcinoma of the pancreas, but this management protocol is applicable to the other periampullary tumours.

Epidemiology[4,5]

Demographic and geographic patterns of pancreatic cancer

In Britain and the USA the annual incidence of pancreatic cancer is approximately 100 per million population. The disease is extremely rare below the age of 40, and approximately 80% of cases occur between 60 and 80 years of age. Although there was a marked rise in the number of cases between 1920 and 1970, recent data suggest a levelling-off in incidence for both men and women in the UK and USA. Throughout the world pancreatic cancer is more common in men than women with a male-to-female ratio of between 1.5 and 2, but recent figures from the UK suggests that this male preponderance has declined in the last two decades to 1.25:1.[3]

The highest incidence of the disease occurs in affluent countries such as Israel, Canada, Sweden, UK and USA. Racial factors influence the incidence of pancreatic cancer; the highest rates are observed in female native Hawaiians, black Americans and Korean Americans. Migrant studies suggest that genetic and environmental factors combine to determine the incidence in specific racial groups.

Dietary factors

Cigarette smoking is the most established risk factor for pancreatic cancer, and smokers are twice as likely to develop the disease as non-smokers. Hyperplastic changes in the pancreatic duct cells and nuclear atypia have been observed among smokers at autopsy, and the extent of such changes appears to increase with the quantity of tobacco smoked. The second most important risk factor is diet, which may help to explain the wide geographical variation in incidence as well as the altered risk in certain migrant populations. There is a significant correlation internationally between pancreatic cancer mortality and per capita fat consumption. A similar association exists with a diet high in meat produce. By contrast, a high intake of dietary fibre may provide some protection against the development of pancreatic cancer. In laboratory animals fed high fat diets, the incidence of nitrosamine-induced pancreatic tumours is enhanced. Although a link with coffee intake has been extensively investigated, there is no evidence that this is an independent risk factor.

Occupational factors

Exposure to β-naphthylene and benzidine causes a fivefold increase in mortality from pancreatic cancer. Similarly, an excess number of cases has been observed in workers exposed to ethylene dichloride.

Medical history

Hereditary factors

Patients with pancreatic cancer are statistically more likely to have close relatives who have developed the disease. Studies have shown that as many as 7.8% of patients with pancreatic cancer have a family history of the disease, as opposed to 0.6% of controls. Therefore, if an individual has a family member affected with pancreatic adenocarcinoma, he or she has a small increase in risk. Although most pancreatic cancers occur sporadically, the disease may occur in family clusters, and often in association with several other specific hereditary disorders: hereditary pancreatitis, ataxia-telangiectasia, hereditary non-polyposis colon cancer and familial atypical mole-malignant melanoma syndrome. Autosomal dominant transmission of pancreatic cancer can occur in isolated families in the absence of a known hereditary syndrome. Although environmental exposure common to affected family members may explain this clustering rather than hereditary factors, identification and study of the gene defects in these families may in the future enable at-risk individuals to be identified by genetic screening.[6]

Diabetes mellitus

Several investigators have demonstrated an increased risk of pancreatic cancer among diabetics, although this is not a consistent finding. The diabetes is often detected within a year of the diagnosis of pancreatic cancer, implying that it is an early symptom rather than a causal relation. Mere destruction of pancreatic tissue by the tumour is an unlikely explanation for the islet cell dysfunction.

Chronic pancreatitis

There may be a weak association between chronic pancreatitis and pancreatic cancer, but the inflammatory changes that are often associated (distal obstructive pancreatopathy) usually reflect ductal obstruction by the tumour.

Gastrectomy

There appears to be a two- to five-fold increased risk of pancreatic cancer 15–20 years after a partial gastrectomy. It has been suggested that reduced gastric acidity allows overgrowth of bacteria that elaborate pancreatic carcinogens, particularly N-nitroso compounds.

Epidemiology of extrahepatic bile duct and ampullary cancer

Carcinoma of the distal common bile duct and carcinoma of the ampulla each account for around 5% of tumours of the pancreatobiliary junction.[7] Each tumour is almost invariably malignant, and most of them occur in patients older than 65 years with a slight male preponderance.[8] An increased incidence of extrahepatic bile duct cancer has been reported in patients with ulcerative colitis, primary sclerosing cholangitis and disorders leading to biliary stasis, such as choledochal cysts.[8] Chronic inflammation may contribute to the development of dysplasia and subsequent carcinoma, and a few bile duct malignancies develop in pre-existing adenomas.[8]

Epidemiology of primary duodenal carcinoma

Adenocarcinoma of the duodenum is an uncommon malignancy which accounts for another 5% of periampullary tumours.[7] Many of these tumours arise in pre-existing villous adenomas, especially in patients with familial polyposis coli, in whom primary duodenal carcinoma is the second commonest malignancy.[9]

Pathology ### Pancreatic cancer (Table 10.1)[10,11]

Ductal adenocarcinoma of the pancreas accounts for more than 90% of all malignant pancreatic exocrine tumours. All demographic, morphological and prognostic data concerning pancreatic cancer relate to this dominant type. Its morphological variants (giant cell carcinoma, adenosquamous carcinoma and mucinous carcinoma) and acinar cell carcinoma all have a similar or worse prognosis than ductal adenocarcinoma. Pancreatic cancer has a propensity for perineural invasion within and beyond the gland and for rapid lymphatic spread. The commonest sites of extralymphatic involvement are the liver, peritoneum and lung.

The rare malignant or potentially malignant cystic tumours of the pancreas include the mucinous cystadenoma/cystadenocarcinoma (mucinous cystic neoplasms), serous cystadenoma and papillary–cystic tumour. They behave quite differently with a good prognosis if completely resected. Primary lymphoma of the pancreas also carries a better prognosis than adenocarcinoma, being amenable to chemotherapy and irradiation. The pancreas may also be the site of secondary deposits from other tumours including breast and lung carcinoma and malignant melanoma. Post-mortem studies have shown that for every primary tumour of the pancreas four metastatic deposits are found.[10] However,

Table 10.1 *Classification of primary malignant tumours of the exocrine pancreas*

Origin	Type of tumour
Ductal epithelium	duct cell adenocarcinoma, giant cell carcinoma, adenosquamous carcinoma, mucinous (colloid) carcinoma, microadenocarcinoma (solid microglandular), mucinous cystadenocarcinoma
Acinar cell	acinar cell carcinoma, acinar cystadenocarcinoma, pancreatoblastoma
Non-epithelial tissue	fibrosarcoma, leiomyosarcoma, histiocytoma, rhabdomyosarcoma, osteogenic sarcoma, malignant schwannoma, liposarcoma, lymphoma
Uncertain histogenesis	papillary-cystic neoplasm

in clinical practice these metastases are rarely the presenting feature and seldom contribute to the differential diagnosis of a pancreatic mass.

Bile duct, ampullary and duodenal cancer

Virtually all periampullary tumours are adenocarcinomas. The papillary variant of bile duct or ampullary carcinoma is associated with the most favourable outcome, whereas mucinous adenocarcinoma has a particularly poor prognosis.[8] Carcinoid tumours and sarcomas of the duodenum are responsible for about 2% of periampullary tumours, and surgical excision of these tumours is often curative.[7] All extrapancreatic cancers in this region have a better prognosis than ductal carcinoma of the pancreas.

Clinical presentation

Carcinoma of the head of pancreas

At least two-thirds of cases of pancreatic cancer arise in the head of the gland. The most frequent symptoms are obstructive jaundice, weight loss and abdominal pain. Anorexia, nausea and vomiting are often present. Weight loss may be prominent and occurs as a result of anorexia, malabsorption (secondary to exocrine insufficiency) and diabetes.

Jaundice is present in at least 90% of cases as a consequence of either invasion or compression of the common bile duct. The jaundice is often painless but tends to be progressive and is frequently accompanied by pruritus. If the tumour originates in the uncinate process or neck of the gland, jaundice is a relatively late feature accompanied by appreciable weight loss.

Pain is present in about 70% of patients at the time of diagnosis and is usually located in the epigastrium or left upper quadrant. It is often vague in nature; it radiates to the back in 25% of patients and is occasionally confined to the back. Back pain is an ominous symptom which usually signifies irresectability.

An episode of acute pancreatitis is occasionally the first presenting feature. In advanced cases duodenal obstruction results in persistent vomiting. Another late manifestation is gastrointestinal bleeding, which may be a consequence of gastroduodenal invasion or may originate from varices secondary to portal or splenic vein occlusion. Hepatomegaly occurs in approximately 80% of patients at the time of presentation. A palpable gall bladder (Courvoisier's sign) is commonly found in jaundiced patients on careful examination.

The other periampullary tumours produce a similar clinical picture (jaundice, epigastric pain, weight loss), but certain clinical features may help to distinguish them from pancreatic cancer. Duodenal carcinoma may present with occult gastrointestinal bleeding causing iron deficiency anaemia, or with epigastric fullness and vomiting as a result of gastric outlet obstruction.[9] Fluctuating jaundice is characteristic of ampullary tumours.

Carcinoma of the body and tail of pancreas

These tumours develop insidiously and are asymptomatic in their early stages. By the time of diagnosis they are generally more advanced than lesions located in the head. There is marked weight loss with back pain in 60% of patients. Jaundice is uncommon and usually reflects an advanced cancer with involvement of the porta hepatis. Vomiting sometimes occurs at a late stage from invasion of the duodenojejunal flexure. An abdominal mass is detected more often than in cancer of the head of pancreas and usually indicates an unresectable tumour.

Trousseau's sign of migratory thrombophlebitis has been reported in 7% of patients with pancreatic cancer, especially those in the body and tail. Frank diabetes mellitus is present in 15% of pancreatic cancer patients, and many more have impaired glucose tolerance. An increase in insulin requirements in a stable diabetic raises the suspicion of pancreatic cancer.

It must be emphasised that the symptomatology described is not specific to pancreatic cancer; patients with periampullary tumours or chronic pancreatitis may present with an identical clinical picture. Since the treatment protocol and the prognosis varies widely with the particular type of neoplasm, a specific diagnosis is important in every patient. There are two principal aims of further investigation in a patient with suspected pancreatic cancer.

1. Confirmation of the diagnosis is sought, with differentiation from other pancreatic or periampullary tumours and chronic pancreatitis.
2. Accurate staging of the disease and assessment of resectability.

Investigations: Diagnosis

Full blood count

Many patients with pancreatic cancer are anaemic as a result of nutritional deficiency and chronic blood loss. Stool examination usually reveals occult blood in patients with carcinoma of the pancreatic head. The occurrence of frank gastrointestinal bleeding suggests the diagnosis of ampullary or duodenal carcinoma.

Biochemistry

A rapid elevation of serum bilirubin and alkaline phosphatase on serial measurements of liver function will suggest a diagnosis of periampullary malignancy. Transaminase levels become elevated to a lesser degree reflecting injury to hepatocytes as a result of unrelieved biliary obstruction. Blood glucose may be elevated.[12]

Pancreatic function tests

Pancreatic exocrine function is impaired in almost all patients with pancreatic cancer as a result of malnutrition, damage to the pancreatic parenchyma and the effects of an obstructed pancreatic duct. Fat malabsorption is compounded by the absence of bile salts within the intestinal lumen in jaundiced patients. These abnormalities of exocrine function are non-specific and do not help to differentiate pancreatic cancer from chronic pancreatitis.

Ultrasonography

Real-time ultrasound scan should be the initial investigation performed on a patient with suspected pancreatic cancer, especially in the presence of jaundice. It is inexpensive, avoids exposure to ionising radiation and may in many cases accurately diagnose and stage the disease.[13] Ultrasonography can detect pancreatic masses, dilatation of the biliary and pancreatic ducts, liver metastases, ascites and extrapancreatic spread. In addition, Doppler ultrasonography can be utilised to image blood flow in the portal vein and superior mesenteric vessels. Satisfactory images of the pancreas are obtained in about 80% of patients; suboptimal examinations are the result of overlying bowel gas, obesity or previous surgery.

Most pancreatic cancers are hypoechoic and are usually accompanied by changes in the contour of the gland. The overall diagnostic sensitivity of ultrasound in detecting pancreatic tumours is around 70%, but this figure falls to below 30% with tumours less than 2 cm in diameter.[14] The diagnostic yield is influenced by the skill and experience of the ultrasonographer, but excellent overall results have been reported.[15] Ultrasonography is not very helpful in locating duodenal tumours.[9]

Computed tomography

Dynamic contrast-enhanced computed tomography (CT) is the most widely used and most useful modality for the diagnosis and staging of periampullary tumours and lesions of the distal pancreas. A positive CT diagnosis of pancreatic cancer is made if (1) a focal or diffuse pancreatic mass (usually of reduced attenuation) is present without evidence of acute or chronic pancreatitis or (2) if a dilated main pancreatic duct and/or common bile duct is present with or without a pancreatic mass.[15–17] Using these criteria the overall sensitivity of CT in diagnosing pancreatic cancer was as high as 97% in a recent large prospective study,[17] but sensitivity is much lower for lesions <2 cm in diameter. CT allows an accurate assessment of local tumour extension, adjacent organ invasion, liver and lymph node metastases, ascites and vascular involvement. Contrast-enhanced CT is also an excellent modality for diagnosing duodenal tumours.[18]

Neither CT nor ultrasonography can differentiate pancreatic adenocarcinoma from other solid tumours of the pancreas. A false positive diagnosis of pancreatic cancer occurs in about 10% of cases with CT scanning[15,16] as a result of focal pancreatitis, variations in normal pancreatic anatomy, other primary or secondary tumours of the pancreas or rarely tuberculosis or sarcoidosis. As these patients have a significantly better chance of survival than patients with pancreatic cancer, it is imperative that a CT or ultrasound diagnosis of pancreatic cancer is confirmed with percutaneous (or open) biopsy in all patients who are not going to undergo surgical resection.

Fibreoptic endoscopy

Although duodenal tumours may be diagnosed by conventional upper gastrointestinal endoscopy, the pancreatobiliary junction is most clearly visualised with endoscopic retrograde cholangiopancreatography (ERCP). ERCP also permits the relief of obstructive jaundice via the insertion of an endoscopic stent. Tumours of the ampulla and duodenum can be biopsied under direct vision. Transpapillary wire-guided brush cytology, needle aspiration or forceps biopsy can also be used to obtain cytology specimens from pancreatic and biliary strictures. Although these tests are highly specific for malignancy and avoid the risk of disseminating tumour, false negative results are frequent.[15]

Over 97% of patients with pancreatic cancer will have an abnormal pancreatogram as a result of obstruction or encasement of the duct.[19] Thus in suspected cases without a pancreatic mass on scanning, ERCP is likely to confirm the clinical suspicion. Chronic pancreatitis may produce similar ERCP findings to pancreatic cancer, but malignant strictures are irregular and often exceed 10 mm in length; benign strictures should not exceed 5 mm.[20]

Tumour markers[15,21]

A wide range of tumour-associated antigens, hormones, enzymes and immunoglobulins have been evaluated for the diagnosis, prognosis and follow-up of pancreatic cancer. At present none has a sufficiently high sensitivity and specificity to be of value in routine screening. The best known serum marker is CA 19-9. Its overall sensitivity in diagnosing pancreatic cancer is greater than 90%, but values are often normal in the early stages of the disease. CA 19-9 has a low specificity (75%); pancreatitis, biliary disease and other gastrointestinal cancers may all produce elevated values. It is of prognostic value because levels fall if the tumour is completely excised. Persistent elevation after tumour resection is an ominous finding. Most other tumour markers are less accurate than CA 19-9. The dismal outlook in pancreatic cancer makes the development of a suitable serum marker for screening highly desirable. The use of monoclonal antibodies to target tumour-associated antigens might provide a breakthrough in this area.[15]

Fine-needle aspiration cytology (FNAC)

Percutaneous aspiration cytology under ultrasound or CT guidance is a useful diagnostic technique. It is highly specific with very few false positive results. However, sampling errors are frequent, so a negative cytological examination certainly does not exclude a diagnosis of pancreatic cancer.[22,23] False-negative cytological results are most likely to occur with potentially curable small tumours. Cytology may fail to differentiate adenocarcinoma from endocrine tumours or lymphoma.[15] Tru-cut® biopsy is more invasive but may increase the diagnostic yield.

It is generally accepted that percutaneous biopsy should not be performed in patients in whom surgical exploration is contemplated as it (rarely) results in tumour seeding along the needle tract.[15] Furthermore, there is an association between the presence of malignant cells in peritoneal washings collected during diagnostic laparotomy and prior percutaneous needle biopsy.[24] Besides potentially compromising the chance of cure, needle biopsy of the pancreas can occasionally cause pancreatitis or pancreatic fistula or injure the stomach or colon; a few deaths have occurred as a direct result of this procedure.[15] Biopsy is particularly useful in the frail, elderly patient in whom resection is not considered but a tissue diagnosis is required to avoid the need for diagnostic laparotomy.

Other investigations

Endoscopic ultrasound scanning enables direct imaging of the pancreas through the gastrointestinal tract. The pancreatic head is visualised with the ultrasonic endoscope placed in the second part of the duodenum, and the body and tail of pancreas are imaged through the stomach wall. This technique employs the use of a fluid interface between the probe and the stomach or intestinal wall, and it avoids the problems of obesity and excessive bowel gas which are encountered in conventional ultrasound examination. It is said to be more accurate than CT in detecting pancreatic masses especially when these are less than 2 cm.[12,25] Although still considered experimental, this investigation may be useful in excluding pancreatic cancer in those patients who have normal conventional imaging but elevated tumour markers.[15]

Magnetic resonance imaging has been evaluated in periampullary tumours but appears to offer no advantage over CT in diagnosis and staging.[15,26] Positron emission tomography (PET) has been recently reported to be more accurate than CT or ultrasound in detecting lymph node metastases from pancreatic cancer, but its role in the diagnosis and staging of the disease remains unclear.[27]

Investigations: Staging

In the recent past surgical exploration was recommended for nearly all patients with pancreatic cancer.[28] Laparotomy enabled confirmation of the diagnosis and assessment of resectability, plus the opportunity to provide palliation for patients with unresectable disease by means of a biliary and/or duodenal bypass. However, advances in preoperative diagnosis and staging and the development of non-operative techniques of palliation has meant that many patients with advanced disease may be spared the trauma associated with surgical exploration. There remains a role for surgical bypass in those whose tumour was potentially resectable on preoperative imaging and in younger patients with an expectation of survival beyond about three months.

The goal of preoperative staging of pancreatic cancer (and other periampullary tumours) is to ensure that each patient receives the most appropriate treatment with minimal morbidity. More specifically the objective is to define which tumours are potentially resectable, which are not resectable but are still localised, and which have already metastasised to distant sites.[20] Staging is of particular importance in pancreatic cancer, because of the prevailing incidence of portal vein involvement and early liver metastases.

The TNM staging classification for exocrine pancreatic cancer recommended by International Union Against Cancer (UICC) (Table 10.2) correlates well with prognosis.

Ultrasonography

Preoperative staging of pancreatic cancer starts with ultrasonography, which is the least invasive test. It may be the only investigation required in a patient who has advanced disease with liver metastases or ascites. In such a patient, percutaneous biopsy or aspiration of ascitic fluid under ultrasound guidance with subsequent cytological examination may confirm the diagnosis. Major vascular invasion may be evident on ultrasound scanning and indicates irresectability for most surgeons.

Computed tomography

Although ultrasound scan may accurately predict vascular invasion,[13,29] corroborative evidence is usually sought from spiral CT scanning and sometimes from angiography as well. CT features of irresectability include contiguous organ invasion, including the portal vein, coeliac axis and superior mesenteric artery, and distant metastases.[17] The accuracy of CT in predicting irresectability is as high as 90–100% in specialist centres, but it is much less accurate in predicting surgical resectability, with a sensitivity of 45–72%.[17,26] Spiral CT scan seems to offer a definite advantage over conventional scanning.

Visceral angiography

It remains our policy for patients with potentially resectable periampullary tumours to undergo visceral angiography as a further staging investigation. These films provide an excellent means of assessing major vessel occlusion or encasement and will also delineate the arterial

Table 10.2   *UICC classification of exocrine pancreatic cancer (1987)*

T: Primary tumour

TX	Primary tumour cannot be assessed
T0	No evidence of primary tumour
T1	Tumour limited to the pancreas
	T1a Tumour 2 cm or less in greatest dimension
	T1b Tumour more than 2 cm in greatest dimension
T2	Tumour extends directly to any of the following: duodenum, bile duct, peripancreatic tissues
T3	Tumour extends directly to any of the following: stomach, spleen, colon, adjacent large vessels

N: Regional lymph nodes

NX	Regional lymph nodes cannot be assessed
N0	No regional lymph node metastasis
N1	Regional lymph node metastasis

M: Distant metastases

MX	Presence of distant metastasis cannot be assessed
M0	No distant metastasis
M1	Distant metastasis

Stage grouping

Stage I	T1	N0	M0
	T2	N0	M0
Stage II	T3	N0	M0
Stage III	Any T	N1	M0
Stage IV	Any T	Any N	M1

anomalies that are so common in the general population.[30] Particular attention is paid to the venous phase of the superior mesenteric angiogram. Clear-cut invasion of the portal vein and its major tributaries or of the superior mesenteric, coeliac or hepatic artery, is taken to indicate an irresectable tumour. Artefactual underfilling of the great veins is a potential trap. Retrograde flow and a collateral circulation confirms portal vein occlusion.

In one report, 28 of 90 patients with 'resectable periampullary tumours' on the basis of dynamic CT had angiographic evidence of major vascular encasement or occlusion; this report emphasises the inadequacy of CT scanning alone in predicting resectability.[31] None of the patients with major vascular occlusion were found to be resectable at operation, but six with evidence of encasement were resectable. In two of these patients a segment of portal vein was excised with the specimen, and in the other four patients the angiogram had yielded false-positive results. The development of spiral CT may reduce the need for angiography in the future. Laparotomy by an experienced surgeon still provides the most accurate assessment of resectability and should be undertaken if there is any doubt, especially in younger patients.

Diagnostic laparoscopy and laparoscopic ultrasound

The presence of liver or peritoneal metastases indicates incurability, and surgical resection is contraindicated. Liver metastases greater than 1–2 cm are usually identified by ultrasonography or CT, but smaller lesions together with omental and peritoneal deposits require direct visualisation. These tiny metastatic lesions are present in 24–41% of periampullary tumours thought to be resectable on the basis of dynamic CT, and in over 90% of cases they can be visualised and biopsied laparoscopically.[26,32–34] Laparoscopy may also identify locally advanced disease invading the ligament of Treitz and transverse mesocolon, which is also considered to be irresectable. Although the routine use of diagnostic laparoscopy avoids unnecessary surgical exploration in an appreciable number of patients, it is an invasive investigation in its own right.

Recently laparoscopy has been combined with laparoscopic ultrasonography for the staging of periampullary tumours.[29,35] Laparoscopic ultrasound can identify and biopsy small metastases within the liver substance which would not normally be seen by laparoscopy alone. Furthermore major vessel involvement by tumour can be assessed accurately by laparoscopic ultrasound, and biopsy of enlarged lymph nodes is also possible. However, visualisation of local tumour extension in major vessels is technically demanding and ultrasonographically guided biopsies are difficult to perform.[29] At present, therefore, trial dissection is still needed, in our experience, to confirm the findings of laparoscopic ultrasound.

Before accurate preoperative staging, resectability rates at laparotomy were between 5 and 25%.[3,28] When CT, visceral angiography and laparoscopy were combined to stage periampullary tumours, rates approached 80%.[26] The complexity of staging tests should be tailored to the surgeon's policy of irresectable cancer. If internal bypass is favoured over non-operative stenting for patients with less advanced disease, then it is necessary only to exclude those with obvious disseminated carcinoma.

Treatment: Resectional surgery

Surgical excision offers the only chance of cure in pancreatic and other periampullary cancers. Unfortunately only about 20% of patients with cancer of the pancreatic head and less than 3% of those with carcinoma of the body or tail have lesions that are suitable for resection.[3,7,28] The resectability rates for other periampullary tumours are more favourable; over 90% of ampullary carcinomas were suitable for 'curative' resection in a recent large series.[12]

Preoperative preparation

In jaundiced patients, coagulopathy should be corrected by the parenteral administration of vitamin K. To prevent the development of postoperative renal failure patients should be well hydrated, and any electrolyte imbalance must be rectified. Prophylactic antibiotics are prescribed routinely, and some patients may benefit from preoperative parenteral nutrition. Although some authors recommend routine preoperative biliary drainage (whether endoscopic or transhepatic), clinical trials have failed to show a reduction in postoperative morbidity and mortality.[36–38] Preoperative drainage will contaminate the biliary tree and can often delay definitive treatment. Therefore, many surgeons prefer to proceed straight to pancreatectomy and reserve biliary drainage for those with evidence of cholangitis, impaired renal function or prolonged jaundice.

Assessment of resectability[39]

A thorough laparotomy is performed to exclude obvious irresectability in the form of widespread metastases, gross posterior fixity and invasion into the transverse mesocolon or small bowel mesentery. Resection is usually not justified unless it is likely to be macroscopically complete, as the presence of residual microscopic or macroscopic tumour precludes long-term survival.[12,40] Lymph node involvement should be confirmed by frozen section examination but does not preclude resection as long as the nodes can be excised *en bloc*. If resection seems to be feasible, attention is focused on carefully developing the plane between the neck of the pancreas and the underlying superior mesenteric and portal vein. The portal vein 'tunnel' is initially exposed by tracing the middle colic vein to its junction with the superior mesenteric vein. If this dissection is difficult, the portal vein is exposed above the neck of the pancreas by deep dissection in the free edge of the lesser omentum. In the event of gross invasion of the portal vein (which usually is evident on preoperative angiography and CT), the resection is abandoned. In selected cases of partial tethering or invasion of the portal vein a small segment of vein may be excised and reconstructed, although long-term survival is unlikely in such patients.[40]

There are four main types of pancreatic resection: proximal pancreatoduodenectomy, regional pancreatectomy, distal pancreatectomy and total pancreatoduodenectomy.

Proximal pancreatoduodenectomy[39,41]

This procedure has received widespread application in the treatment of periampullary tumours and cancer of the pancreas when the lesion is confined to the head or uncinate process of the gland. Conventional or standard proximal pancreatoduodenectomy involves resection of the distal stomach, duodenum and head of pancreas en bloc. The line of resection is generally through the pancreatic neck in the line of the portal vein, and the absence of tumour at the site of pancreatic transection is sought by sending tissue for frozen section examination.

Historically a distal gastrectomy was performed to reduce gastric acidity and prevent the lethal complication of stress ulceration and bleeding in the early postoperative period. In recent years, however, numerous authors have challenged the need to perform a gastrectomy and have advocated a modification of the Whipple operation with preservation of the stomach, pylorus and proximal duodenum (pylorus-preserving proximal pancreatoduodenectomy, PPPP). This procedure retains the entire stomach as a reservoir; as a result, postgastrectomy complications are minimised, the incidence of marginal ulceration is low and enterogastric reflux is less common.[42–45] The evidence suggests that PPPP is associated with better postoperative nutritional status and weight gain than the Whipple's operation, i.e. standard pancreatoduodenectomy.[46] The main concern with PPPP is its oncological adequacy for treating periampullary and pancreatic malignancy. The two potential drawbacks are tumour involvement of the duodenal transection line and incomplete removal of regional lymph nodes.[46] Infiltration of the duodenal resection margin has been reported[47] but is extremely uncommon. We routinely perform frozen section examination of the duodenal transection margin but it is scarcely ever positive. If it were, the procedure would be converted into a Whipple's pancreatoduodenectomy.

In a recent study of 90 carcinomas of the pancreatic head, the perigastric lymph nodes were involved in 13 patients[48] and PPPP might have been inadequate in some of these. It is only the nodes along the greater and lesser curves of the antrum that are spared, and these are rarely involved at an early stage. Large series have reported equivalent or better long-term survival figures for PPPP compared to Whipple's resection for carcinoma of the head of pancreas.[41] Ampullary and distal bile duct carcinoma seldom metastasise to the perigastric lymph nodes, so PPPP does not transgress oncological principles.[48,49] It is our policy to perform PPPP for most periampullary and pancreatic tumours except those that arise close to the pylorus or proximal duodenum, in which there is a risk of incomplete excision.[39]

Various options exist for restoring gastrointestinal continuity after either Whipple's resection or PPPP. Regarding the pancreatic stump, options include oversewing or ductal blockage without anastomosis, pancreatojejunostomy and pancreatogastrostomy.[41,46] Simple oversewing risks fistula formation. Ductal blockage is probably safer, but it necessitates postoperative pancreatic enzyme supplementation and is not favoured by many surgeons. Pancreatojejunostomy may be performed as an end-to-end or end-to-side procedure, whereas pancreatogastrostomy is usually performed in an end-to-side fashion. Particular care must be taken with the pancreatic anastomosis to prevent the development of a pancreatic fistula. We favour non-absorbable sutures, an invaginating end-to-end technique and the use of transanastomotic stents. The biliary anastomosis is most frequently performed as an end-to-side choledochojejunostomy. If a partial gastrectomy is performed, a Hoffmeister modification with a side-to-side gastrojejunostomy is the most common procedure.[41] After PPPP, the duodenojejunostomy is normally performed in an end-to-side fashion. Our usual reconstructive technique anastomoses the proximal jejunum to pancreas first, followed by the bile duct and then the duodenal cap[39,41] (Fig. 10.1).

During recent years the mortality and morbidity rates of pancreato-duodenectomy have steadily declined. The mortality rate has fallen from as high as 20–40% in the 1960s and early 1970s to 5% or less.[3,39,40,50] This improvement has been the result of increased surgical experience in referral centres plus advances in the intensive care management of postoperative patients. However, complications are still common and include delayed gastric emptying, pancreatic fistula, intra-abdominal abscess, pancreatitis and bile leak. The most feared complication is pancreatic fistula, which is seen in up to 25% of all patients and may lead to intra-abdominal abscess, haemorrhage and death. However, careful monitoring of drain amylase levels resulting in early diagnosis

Figure 10.1
Reconstruction following pylorus preserving pancreatoduo-denectomy

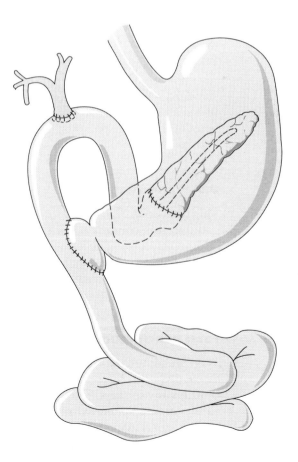

coupled with percutaneous drainage of intra-abdominal fluid collections, prophylactic use of the somatostatin analogue octreotide and total parenteral nutrition have greatly reduced the fatalities from this complication.[41,51] The complications of pancreatoduodenectomy and their management are discussed in detail in a recent review article.[51]

Regional (radical) pancreatectomy[52]

Detailed analysis of surgical specimens has identified the lymph node groups that may be involved in pancreatic cancer.[48,53] Many affected patients have nodal metastases in sites not normally resected with the standard Whipple resection. In an attempt to remove these areas of tumour spread a more radical pancreatic resection was developed, in which pancreatic resection is accompanied by extensive retroperitoneal lymph node and soft tissue resection. Resection of the superior mesenteric-portal vein and even the superior mesenteric artery is often performed with vascular reconstruction (usually achieved by end-to-end anastomosis). The retroperitoneal lymph node dissection extends from the coeliac trunk to the inferior mesenteric trunk and from the right margin of the inferior vena cava to the left margin of the abdominal aorta.[48] The extended pancreatic resection has gained most popularity in Japan and in expert hands has an operative mortality of around 6%, which is comparable with the standard pancreatoduodenectomy. Whether it confers any survival advantage over conventional pancreatic resection is uncertain as no prospective randomised trials between standard and radical resection have been performed.[52] Hepatic micrometastases are likely to thwart such extensive procedures in an appreciable number of patients, and a high complication rate could be anticipated with the routine adoption of supraradical surgery.

Distal pancreatectomy

This resection is indicated for lesions located in the body and tail of the gland and is combined with splenectomy. Typical ductal carcinoma is seldom resectable due to the advanced nature of these lesions at the time of presentation, but distal pancreatectomy is often feasible for the rare slow-growing malignant tumours which include cystadenocarcinoma and papillary-cystic neoplasm.

Total pancreatoduodenectomy

This procedure has been advocated to avoid the serious problems associated with the pancreatojejunal anastomosis and to remove multicentric disease (reported in up to one-third of resection specimens).[5] However, total pancreatectomy results in rather brittle diabetes, and the overall operative mortality is actually higher than for the standard Whipple's resection.[41] Furthermore, there is no survival advantage with this procedure.[41] Thus total pancreatectomy is reserved for the following indications:[5]

1. Pancreatic cancer in an insulin-dependent diabetic;
2. Diffuse involvement of the whole pancreas by tumour without evidence of spread;
3. Cancer at the site of pancreatic transection demonstrated on frozen section during proximal pancreatoduodenectomy;
4. Perhaps when the residual pancreas is friable and the risk of a pancreatojejunal anastomotic leak is especially high.

Long-term survival

Pancreatic cancer

Sperti *et al.*[40] recently reviewed all the major series of pancreatic resection published since 1990. The average rate of resectability was 20%, and the mean operative mortality rate was 9% (range 2–20%). The 5-year actuarial survival rate was 12%, but only 77 of the 2075 patients reviewed were alive 5 years after resection. These figures make rather depressing reading; although operative mortality is now greatly reduced, the overall survival following surgical resection of pancreatic cancer has remained virtually unchanged in the last 50 years.[54]

One of the most important factors influencing survival following surgical resection is tumour biology.[41] Small (<2 cm), well-differentiated, node-negative tumours have the best prognosis but unfortunately only represent a small percentage of resectable lesions. DNA content of pancreatic tumour cells as determined by image cytology is also an important determinant of survival. Thus, patients with tumours containing a diploid number of chromosomes had a 5-year survival of 39%, as compared to those with aneuploid tumours who had a 5-year actuarial survival of only 8%.[41] In a multivariate analysis, aneuploidy, tumour diameter and lymph node status were all independent predictors of survival.[41] Expression of the procoagulant tissue factor is also associated with poor histological differentiation.[55] Possibly the most important determinant of long-term survival is positivity of resection margins.[56] This problem occurs more frequently than previously thought and relates particularly to the posterior tumour margin, which can usually be cleared macroscopically without difficulty only to be found later to be microscopically involved.[57] Posterior spread occurs especially as a result of cancer cells tracking along perineural sheaths or individual lymphatics, rather than through the pancreatic parenchyma.

Although extended (radical) resection may increase surgical resectability rates, the incidence of local recurrence and 5-year survival figures are no better than for conventional resection.[40,41,52,58] Although the overall outlook is bleak, some centres have reported an improvement in long-term survival following pancreatoduodenectomy, which is attributed to a lower hospital mortality rate, less intraoperative blood transfusion and the increased use of adjuvant radiation and chemotherapy.[41]

Periampullary tumours

Other periampullary adenocarcinomas have a much more favourable long-term outlook. Most of these lesions can be resected for cure, and 5-year actuarial survival rates of 21–56% have been reported for carcinoma of the periampullary region.[7,36,49,59,60] Duodenal carcinoid tumours and sarcomas have a better prognosis than adenocarcinoma.[7]

Adjuvant therapy following 'curative surgery'

After apparently curative resection of pancreatic ductal carcinoma, subsequent metastases are frequently found in the liver (23–52%), peritoneal cavity (27–62%) and extra-abdominal sites (8–29%).[57] Recent studies have attempted to assess whether adjuvant radiotherapy and chemotherapy will reduce the incidence of recurrent disease and thus prolong survival following surgical resection. An early study performed by the North American Gastrointestinal Tumour Study Group (GITSG) randomised patients who underwent curative resection to receive supportive care or adjuvant treatment.[61] The latter consisted of post-operative external beam radiotherapy combined with chemotherapy (5-fluorouracil), and treatment was continued for 2 years or until the development of recurrence. Although the number of patients recruited into the study was small, adjuvant therapy was well tolerated and conferred a definite survival advantage. However, this study failed to convince many surgeons of the merits of adjuvant therapy. Other studies have attempted to assess the role of adjuvant radiotherapy and/or chemotherapy, but patient recruitment has been small and many trials have not been randomised.[57] Nevertheless two multicentre European studies are nearing completion, and these should contain enough patients to determine whether adjuvant therapy confers a definite survival advantage.[57]

Neoadjuvant therapy

Chemotherapy and radiotherapy have also been given to patients with pancreatic cancer prior to surgical resection in an attempt to increase the chance of successfully resecting locally advanced tumours and/or to reduce the proportion of cancers with positive surgical resection margins.[57] Although this approach has shown encouraging results, its potential benefit has not been assessed in randomised trials.

Palliative treatment

Since fewer than 20% of patients with pancreatic cancer are suitable for curative resection, good palliative therapy is of great importance. Palliative treatments are aimed at alleviating obstructive jaundice and pruritus, relieving or preventing duodenal obstruction and controlling pain. Furthermore, radiotherapy and/or chemotherapy may prolong survival in patients with unresectable disease.

Relief of jaundice

Obstructive jaundice is the dominant clinical feature in periampullary tumours. Untreated, it results in progressive liver dysfunction, culminating in liver failure and early death. In addition it causes intolerable itching and anorexia and has a deleterious effect on most organ systems. Relief of biliary obstruction normalises liver function, reverses coagulopathy, corrects metabolic arrangements and improves nutritional status and overall well-being. Palliation of jaundice may be achieved by endoscopic transpapillary stenting or percutaneous transhepatic stenting as well as by the more traditional surgical approaches.

Endoscopic biliary stenting[62]

This technique of palliating malignant obstructive jaundice was first described in 1980 and is now well standardised and widely available. When performed regularly, it carries a technical success rate of 85–90%; relief of jaundice and pruritus occurs in around 90% of such patients. The procedure for endoscopic insertion of biliary endoprosthesis follows ERCP and is performed under sedation. Prophylactic antibiotics are administered and clotting abnormalities are corrected. When the location and length of the bile duct stricture is defined, a guidewire is manipulated across the stricture to the level of the right or left hepatic duct. The endoprosthesis is then placed over the guidewire and positioned across the stricture using a variety of delivery systems.

The original endoprostheses were made of plastic (polyethylene) and had an internal diameter of 8 to 12 Fr. Complications of plastic stent placement include the acute problems related to ERCP such as cholangitis, pancreatitis, bile duct and duodenal perforation, and delayed complications directly related to the endoprosthesis including cholecystitis, duodenal perforation, and stent migration, fracture or occlusion. Most of these complications are uncommon except for stent occlusion, which may occur from days to years after placement with a mean interval of 6–8 months. Many patients with advanced disease will die before stent occlusion occurs, and only about 20–30% of patients with pancreatic cancer will require stent exchange. In an attempt to solve the problem of plastic stent occlusion, larger-diameter expandable metallic stents (30Fr) have been developed which can be delivered on a relatively small diameter catheter (7Fr) and expanded within the biliary tree to a diameter of up to 1 cm (30Fr). Randomised trials have confirmed that these endoprostheses have a superior long-term patency when compared to plastic stents. In addition metal stents expand tightly against the wall of the bile duct and eventually become incorporated within it; they are therefore not associated with the complication of migration. Obstruction of metal stents may occur due to overgrowth of tumour proximal or distal to the ends of the prosthesis or sometimes due to ingrowth through the mesh. The incidence of this complication may be reduced by placing the ends of the stent well beyond the site of the tumour.

Percutaneous biliary drainage[63]

For most periampullary tumours percutaneous biliary drainage has been surpassed by endoscopic techniques. Speer *et al.*[64] compared endoscopic and percutaneous stenting in 75 patients with malignant obstructive jaundice and concluded that the endoscopic approach was more likely to be successful and was associated with fewer complications. Nevertheless, technical difficulties, variations in biliary anatomy or extrinsic invasion of the ampulla by large cancers in the head of pancreas may preclude endoscopic drainage, and percutaneous stent placement provides a valuable alternative means of palliating obstructive jaundice. It is also indicated in patients with recurrent jaundice after surgical bypass.

Percutaneous biliary decompression can be achieved by the use of internal–external biliary drainage catheters or by employing endoprostheses. Patients with distal bile duct strictures whose life expectancy is less than 6 months are best served by percutaneous or endoscopic biliary stents. Percutaneous drainage catheters are usually reserved for patients with obstruction at the level of the liver hilum, where endoscopic endoprostheses are less effective. Percutaneous transhepatic stenting is usually performed in two stages. Initially an internal–external drainage catheter is placed through the liver (under local anaesthetic) and across the malignant stricture into the duodenum. The second stage of the procedure is carried out 2–3 days later and comprises dilatation of the tract to an appropriate size and insertion of the endoprosthesis. As with endoscopic stents, either plastic or expandable metal stents are available. Metal stents are associated with fewer early complications as they can be delivered on a 7Fr introducing catheter, whereas plastic stents produce large calibre tracts (12–14 Fr) with a higher risk of haemobilia and bile peritonitis.

Surgical biliary bypass

Cholecystojejunostomy is the simplest biliary–enteric bypass carried out for irresectable pancreatic cancer, but it is seldom appropriate. In patients likely to survive more than a few weeks there is a risk of about 20% of further jaundice or cholangitis.[65] If the gall bladder is selected for the anastomosis, then intraoperative cholangiography (through the gall bladder) must be performed to ensure patency of the cystic duct and to make sure that the cystic duct–common duct junction is at least 2–3 cm above the tumour mass. Although choledochojejunostomy is a little more difficult and takes longer to perform than cholecystojejunostomy, it has a higher initial success rate (97% vs 89%) with an equivalent operative mortality of less than 10%.[66] Furthermore, the risk of recurrent jaundice or cholangitis is less than 10%.[65] For these reasons we advocate choledochojejunostomy in most patients with biliary obstruction. For those with disseminated cancer the greater simplicity of a gall bladder anastomosis is attractive, but we prefer to avoid operation altogether in such cases. Our own practice is to combine the choledochojejunostomy

Figure 10.2 *Single loop biliary bypass for irresectable carcinoma of the pancreas*

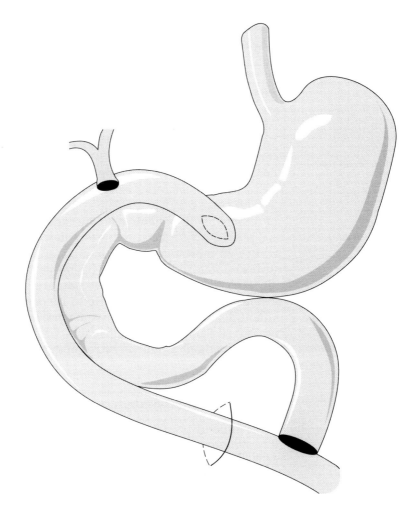

with a gastroenterostomy to form a single loop biliary and gastric bypass (Fig. 10.2).[67]

Surgical bypass versus endoprosthesis

The choice of palliative approach varies with each individual and will depend on the presentation and prognosis of the disease as well as the general health of the patient. It may also be influenced by the local availability of surgical, endoscopic and radiological expertise.

Randomised studies conducted on patients with malignant obstructive jaundice have concluded that operative and non-operative methods of biliary drainage are equally effective in the short-term relief of jaundice.[65] Operation has several advantages over endoscopic approaches. First, it enables an unequivocal assessment of resectability, which may be in doubt despite sophisticated imaging. Secondly, there is a lower incidence of recurrent jaundice, which occurs in up to 30% of patients with biliary stents.[66] Thirdly, surgical drainage is also associated with a lower risk of cholangitis than endoprosthesis insertion.[66] Fourthly, it may be combined with a gastric bypass to provide prophylaxis against future duodenal obstruction, which occurs in about 2% of patients.[68]

To set against these benefits, clinical trials have shown that operation is associated with a higher 30-day mortality and greater morbidity than stent insertion.[65,69] Proponents of the surgical approach argue that the mortality rates of 19–24% reported in these studies are unacceptably high, and in other series of surgical bypass the operative mortality has been less than 5%.[70] A sensible approach would be to reserve operation for reasonably fit patients who are expected to survive at least 6 months as it provides the most durable long-term palliation. In patients unlikely to survive more than a few months and in the elderly or those with cardiorespiratory disease, non-operative palliation is preferred. Recent advances in minimally invasive surgery have enabled cholecystojejunostomy and gastrojejunostomy to be performed laparoscopically.[71,72] Although these reports demonstrate that laparoscopic biliary and gastric bypass is feasible in selected patients, large series have not been reported and this method cannot yet be recommended.

Relief of duodenal obstruction

At the time of presentation 30–50% of patients with pancreatic cancer have symptoms of nausea and vomiting, although the incidence of actual mechanical obstruction demonstrated on radiographic or endoscopic examination is only about 5%. Periampullary tumours quite often obstruct the second part of the duodenum, whereas lesions of the body and tail may occasionally involve the fourth part. As the tumour enlarges, the risk of duodenal invasion and obstruction increases. Thus following biliary bypass alone, 17% of patients will develop duodenal obstruction and require subsequent gastric bypass, which carries an average mortality rate of 22%.[65] A retrospective review of published series revealed that the mortality rate of biliary bypass is not increased by adding a gastroenterostomy.[65] For these reasons it is recommended that biliary bypass is combined with gastric bypass ('double bypass') in most patients with irresectable cancer of the pancreatic head. Some authors argue against this policy because of the high incidence of delayed gastric emptying that follows the combined procedure. However, this complication usually resolves following varying periods of nasogastric intubation, and its incidence may be reduced by fashioning the gastroenterostomy proximal to the biliary anastomosis.[73]

Rarely gastric outlet obstruction may occur due to tumour invasion of the gastrojejunostomy or duodenojejunostomy which may follow either palliative bypass or pancreatoduodenectomy. This complication poses a difficult management problem as reoperation carries a high risk in the terminally ill patient. One possible but not very satisfactory approach involves gastric decompression via a percutaneous endoscopic gastrostomy (PEG), with jejunostomy feeding to provide simultaneous nutritional support. Recently endoscopic stenting of both duodenal strictures and obstructed gastrojejunostomies has been described using expandable metal prostheses. This superior technique enables patients to resume enteral nutrition. Early results are encouraging, but the method requires further assessment.[62]

Relief of pancreatic pain

Pain is a presenting symptom in almost all patients with pancreatic cancer, although it is usually mild and settles after bypass surgery or stenting. More severe pain, which is frequently located in the back, is typical of carcinoma of the body and tail and invasive lesions of the head. The intensity of pain is related to the stage of disease, being most severe in advanced cases. Factors thought to produce pancreatic pain include increased parenchymal pressure secondary to pancreatic ductal obstruction, neural infiltration, superimposed pancreatic inflammation and distal common bile duct stenosis.[62] Pancreatic pain may occasionally be intolerable and provides a major therapeutic challenge.

Pancreatic duct dilatation secondary to duct obstruction is frequently evident on CT scanning and/or ERCP and is a characteristic feature of pancreatic cancer. The association between this finding and the presence of pancreatic pain is variable. However, limited experience with 5 or 7 Fr pancreatic stents placed across the malignant pancreatic stricture in such patients has produced useful abatement of pain. In some patients dramatic pain relief was achieved within 48 h after endoscopic stenting.[62] At the time of laparotomy pancreatic duct decompression over a T-tube into the stomach or jejunum may also be performed in an attempt to alleviate pancreatic pain.[66] Although biliary or gastrointestinal obstruction may contribute to the pain of pancreatic cancer, an appropriate bypass is unlikely on its own to relieve severe pancreatic pain.[68,74]

In patients undergoing laparotomy, peroperative chemical ablation of the coeliac ganglia is a proven method of relieving pancreatic pain. Splanchnicectomy may be achieved with 5% phenol in almond oil or 50% ethanol and produces effective palliation of pain in about 70% of patients.[65] In patients who are managed non-operatively, percutaneous coeliac nerve block may be performed with either fluoroscopic or CT guidance with equivalent success rates.[75] Similarly, thoracoscopic division of the splanchnic nerves has been successful in alleviating pancreatic pain and provides an alternative method of percutaneous nerve block.[76]

Pancreatic pain may also be effectively palliated with external beam radiotherapy,[65] and this should certainly be considered in patients with recurrent pain following percutaneous coeliac block.

Adjuvant therapy for advanced pancreatic cancer

Combined external beam radiotherapy and 5-fluorouracil (5-FU) administered to patients with locally advanced pancreatic cancer may confer an overall survival advantage.[77–79] In the largest of these studies by the Gastrointestinal Tumor Study Group, radiotherapy and 5-FU prolonged median survival time was from 23 weeks (radiotherapy alone) to 40–42 weeks.[78] However, even with combined therapy 2-year survival is in the region of only 10–20%, and 5-year survivors are exceptional.[80] Patients usually succumb to either uncontrolled local disease or the subsequent development of liver or peritoneal metastases. Intraoperative radiotherapy in addition to external beam radiation and 5-FU results in an improvement in local control but does not affect the incidence of metastases and does not translate into an overall survival advantage.[20,80] Pilot studies are being conducted in an attempt to decrease the incidence of liver and peritoneal failures by utilising more aggressive chemotherapy regimes, and the results are eagerly awaited.[80] External beam radiotherapy plus 5-FU is remarkably well tolerated, with a low incidence of side effects and toxicity.[79] However, the overall benefit of such treatment is questionable as the modest survival advantage must be weighed against the added burden of frequent hospital visits.

On the basis of evidence linking pancreatic cancer to sex hormones, the effect of both antioestrogens and antiandrogens on the survival of patients with advanced disease has been investigated.[81,82] Neither the antioestrogen tamoxifen nor cyproterone acetate (an antiandrogen) has been shown statistically to prolong life, but occasional instances of long-term survival with tamoxifen have been documented.[82–84] These isolated cases suggest that there may be a small subgroup of patients who benefit from this treatment, which has few side effects.[20]

Palliative surgical resection

A substantial proportion of pancreatoduodenectomies are subsequently labelled non-curative because residual microscopic disease is left *in situ*.[36,85,86] As the survival of these patients may exceed that of palliative bypass procedures, it has been suggested that non-radical resection may benefit selected patients.[36] This approach is probably only justified for young patients in centres with a low operative mortality rate for pancreatoduodenectomy.

Summary of management
An algorithm for the management of patients with pancreatic cancer and periampullary tumours is given in Fig. 10.3.

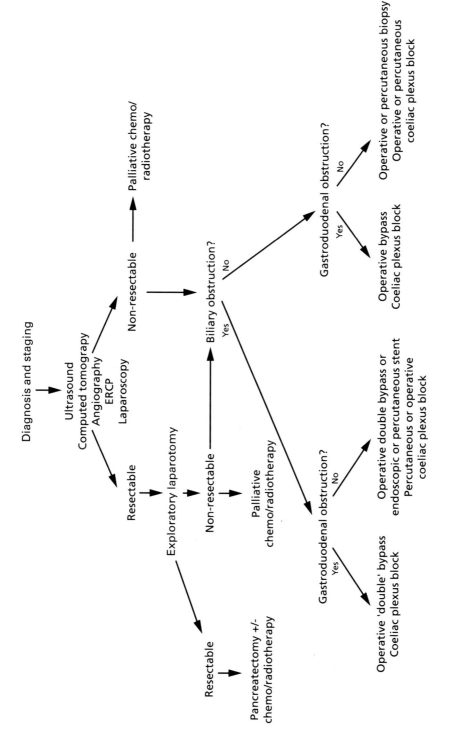

Figure 10.3 *Algorithm for the management of patients with pancreatic cancer and periampullary tumours*

Future developments in the treatment of pancreatic cancer

Although the last decade has brought improvements in diagnosis and staging, a significant reduction in the mortality rate associated with pancreatic resection and advances in the palliative treatment of inoperable disease, the overall prognosis of pancreatic cancer remains very poor for two reasons. First, the high incidence of local, peritoneal and hepatic recurrence even after apparently curative resection implies that widespread dissemination of malignant cells occurs at an early stage of the disease during the preclinical phase. Thus treatments such as resection and radiotherapy that are primarily directed at localised disease have a limited chance of achieving cure.[87] Earlier detection of pancreatic cancer would surely prove beneficial as 5-year survival rates of 30% have been obtained after resection of tumours of less than 2 cm in diameter.[88] The second factor responsible for the poor outlook in adenocarcinoma of the pancreas is that most patients present with advanced irresectable disease for which there is no effective therapy.

Although the idea of screening is appealing, a suitable screening test for pancreatic cancer remains elusive. Even if a screening test with 99% sensitivity and specificity existed, it would yield 99 false-positive results for each true positive result because the prevalence of pancreatic cancer is only 0.01%.[89]

Attempts to decrease the incidence of locoregional recurrence after 'curative' resection by means of adjuvant chemoradiation have achieved some success. Neoadjuvant chemotherapy regimes may confer an even greater benefit, although randomised trials confirming this are not yet available. Even more exciting is the prospect that selective gene therapy may boost the cytotoxicity of chemotherapeutic agents against pancreatic cancer cells 100-fold.[57] Intraoperative photodynamic therapy is an experimental technique in which surface malignant cells are destroyed by their uptake of photosensitive haematoporphyrin derivatives, which are subsequently activated by exposure to light of specific wavelength and intensity.[87] This treatment may be effective in destroying microscopic foci of residual disease.

About 80% of cases of pancreatic cancer are irresectable at presentation, and unfortunately no potential cure for advanced disease is on the horizon.[90] Probably the best hope for the future lies in the understanding of the molecular genetic changes that occur in pancreatic cancer cells, an area of research under active pursuit.[91]

Cystic neoplasms of the pancreas[92]

Cystic tumours of the pancreas account for less than 1% of all pancreatic neoplasms. This heterogeneous group of tumours is important because of their high cure rate as well as frequent confusion with the commoner pancreatic pseudocyst. Neoplasms account for about 10% of cystic lesions of the pancreas. Approximately 50% of these are mucinous cystic neoplasms and 30% are serous cystadenomas. Mucinous ductal ectasia, papillary cystic tumours and cystic neuroendocrine tumours account for the remaining 20%. Cystic tumours are frequently large and can reach up to 25 cm in diameter.

Most patients with cystic neoplasms present with vague symptoms of mild upper abdominal pain or discomfort. Other symptoms include weight loss, a palpable mass, postprandial fullness, nausea and vomiting. Investigation reveals a cystic lesion on ultrasound and/or CT scan.

Cystic tumours can usually be differentiated preoperatively from pancreatic pseudocysts by a combination of clinical, biochemical and radiological features. A pancreatic pseudocyst either follows an episode of acute pancreatitis or occurs in a patient with chronic pancreatitis, most of whom are men who abuse alcohol, have a long history of pancreatic pain and/or symptoms of pancreatic insufficiency. By contrast, cystic neoplasms are commoner in women and have no preceding factors. Serum amylase is frequently elevated in patients with pseudocysts, whereas it is normal in those with cystic tumours. CT scanning usually accurately discriminates cystic neoplasms from pseudocysts by showing solid components, septa and loculations. Occasionally cystic neoplasms cannot be differentiated from pseudocysts before surgical exploration. At operation most cystic tumours are seen to be discrete lesions, with adjacent normal pancreas and a loose attachment to neighbouring structures. In sharp contrast pseudocysts are thick-walled inflammatory masses, which are usually adherent to omentum and/or adjacent viscera. The remaining pancreas is markedly indurated. A frozen section biopsy taken from the wall of the lesion clinches the diagnosis of a cystic neoplasm.

Cystic tumours are all potentially malignant and should be excised whenever possible. Resection may involve a PPPP (or Whipple procedure) if the lesion is in the head of the gland, or distal pancreatectomy with splenectomy if it is located in the tail. If there is any doubt as to the nature of a cystic lesion at operation, it should be excised. It is better to resect a pseudocyst than leave behind or drain a cystic neoplasm. These lesions have a very high cure rate unless malignant change supervenes.

References

1. Review of the national cancer registration system. Office of Population Censuses and Surveys. Series MB 1, No. 17. London: HMSO, 1990.
2. Andersson A, Bergdahl L. Carcinoma of the exocrine pancreas. Am Surg 1976; 42: 173–7.
3. Bramhall SR, Allum WH, Jones AG, Allwood A, Cummins C, Neoptolemos JP. Treatment and survival in 13560 patients with pancreatic cancer, and incidence of the disease, in the West Midlands: an epidemiological study. Br J Surg 1995; 82: 111–15.
4. Gold EB. Epidemiology of and risk factors for pancreatic cancer. Surg Clin North Am 1995; 75: 819–43.
5. Watanapa P, Williamson RCN. Cancer of the exocrine pancreas. In: Bouchier IAD, Alan RN, Hodgson HJF, Keighley MRB (eds) Gastroenterology: clinical science and practice, 2nd edn. London: WB Saunders, 1993, pp. 1635–56.
6. Lumadue JA, Griffin CA, Osman M, Hruban RH. Familial pancreatic cancer and the genetics of pancreatic cancer. Surg Clin North Am 1995; 75: 845–55.
7. Michelassi F, Erroi F, Dawson PJ et al. Experience with 647 consecutive tumours of the duodenum, ampulla, head of pancreas and distal common bile duct. Ann Surg 1989; 210: 544–54.

8. Carriaga MT, Henson DE. Liver, gall bladder, extra-hepatic bile ducts and pancreas. Cancer 1995; 75(suppl 1): 171–90.

9. Scott-Coombes D, Williamson RCN. Surgical treatment of primary duodenal carcinoma: a personal series. Br J Surg 1994; 81: 1472–4.

10. Cubilla AL, Fitzgerald PJ. Tumours of the exocrine pancreas. In: Atlas of Tumour Pathology, Second series, fascicle 19. Washington, DC: Armed Forces Institute of Pathology, 1984.

11. Morohoshi T, Held G, Kloppel G. Exocrine pancreatic tumours and their histological classification. A study based on 167 autopsy and 97 surgical cases. Histopathology 1983; 7: 645–61.

12. Klempnauer J, Ridder GJ, Pichlmayr R. Prognostic factors after resection for ampullary carcinoma: multivariate survival analysis in comparison with ductal carcinoma of the pancreatic head. Br J Surg 1995; 82: 1686–91.

13. Campbell JP, Wilson SR. Pancreatic neoplasms: how useful is evaluation with ultrasound? Radiology 1988; 167: 341–4.

14. Yasuda K, Mukai H, Fujimoto S et al. The diagnosis of pancreatic cancer by endoscopic ultrasonography. Gastrointest Endosc 1988; 34: 1–8.

15. Moossa AR, Gamagami RA. Diagnosis and staging of pancreatic neoplasms. Surg Clin North Am 1995; 75: 871–90.

16. Freeny PC, Marks WM, Ryan JA, Traverso LW. Pancreatic ductal adenocarcinoma: diagnosis and staging with dynamic CT. Radiology 1988; 166: 125–33.

17. Freeny PC, Traverso LW, Ryan JA. Diagnosis and staging of pancreatic adenocarcinoma with dynamic computed tomography. Am J Surg 1993; 165: 600–6.

18. Kusumoto H, Takahashi I, Yorhida M et al. Primary malignant tumours of the small intestine: an analysis of 40 Japanese patients. J Surg Oncol 1992; 50: 139–43.

19. Freeny PC. Radiologic diagnosis and staging of pancreatic ductal adenocarcinoma. Radiol Clin North Am 1989; 27: 121–8.

20. Warshaw AL, Fernández-Del Castillo C. Pancreatic carcinoma. N Engl J Med 1992; 326: 455–65.

21. Steinberg W. The clinical utility of CA 19-9 tumor-associated antigen. Am J Gastroenterol 1990; 85: 350–5.

22. Paksoy N, Lilleng R, Hagmar B et al. Diagnostic accuracy of fine needle aspiration cytology in pancreatic lesions. Acta Cytol 1993; 37: 8890–3.

23. Pinto MM, Avila NA, Criscuolo EM. Fine needle aspiration of the pancreas. Acta Cytol 1988; 32: 39–42.

24. Warshaw AL. Implications of peritoneal cytology for staging of early pancreatic cancer. Am J Surg 1991; 161: 26–9.

25. Nakaizumi A, Uehara H, IIshi H et al. Endoscopic ultrasound in diagnosis and staging of pancreatic cancer. Dig Dis Sci 1995; 40: 696–700.

26. Warshaw AL, Gu Z-U, Wittenberg J, Waltman AC. Preoperative staging and assessment of resectability of pancreatic cancer. Arch Surg 1990; 125: 230–3.

27. Bares R, Klever P, Hauptmann S et al. F-18 fluorodeoxyglucose PET in vivo evaluation of pancreatic glucose metabolism for the detection of pancreatic cancer. Radiology 1994; 192: 79–86.

28. Connolly MM, Dawson PJ, Michelassi F, Moosa AR, Lowenstein F. Survival in 1001 patients with carcinoma of the pancreas. Ann Surg 1987; 206: 366–73.

29. Bemelman WA, De Wit LT, Van Delden OM et al. Diagnostic laparoscopy combined with laparoscopic ultrasonography in staging of the pancreatic head region. Br J Surg 1995; 82: 820–4.

30. Appleton GVN, Bathurst NGC, Virjee J, Cooper MJ, Williamson RCN. The value of angiography in the surgical management of pancreatic disease. Ann R Coll Surg Engl 1989; 71: 92–6.

31. Dooley WC, Cameron JL, Pitt HA et al. Is preoperative angiography useful in patients with peri-ampullary tumours? Ann Surg 1990; 211: 649–53.

32. Warshaw AL, Tepper JE, Shipley WU. Laparoscopy in the staging and planning of therapy for pancreatic cancer. Am J Surg 1986; 151: 76–9.

33. Fernández-Del Castillo C, Rattner DW, Warshaw AL. Further experience with laparoscopy and peritoneal cytology in the staging of pancreatic cancer. Br J Surg 1995; 82: 1127–9.

34. Cuschieri A. Laparoscopy for pancreatic cancer: does it benefit the patient? Eur J Surg Oncol 1988; 14: 41–4.

35. John TG, Grieg JD, Carter DC, Garden OJ. Carcinoma of the pancreatic head and periampullary region: tumor staging with laparoscopy and laparoscopic ultrasonography. Ann Surg 1995; 221: 156–64.

36. Klinkenbijl JHG, Jeekel J, Schmitz PIM et al. Carcinoma of the pancreas and peri-ampullary region: palliation versus cure. Br J Surg 1993; 80: 1575–8.

37. Pitt HA, Gomes AS, Lois JF et al. Does preoperative percutaneous biliary drainage reduce operative risk or increase hospital cost? Ann Surg 1985; 201: 545–53.

38. Hatfield ARW, Terblanche J, Fataar S et al. Preoperative external biliary drainage in obstructive jaundice. Lancet 1982; ii: 896–9.

39. Watanapa P, Williamson RCN. Resection of the pancreatic head with or without gastrectomy. World J Surg 1995; 19: 403–9.

40. Sperti C, Pasquali C, Piccoli A, Pedrazzoli S. Survival after resection for ductal adenocarcinoma of the pancreas. Br J Surg 1996; 83: 625–31.

41. Pitt HA. Curative treatment for pancreatic neoplasms: Standard resection. Surg Clin North Am 1995; 75: 891–904.

42. Braasch JV. Pancreaticoduodenal resection. Curr Probl Surg 1988; 25: 323–63.

43. Fink AS, DeSouza LR, Mayer EA et al. Long-term evaluation of pylorus preservation during pancreatoduodenectomy. World J Surg 1988; 12: 663–70.

44. McLeod RS, Taylor BR, O'Connor BI et al. Quality of life, nutritional status, and gastrointestinal hormonal profile following the Whipple procedure. Am J Surg 1995; 169: 179–85.

45. Williamson RCN, Bliouras N, Cooper MJ et al. Gastric emptying and enterogastric reflux after conservative and conventional pancreatoduodenectomy. Surgery 1993; 114: 82–6.

46. Zerbi A, Balzano G, Patuzzo R et al. Comparison between pylorus-preserving and Whipple pancreatoduodenectomy. Br J Surg 1995; 82: 975–9.

47. Sharp KW, Ross CB, Halter SA et al. Pancreatoduodenectomy with pyloric preservation for carcinoma of the pancreas: a cautionary note. Surgery 1989; 105: 645–53.

48. Nakao A, Harada A, Nonami T et al. Lymph node metastases in carcinoma of the head of the pancreas region. Br J Surg 1995; 82: 399–402.

49. Roder JD, Stein HJ, Hüttl W, Siewert JR. Pylorus-preserving versus standard pancreatico-duodenectomy: an analysis of 110 pancreatic and peri-ampullary carcinomas. Br J Surg 1992; 79: 152–5.

50. Cameron JL. Long term survival following pancreaticoduodenectomy for adenocarcinoma of the head of the pancreas. Surg Clin North Am 1995; 75: 939–51.

51. Yeo CJ. Management of complications following pancreaticoduodenectomy. Surg Clin North Am 1995; 75: 913–24.

52. Reber HA, Ashley SW, McFadden D. Curative treatment for pancreatic neoplasms: radical resection. Surg Clin North Am 1995; 75: 905–12.

53. Cubilla AL, Fortner J, Fitzgerald PJ. Lymph node involvement in carcinoma of the pancreas area. Cancer 1978; 41: 880–7.

54. Gudjonsson B. Cancer of the pancreas. 50 years of surgery. Cancer 1987; 60: 2284–303.

55. Kakkar AK, Lemoine NR, Scully MF, Tebbutt S, Williamson RCN. Tissue factor expression correlates with histological grade in human pancreatic cancer. Br J Surg 1995; 82: 1101–4.

56. Willett CG, Lewandrowski K, Warshaw AL et al. Resection margins in carcinoma of the head of the pancreas. Implications for radiation therapy. Ann Surg 1993; 217: 144–8.

57. Neoptolemos JP, Kerr DJ. Adjuvant therapy for pancreatic cancer. Br J Surg 1995; 82: 1012–14.

58. Kayahara M, Nabakawa T, Ueno K et al. An evaluation of radical resection for pancreatic cancer based on the mode of recurrence as determined by autopsy and diagnostic imaging. Cancer 1993; 72: 2118–23.

59. Wade TP, El-Ghazzawy AG, Virgo KS, Johnson FE. The Whipple resection for cancer in US Department of Veterans Affairs Hospitals. Ann Surg 1995; 221: 241–8.

60. Sperti C, Pasquali C, Piccoli A et al. Radical resection for ampullary carcinoma: long-term results. Br J Surg 1994; 81: 668–71.

61. Gastrointestinal Tumor Study Group. Further evidence of effective adjuvant combined radiation and chemotherapy following curative resection of pancreatic cancer. Cancer 1987; 59: 2006–10.

62. Lichtenstein DR, Carr-Locke DL. Endoscopic palliation for unresectable pancreatic carcinoma. Surg Clin North Am 1995; 75: 969–88.

63. Kaufman SL. Percutaneous palliation of unresectable pancreatic cancer. Surg Clin North Am 1995; 75: 989–99.

64. Speer AG, Cotton PB, Russell RCG *et al.* Randomised trial of endoscopic versus percutaneous stent insertion in malignant obstructive jaundice. Lancet 1987; ii: 1149–52.

65. Watanapa P, Williamson RCN. Surgical palliation for pancreatic cancer: developments during the past two decades. Br J Surg 1992; 79: 8–20.

66. Boyle TJ, Williamson RCN. Mini-symposium – pancreatic cancer: bypass procedures. Curr Pract Surg 1994; 6: 154–60.

67. Watanapa P, Williamson RCN. Single-loop biliary and gastric bypass for irresectable pancreatic carcinoma. Br J Surg 1993; 80: 237–9.

68. Singh SM, Reber HA. Surgical palliation for pancreatic cancer. Surg Clin North Am 1989; 69: 599–611.

69. Lillemoe KD, Barnes SA. Surgical palliation of unresectable pancreatic carcinoma. Surg Clin North Am 1995; 75: 953–68.

70. Lillemoe KD, Sauter PK, Pitt HA *et al.* Current status of surgical palliation of peri-ampullary carcinoma. Surg Gynecol Obstet 1993; 176: 1–10.

71. Shimi S, Banting S, Cuschieri A. Laparoscopy in the management of pancreatic cancer: endoscopic cholecystojejunostomy for advanced disease. Br J Surg 1992; 79: 317–19.

72. Brune IB, Schonleben K. Laparoskopische seit-zu-seit-gastro-jejunostomies. Chirurg 1992; 63: 577–80.

73. Doberneck RC, Berndt GA. Delayed gastric emptying after palliative gastroenterostomy for carcinoma of the pancreas. Arch Surg 1987; 122: 827–9.

74. Singh SM, Longmire WP, Reber HA. Surgical palliation for pancreatic cancer. The UCLA experience. Ann Surg 1990; 212: 132–9.

75. Sharfman WH, Walsh TD. Has the analgesic efficacy of neurolytic celiac plexus block been demonstrated in pancreatic cancer pain. Pain 1990; 41: 267–71.

76. Worsey J, Ferson PF, Keenan RJ, Julian TB, Landreneau RJ. Thoracoscopic pancreatic denervation for pain control in irresectable pancreatic cancer. Br J Surg 1993; 80: 1051–2.

77. Moertel CG, Childs DS Jr, Reitemeier RJ, Colby MY Jr, Holbrook MA. Combined 5-fluorouracil and supervoltage radiation therapy of locally unresectable gastrointestinal cancer. Lancet 1969; ii: 865–7.

78. The Gastrointestinal Tumor Study Group. Therapy of locally unresectable pancreatic carcinoma: a randomised comparison of high dose (6000 rads) radiation alone, moderate dose radiation (4000 rads + 5-fluorouracil), and high dose radiation + 5-fluorouracil. Cancer 1981; 48: 1705–10.

79. Kaln PJ, Skornick Y, Inbar M, Caplan O, Chaichik S, Rozin R. Surgical palliation combined with synchronous therapy in pancreatic carcinoma. Eur J Surg Oncol 1990; 16: 7–11.

80. Gunderson LL, Nagorney DM, Martenson JA *et al.* External beam plus intraoperative irradiation for gastrointestinal cancers. World J Surg 1995; 19: 191–7.

81. Greenway BA. Carcinoma of the exocrine pancreas: a sex hormone responsive tumour. Br J Surg 1987; 74: 441–2.

82. Keeting JJ, Johnson PJ, Cochrane AMG *et al.* A prospective randomised controlled trial of tamoxifen and cyproterone acetate in pancreatic carcinoma. Br J Cancer 1989; 60: 789–92.

83. Bakkevold KE, Pettersen A, Arnesjo B, Espehaug B. Tamoxifen therapy in unresectable adenocarcinoma of the pancreas and the papilla of Vater. Br J Surg 1990; 77: 725–30.

84. Wong A, Chan A, Arthur K. Tamoxifen therapy in unresectable adenocarcinoma of the pancreas. Cancer Treat Rep 1987; 71: 749–50.

85. Manabe T, Tobe T. Progress in the diagnosis and treatment of pancreatic cancer – the Kyoto University experience. Hepatogastroenterology 1989; 36: 431–6.

86. Lygidakis NJ, Van Der Hyde, Houtheff HJ *et al.* Resectional surgical procedures for carcinoma of the head of the pancreas. Surg Gynecol Obstet 1989; 168: 157–65.

87. Ettinghausen SE, Schwartzentruber DJ, Sindelar WF. Evolving strategies for the treatment of adenocarcinoma of the pancreas. J Clin Gastroenterol 1995; 21: 48–60.

88. Tsuchiya R, Tomioka T, Kunihide I *et al.* Collective review of small carcinomas of the pancreas. Ann Surg 1986; 203: 77–81.

89. Warshaw AL, Swanson RS. Pancreatic cancer in 1988; possibilities and probabilities. Ann Surg 1988; 208: 541–53.

90. Williamson RCN. Pancreatic cancer: the greatest oncological challenge. Br Med J 1988; 296: 445–6.

91. Hahn SA, Kern SE. Molecular genetics of exocrine pancreatic neoplasms. Surg Clin North Am 1995; 75: 857–69.

92. Fernández-del Castillo C, Warshaw AL. Cystic tumours of the pancreas. Surg Clin North Am 1995; 75: 1001–16.

11 Hepatobiliary and pancreatic trauma

Ajith Siriwardena
O. James Garden

Introduction

In contemporary society, trauma to the liver and pancreas has two major causes: first, motor vehicle accidents, which account for the majority of blunt liver and pancreatic trauma; and second, knife and gunshot wounds which are the major cause of penetrating injuries to the liver and pancreas. The proportion of blunt to penetrating trauma varies, but in the UK blunt trauma predominates and in our institution the ratio of blunt to penetrating liver trauma in a series of 75 patients over a 10-year period was 1.5:1.[1] In contrast, penetrating wounds were present in 86.4% of 1000 patients treated in a trauma centre in Houston, Texas from 1979 to 1984.[2] The spleen and the liver are the most frequently damaged structures in blunt abdominal trauma.[3] The small intestine, colon and liver are the most frequently injured viscera in patients with penetrating trauma. It should be borne in mind that reports from North American trauma centres represent patterns of injury which may vary considerably from those seen in casualty departments in Europe. The overall mortality after liver and pancreatic injury is related to the severity of the injury and to the presence of multi-organ injury.

This chapter will discuss the presentation and initial assessment of patients with liver injury. The indications for conservative management will be discussed and the arguments in favour of operative intervention considered. The factors guiding operative decision making and the available therapeutic options at operation will be examined. The detection and management of patients with pancreatic injury and traumatic (non-iatrogenic) injury to the extrahepatic bile duct system will be reviewed. This chapter will conclude with a discussion of complications after liver trauma together with a consideration of the outcome in patients with hepatic injury.

Mechanisms of liver injury

Blunt trauma to the liver in motor vehicle accidents can be sustained as a result of a deceleration injury in which there is shearing of the liver on its ligamentous attachments. A compression injury can result from contact with the steering wheel. The two types of injury may co-exist but tend to produce somewhat different types of liver injury. Shearing injuries create fissures in the hepatic parenchyma which can extend to involve major vessels. Compression injuries can rupture Glisson's capsule and can also lead to subcapsular haematoma formation. In contrast, penetrating trauma to the liver may not be associated with extensive parenchymal disruption but life-threatening haemorrhage can occur if a major vessel is transected. Significant bile leaks may occur after both blunt and penetrating trauma if the injury results in damage to segmental or major bile ducts.

Injury to the hepatic veins and juxtahepatic vena cava can occur as a result of shearing stress in blunt trauma. It is worth noting that there may not be initial exsanguinating haemorrhage as the weight of the liver may provide some compression.[4] Embolisation of air and of detached fragments of liver parenchyma are special risks associated with major injuries to the hepatic veins or vena cava.[4]

Classification of liver injury

The classification of liver injury described by Moore et al.[5] has been adopted for general use by the American Society for the Surgery of Trauma (Table 11.1). The hepatic injury grade is calculated from assessment of the liver injury using information derived from radiological study, operative findings or autopsy report. Where there are multiple injuries to the liver the grade is advanced by one stage. Greater use of this classification system would permit more objective comparison of outcome in liver trauma between centres. Schweizer et al.[6] describe a protocol-based liver trauma management system employing this system of classification that permitted lesser injuries to be treated non-operatively and allowed improved selection of patients for operative treatment.[6]

Initial assessment and diagnosis of liver injury

Initial assessment

The initial assessment of the patient with suspected trauma to the liver is the initial management of any major trauma patient. Following Advanced Trauma Life Support course principles,[7] the initial focus of attention is on the patient's airway, breathing and circulation. The airway is secured, intravenous access established and fluid resuscitation commenced. There has been recent controversy regarding the role of aggressive fluid replacement in trauma victims with evidence suggesting that over-aggressive fluid replacement is associated with an adverse outcome.[8] As this evidence came from an American series which included a large proportion of relatively young, previously fit adults suffering from penetrating trauma to the torso, with ready access to trauma centres, the results may not be applicable to practice in other countries such as the UK. A detailed discussion of volume fluid replacement is outwith the scope of this chapter but it should be borne in mind

Table 11.1 *Hepatic injury scale used by the American Association for the Surgery of Trauma*

Grade I	Haematoma	Subcapsular, non-expanding, <10% of surface area
	Laceration	Capsular tear, non-bleeding, <1 cm parenchymal depth
Grade II	Haematoma	Intraparenchymal, subcapsular, non-expanding, 10–50% of surface area, <2 cm in diameter
	Laceration	Capsular tear, active bleeding; 1–3 cm parenchymal depth, <10 cm in length
Grade III	Haematoma	Subcapsular, >50% of surface area or expanding; ruptured subcapsular haematoma with active bleeding, intraparenchymal haematoma >2 cm or expanding
	Laceration	>3 cm in parenchymal depth
Grade IV	Haematoma	Ruptured intraparenchymal haematoma with active bleeding
	Laceration	Parenchymal disruption involving 25–50% of hepatic lobe
Grade V	Laceration	Parenchymal disruption involving over 50% of hepatic lobe
	Vascular	Juxtahepatic venous injuries – retrohepatic vena cava or major hepatic vein injury
Grade VI	Vascular	Hepatic avulsion

that over-aggressive fluid replacement may increase the risk of pulmonary complications and in patients with liver injury may increase the risk of coagulopathy-related bleeding.

Diagnosis

In penetrating abdominal trauma, hepatic injury should be considered in any patient with a wound to the abdomen. Hepatic injury should also be considered in patients with penetrating low thoracic wounds and also in posterior penetrating wounds below a coronal plane at the tips of the scapulae.[4]

Patients with major hepatic injury (grades IV, V and VI) present with profound clinical shock and abdominal distension. Hypotension resistant to fluid resuscitation combined with gross abdominal distension constitutes an indication for immediate operation. The management options for patients in this situation will be discussed in detail subsequently. Emergency room thoracotomy with cross clamping of the descending thoracic aorta is a dramatic intervention but even in centres where this technique is advocated the outcome is poor. For example, in Feliciano's series of 1000 patients with liver trauma treated during a 5-year period, 45 patients underwent emergency room thoracotomy for control of haemorrhage related to their liver injury and all died.[2] Emergency room thoracotomy remains a potentially life-saving manoeuvre in patients with significant intrathoracic injury with co-existent liver injury. However, there is little place for this intervention in patients with isolated liver injury or in patients with abdominal injury as the predominant injury. These patients are better served by rapid assessment and transport to a formal operating theatre.

In less dramatic situations, with a patient who is haemodynamically stable or responds to fluid resuscitation, appropriate investigations can be employed to obtain more information regarding the liver injury and to ascertain whether there is co-existing intra-abdominal visceral injury. During the initial survey a detailed clinical history is taken. In blunt motor vehicle trauma particular attention is paid to the mechanism of the accident with supplemental information from ambulance crew, witnesses or police being used to piece together a picture of the accident. Speed of vehicle, position of occupant in vehicle, use of seatbelts, use of supplemental airbag restraint systems and a history of ejection of the patient from the vehicle are important items of information. Conscious patients may complain of abdominal pain. Shoulder tip pain may arise from blood in the subhepatic space causing phrenic nerve irritation.

As resuscitation proceeds, a detailed physical examination is carried out. On inspection, attention is paid to the presence of anterior abdominal wall bruising which may indicate compression from a seatbelt and flank bruising which may indicate retroperitoneal extravasation of blood. Signs of localised or generalised peritonitis are recorded in the conscious patient. In this context it should be noted that although there is evidence that in patients with acute abdominal pain the use of opiate analgesia will not significantly obscure physical signs[9] this has not been established in abdominal trauma patients where the situation may be complicated by head injury, alcohol intoxication or the requirement for assisted ventilation.

Baseline investigations consist of blood count (for haemoglobin and haematocrit), blood for cross-matching, serum urea and electrolytes, serum amylase and coagulation screen. An erect chest radiograph and a plain abdominal film can be taken if the patient is sufficiently stable. In the context cf diagnosing liver injury, features that may be of relevance include fractures of the lower ribs, elevation of the right hemi-diaphragm and loss of the psoas shadow suggesting retroperitoneal bleeding. Retroperitoneal perforation of the duodenum may give rise to soft tissue shadowing in the right upper quadrant, loss of the psoas shadow and extraluminal gas may occasionally be noted.

Diagnostic peritoneal lavage (DPL) is a widely used investigative modality but a major criticism of this technique is that it is oversensitive in detecting intra-abdominal blood and provides no information regarding either the site or the nature of the injury. This oversensitivity may in turn lead to patients undergoing surgery where they may be better treated non-operatively.

As a result of these major limitations attention has focused on ultrasound scanning and computed tomographic (CT) scanning. Ultrasound and CT have the advantage of being non-invasive and of allowing a greater degree of evaluation of the extent of liver injury. Contrast-enhanced CT has the further advantage of allowing non-perfused areas of hepatic parenchyma to be visualised and contrast can be seen in the renal collecting systems if the kidneys are perfused. The contrast-enhanced CT scan is the 'gold standard' imaging modality for the assessment of liver trauma.[10]

Although contrast-enhanced CT will accurately demonstrate hepatic parenchymal injury it is not an accurate tool for assessing injury-related blood loss and this may be over- or underestimated.[11] In a series of 37 patients with liver trauma undergoing CT followed by laparotomy, Croce et al.[11] reported that the CT-defined grade of injury differed from the grade of liver injury described at operation in 31 patients (84%). In four patients, preoperative CT demonstration of parenchymal haematoma was not confirmed at operation and in the other 27 patients there was discrepancy between CT grading and operator grading of liver lacerations. However, a more detailed analysis of this report reveals that of the 37 patients undergoing laparotomy, 15 required no liver-related intervention (thus CT over- or under-diagnosis of the extent of a laceration becomes less relevant) and it is possible to interpret the unconfirmed intraparenchymal haematomas as being missed by the surgeon at operation rather than as CT over-diagnosis. Croce et al. concluded that limitations of CT were that it should not be used in isolation to estimate blood loss and that CT may not provide an accurate assessment of the extent of a liver laceration in some areas of the liver – specifically in the vicinity of the falciform ligament. However, CT will accurately indicate the presence of a liver laceration, it will demonstrate parenchymal injury and the use of serial CT scanning will allow the course of the injury to be carefully monitored (Fig. 11.1).

Refinements in equipment such as the development of spiral CT and three-dimensional image reconstruction have improved the diagnostic accuracy of the CT scan. The technique of 3D image reconstruction was used in a small series of eight trauma patients by Goodman et al.,[12] who reported that this technique permitted precise anatomical delineation of damaged areas of liver parenchyma. Increasing use of CT in liver trauma has led to the better recognition of CT features of liver injury. Specific signs such as periportal tracking have been reported to correlate with specific patterns of liver injury. Yokota and Sugimoto[13] defined periportal tracking as the presence of a circumferential area of low attenuation around the portal triad on contrast-enhanced CT. Periportal tracking is thought to represent blood or fluid within the condensation of the Glissonian sheath around the portal structures and thus indicates the presence of injury to structures in the portal triad. If the sign is present in

Figure 11.1 *CT scan of a 25-year-old male who sustained a blunt injury to the right chest wall but was admitted to hospital haemodynamically stable. The scan shows a substantial subcapsular haematoma associated with an intraparenchymal laceration. This patient was managed successfully without operation.*

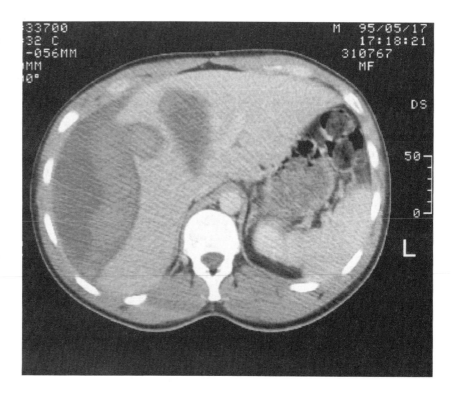

the periphery of the liver it may alert the clinician to the presence of peripheral bile duct injury which in turn may present as a bile leak. Central periportal tracking – around the porta hepatis – correlates to the presence of central or extrahepatic pedicle injury.

There has been little work to directly compare DPL and CT in the assessment of liver injury. Davis et al.[14] reported a small series of 19 patients with blunt abdominal trauma who underwent CT followed by DPL. In their series one patient underwent a laparotomy because of a positive DPL with a normal CT with operative findings of a liver injury. At operation this patient was found to have a hepatic laceration which required no specific intervention. It could be argued that contemporary management of such a patient with a liver laceration without evidence of parenchymal injury on CT would be non-operative. In addition, two further patients underwent laparotomy because of a positive DPL in the presence of a negative CT. They were both found to have splenic lacerations. As the operative management of these patients is not reported it is difficult to ascertain how significant these splenic injuries were. On the basis of these three positive DPL results in patients with negative CT findings the authors state that DPL is more sensitive in detecting free intraperitoneal blood than CT. However, the crucial question raised by the findings of this study – is there any advantage to the patient in the extra sensitivity of DPL in detecting free intra-peritoneal blood? – is not addressed by their results. The use of laparoscopy to evaluate patients with a post-traumatic haemoperitoneum has recently been reported.[15] The authors found this to be a useful technique in evaluating patients with a known haemoperitoneum who were haemodynamically stable. As these haemodynamically stable patients could also be investigated by ultrasound scanning and/or CT, and as their report made no comparison to these techniques, the precise role of laparoscopy as a diagnostic/therapeutic modality is yet to be established.

Endoscopic retrograde cholangiopancreatography (ERCP) has been used as an early diagnostic aid in liver trauma. Sugimoto *et al.*[16] reported the use of this technique in 28 of 64 (44%) patients with blunt liver trauma treated non-operatively. Bile duct injuries were detected in six (9%). As five of these patients developed clinically apparent bile leaks the value of this technique in the routine management of blunt liver trauma also remains to be established. The case summaries included with their report make clear that patients underwent ERCP in the acute phase of their liver injury, often on the day of admission. Although this policy is logical, the practical difficulties of obtaining an ERCP in a patient with liver injury within 24–48 h of admission and at a time when careful haemodynamic monitoring is crucial mean that ERCP in the acute phase of liver injury is unlikely to be widely applicable.

Newer non-invasive imaging techniques such as magnetic resonance imaging have the advantage of being free of ionising radiation but increased cost aside, the time taken to produce a scan means that this technique is as yet not widely used in the trauma setting.[17]

In summary, baseline haematological investigations and baseline radiographs will be taken. Resuscitation room ultrasound scan followed by contrast-enhanced CT scan without recourse to DPL is the preferred sequence of investigations for the assessment of a patient with suspected liver trauma.

Management options

Operative management versus non-operative management

Operative intervention is the standard management policy for patients with gunshot injury with a selective operative management policy being increasingly employed in patients with stab wounds.[4] Selective operative intervention policies are recognised for patients with blunt trauma.

It has long been appreciated that not all intrahepatic haematomas require surgical treatment. Richie and Fonkalsrud[18] described successful conservative management of four patients with liver injury in an era before the availability of the CT scan. Indirect evidence for the feasibility of a non-operative approach came from a report published by White and Cleveland[19] in the same year as that of Richie and Fonkalsrud.[18] White and Cleveland reported a consecutive series of 126 patients with liver trauma, all of whom underwent laparotomy. There were eight deaths (6%). Of interest is that 67 patients in this series (53%) had placement of a drain to the subhepatic space as their only liver-related surgical intervention at laparotomy. With the benefit of hindsight, if the policy of mandatory laparotomy for suspected liver trauma is questioned, it is possible to argue that the majority of these 67 patients could have been successfully managed non-operatively.

In a contemporary report, Schweizer et al.[6] indicated that patients with grade I and grade II injuries as assessed by CT scan could be successfully treated non-operatively. In a series of 128 consecutive adult patients sustaining blunt hepatic trauma, it was reported that 62 patients were treated initially by operation based on physical findings and peritoneal lavage.[20] A total of 66 were haemodynamically stable and underwent CT scanning, of whom 46 were successfully managed non-operatively. It is of note that 51% of patients in their series sustaining grade III and IV injuries were treated conservatively. In contrast, 92% of patients with grade V injuries required laparotomy as they were haemodynamically unstable. Of the 46 patients treated non-operatively 26 had injuries to the posterior lateral sector of the right lobe of the liver (segments VI and VII). It was concluded that haemodynamic stability and the anatomical pattern of injury were important factors in successful non-operative management of liver injury. In addition, of the 82 patients undergoing laparotomy in this series only 42 required any liver-related intervention with a 20% incidence of non-hepatic injury and a 20% incidence of non-therapeutic laparotomy. This last group of 16 patients included 13 patients with a positive DPL who subsequently had a negative laparotomy. In order to present a balanced perspective it should be pointed out that four of the 46 patients treated non-operatively subsequently required a laparotomy (two for bleeding, one for a bile leak and one negative laparotomy). Thus even in this subgroup of patients operated on after initial conservative management there was a non-therapeutic laparotomy.

A prospective study of non-operative treatment of blunt hepatic trauma has been reported from Memphis.[21] Over a 22-month period, patients with blunt hepatic trauma were treated non-operatively if they were haemodynamically stable. CT scanning was used to evaluate the extent of hepatic injury and the results were compared to outcome in a haemodynamically matched cohort of blunt hepatic trauma patients treated operatively. The study reported that of 136 patients with blunt trauma, 24 (18%) underwent emergency surgery. Of the remaining 112 patients, 12 (11%) failed conservative management (for causes not related to the liver injury in seven) and the remaining 100 patients were successfully treated without operation. Of these, 30% had minor injuries (grades I–II) but 70% had major injuries (grades III–V). This study concluded that non-operative management is safe for haemodynamically stable patients and that this was independent of the CT-delineated grade of the liver injury. The blood transfusion requirement was lower in the non-operatively treated group as was the incidence of abdominal complications. In keeping with other reports it is possible to infer from the results of this study that successful selection of patients for conservative treatment cannot be carried out by CT scanning alone but that an overall assessment of suitability for conservative management must take into account haemodynamic stability and the findings of careful, repeated, clinical examination.

Further support for non-operative treatment of hepatic trauma – even when associated with splenic trauma – has come from a report of patients under the age of 19 years.[22] In this retrospective series non-operative treatment was successful in 94% of patients.

An increasing number of reports attest to non-operative treatment following accurate assessment of the injury by CT scanning as a safe option in haemodynamically stable patients with blunt hepatic trauma.[23-25] If such a policy is to be pursued, awareness of the possibility of missing associated visceral injury should be high[26] and serial clinical examination supported by serial scanning is essential to detect the early manifestation of other injuries. The predominant indication for operative intervention in the initial management of blunt liver injury is haemodynamic instability.[20] A cautionary note in the current trend for conservative management of liver injury comes in a report from Paris.[27] They reported a series of 103 patients with severe blunt hepatic trauma (grades III–V) treated over a period of 18 years. From 1973 to 1981 hepatic resection was carried out in 56% of patients with liver trauma with a perioperative mortality of 24%. From 1982 to 1990 a more conservative policy was adopted (71% of patients being treated without operation) and this was associated with a mortality of 34% in patients undergoing surgery during this period. The authors attributed this apparent increase to a rise in the proportion of severe liver injuries seen and also in the proportion of patients with multiple injuries. However, an important conclusion that they make is that operative intervention is an important strategy in patients with major hepatic vascular injury.

In summary, operative management is indicated in all patients with gunshot wounds of the liver. In patients with hepatic stab wounds and blunt liver injuries there is good evidence to justify a selective non-operative management policy with patients being carefully assessed by repeated clinical examination, haemodynamic monitoring and serial CT scanning. In the early phase haemodynamic instability is the predominant indication for intervention and later on in the course of the injury intervention may be required in order to treat complications such as bile leaks.

Operative management

General strategy

Primary operative intervention is indicated in gunshot injuries of the liver[28] and in other types of liver injury if the patient is haemodynamically unstable despite adequate initial resuscitation.

There are three main principles that guide operative strategy in liver trauma:

1. Arrest of haemorrhage
2. Resectional debridement of devitalised liver tissue
3. Control of bile leaks.

Patients with liver trauma may present initially to surgeons without specialist hepatobiliary experience and without the facilities available in liver surgery units. The surgeon operating on a patient in this situation will attempt to achieve the above goals in treatment but if this cannot be achieved the treatment priority will be to arrest or reduce the rate of bleeding without causing further complications. It is in this context that there is a clear role for packing of the liver. This was popularised in Britain by Calne who advocated primary packing followed by transfer of the patient to the care of a specialist hepatobiliary surgeon.[29] The techniques developed for liver transplantation such as veno-venous bypass, *ex-vivo* surgery, use of the cell saver device for autologous transfusion and use of the ultrasonic dissector and argon beam coagulator are of vital importance in the treatment of patients with complex liver injury.

Choice of incision
A long midline incision is widely employed in emergency laparotomy. It has the advantages that it can be made rapidly, extended proximally (to enter the chest after median sternotomy) or distally as required and access to the liver can be improved by converting the incision into a 'T' by adding a right transverse component or a 'Y' by adding a right lateral thoracotomy. In our experience, extension of the incision into the chest is exceptional. In situations where operation is being carried out after initial conservative management, for example for treatment of bile leakage or resectional debridement, then a primary subcostal incision with fixed costal margin retraction affords excellent access to the liver and in particular to the retrohepatic vena cava and hepatic veins.

Intraoperative decision making
Once the abdomen has been entered a thorough laparotomy is performed in a systematic manner. Bleeding from the liver can be controlled initially by direct pressure using large packs and, if required, by temporary digital compression of the free edge of the lesser omentum. The packs can be gently removed to allow a detailed evaluation of the extent of the injury. It should be borne in mind that a subcapsular haematoma may cover an area of ischaemic tissue and that parenchymal injuries may be associated with damage to segmental bile ducts.[30] As described earlier, in situations where it is thought that definitive control of haemorrhage cannot be obtained, the liver wound can be packed, the incision closed and the patient transferred for definitive treatment. Packing can also be employed as a holding manoeuvre in patients who are critically unstable and will not tolerate a prolonged operative procedure. As packing is thus a widely applicable procedure, some attention should be devoted to technical considerations. Packs consisting

of standard laparotomy pads with radio-opaque marker strips should be placed around the liver to compress the parenchymal tears (Fig. 11.2). The pack should not be inserted into the liver substance itself as this will tend to distract the edges of the parenchymal tear and encourage continued bleeding. Krige *et al.*[31] reported that packing controlled haemorrhage in 18 of 22 patients with major haemorrhage from liver injuries. The four patients in whom packing did not control bleeding were found to have major vascular injury. They also reported that leaving the packs *in situ* for more than three days was associated with a high incidence of infective complications.

If laparotomy reveals grade I or grade II injuries which are not actively bleeding these can be left alone. A large or expanding subcapsular haematoma should be opened as there may be a considerable amount of devitalised tissue underneath. However, the decision to de-roof such a haematoma should be guided by the availability of a suitably trained surgeon and also by the ready availability of specialist liver surgery equipment. If these two criteria cannot be met it may be safer to leave the haematoma unopened, place packs over the surface of the liver to provide compression, close the abdomen and arrange transfer.

If there is hepatic injury with active bleeding and a decision has been made to obtain definitive control rather than pack then the principles which govern the approach are as follows. First ensure good exposure – by extending the incision and by the use of fixed costal margin retractors. Second, control hepatic inflow. The Pringle manoeuvre describes manual occlusion of the structures in the portal triad between index finger and thumb at the foramen of Winslow (Fig. 11.3). A more prolonged occlusion can be achieved by the use of a non-crushing vascular clamp (Fig. 11.4). A normal liver can tolerate inflow occlusion for up to 1 h[32] or 2 h if clamping is used in 20 min periods interspaced by re-perfusion periods of 20 min.[33] However, it should be borne in mind that the ability of a damaged liver to tolerate ischaemia may be impaired. Rather than occluding the entire portal triad it may be possible to dissect out and occlude only the common hepatic artery and portal vein or to occlude selectively either right or left branches using the techniques popularised by Makuuchi.[34] Anomalous blood supply – most commonly in the form of a right hepatic artery arising from the superior mesenteric artery or a left hepatic artery arising from the left gastric artery – may require these vessels to be controlled individually.

Third, hepatic outflow control may also be required. Access to the suprahepatic cava can be gained and it can be controlled by slings following mobilisation of the liver from its peritoneal attachments. Total vascular occlusion of the liver requires control of the inferior vena cava below the liver in addition to the suprahepatic cava[35] and is likely to be poorly tolerated by an injured liver. Elias *et al.*[36] have reported a technique of intermittent vascular occlusion of the liver without vena cava clamping during major hepatectomy by clamping the hepatic pedicle and the terminal portions of the hepatic veins just prior to their

Figure 11.2
(a) *Placement of gauze packs around the liver to compress the fracture.*
(b) *Closure of the incision provides additional compression.*

Reproduced with permission from Blumgart LH (ed.) *Surgery of the liver and biliary tract*, 2nd edn. Edinburgh: Churchill Livingstone, 1994.

(a)

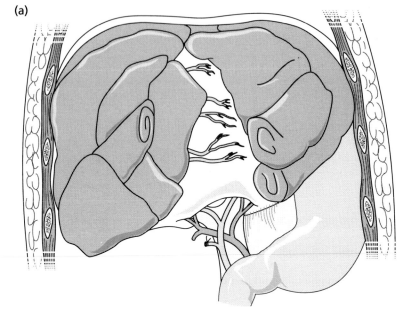

(b)

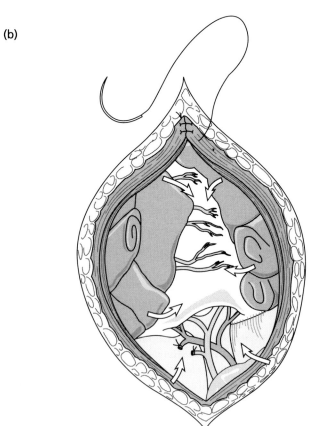

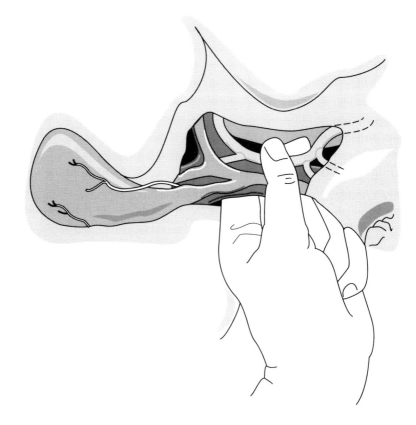

termination in the vena cava. This technique can be used in trauma to reduce the risk of air or liver parenchyma embolisation whilst preserving caval flow.

Surgical haemostasis

Surgical haemostasis is achieved by ligating bleeding vessels or occluding them with clips. The ultrasonic dissector and water jet dissector are useful in removing damaged and non-viable hepatic parenchyma while exposing blood vessels. Diathermy coagulation can also be used and in this context the argon beam coagulator which 'sprays' the diathermy current on an argon beam is invaluable as it produces surface eschar without the diathermy probe becoming adherent to the liver surface. The argon beam coagulator also has the advantage of producing less hepatic tissue necrosis than conventional diathermy[37] which is an advantage in a potentially contaminated operative field. A detailed discussion of these techniques is outwith the remit of this chapter.

Other substances that have been used to obtain haemostasis include fibrin glue[38] and as this substance can be applied at laparoscopy a recent report has described the use of laparoscopically applied fibrin glue in the treatment of liver and splenic injury.[39] As in the area of diagnostic laparoscopy, the use of therapeutic laparoscopy in this field is at an early

Figure 11.4
Occlusion of the structures in the portal triad using a soft non-crushing clamp.

Reproduced with permission from *Rob and Smith's Operative Surgery – Hepatobiliary Surgery.* London: Chapman & Hall, 1996.

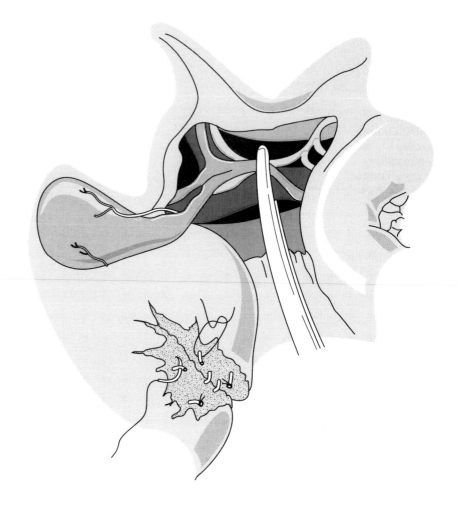

stage and cannot be generally recommended at present. Fibrin glue consists of non-autologous concentrated human fibrinogen and clotting factors to which aprotinin, a fibrinolysis inhibitor is added.[40] There are concerns about its use in man. These relate to the possibility of allergic reactions and fatal hypotension thought to be related to insertion of fibrin glue into deep hepatic lacerations has been reported.[41]

Liver sutures – absorbable sutures on a curved blunt-tipped needle often used in conjunction with a bolster of haemostatic material[42] can be used to approximate a fissured parenchymal injury and thus control haemorrhage as an alternative to exploration of the depths of the injury. The disadvantages of this technique are that vessels may continue to bleed resulting in a cavitating haematoma, bile duct injuries may not be detected and the suture itself may cause further bleeding, ischaemia or intrahepatic bile duct injury.

Stone and Lamb[43] reported that the greater omentum could be employed as a pedicled flap to fill a defect in the liver parenchyma. This technique involves dissection of the omentum from the transverse colon followed by ligation of the omental branches of the left gastroepiploic vessels by dividing the left portion of the gastrocolic omentum. Stone and Lamb reported the use of this technique in 37 patients and although the technique has a role in hepatic trauma it is not widely used as a means of arresting haemorrhage.

The use of a polyglactin perihepatic mesh instead of a pack has been reported.[44] Advocates of mesh hepatorraphy claim that it can provide the benefits of packing without the disadvantages normally associated with the use of gauze packs – in particular that a second laparotomy can be avoided as the mesh is absorbable.[45] However, there is as yet insufficient general experience with this technique.

Selective ligation of the hepatic artery

Selective ligation of the hepatic artery is indicated when intrahepatic manoeuvres have failed and when persistent re-bleeding occurs on unclamping the hepatic pedicle. Mays[46] reported the use of this technique in 60 patients. In this series the right hepatic artery was selectively ligated in 36 patients, the left hepatic artery in 15 and the main hepatic artery in nine. No cases of liver failure or necrosis were observed. Hepatic arterial ligation to control haemorrhage should only be performed when other manoeuvres have failed, when selective ligation has failed and when pedicle clamping has been demonstrated to arrest haemorrhage. Acute gangrenous cholecystitis is a well-recognised complication of hepatic artery ligation and cholecystectomy should be considered if the main hepatic artery or right hepatic artery are to be ligated.[4]

When anatomical variants have been considered and their presence excluded, persistent bleeding despite clamping of the portal pedicle can indicate the presence of juxtahepatic venous injury.

Juxtahepatic venous injury

If the Pringle manoeuvre fails to arrest haemorrhage there may be bleeding from the left liver due to the presence of a left hepatic artery arising from the left gastric artery or due to an aberrant right hepatic artery. The commonest anatomical variation in the origin of the right hepatic artery is the persistence of the right primordial hepatic artery – where the right hepatic artery arises from the superior mesenteric artery.[47] This is present in approximately 10% of cases and the aberrant right hepatic artery can usually be found running just to the right and slightly posterior to the structures in the porta hepatis.

These anatomical variants should be considered and excluded. Persistent bleeding may then indicate the presence of juxtahepatic vein injury.

Chen et al.[48] reported on a series of 19 patients with blunt juxtahepatic venous injury from a group of 92 patients with blunt liver trauma over a 2-year period. Five patients with isolated left hepatic vein injuries were treated with the use of veno-venous bypass with no mortality. Ten of the 20 patients with isolated right hepatic vein injury were treated using an atriocaval shunt but the mortality in these 20 patients was 18 (80%) with one survivor in both the shunted and non-shunted groups. Of four patients with combined right and left hepatic vein injury, one was treated by liver transplantation but all four patients in this group died. The overall mortality rate in patients with juxtahepatic vein injury was 63%. The opportunity to optimise the outcome in patients with these serious injuries probably lies in packing followed by transfer to a specialist liver surgery unit.

Debridement of devitalised liver parenchyma

Anatomic hepatic resections for removal of devitalised parenchyma are utilised less frequently because of the high mortality encountered with this policy and because a formal resection is often unnecessary in order to obtain haemostasis. Instead, non-anatomic or atypical resections aimed at removing devitalised tissue are more frequently practised – the technique of resectional debridement. If specialist liver surgery equipment such as the ultrasonic dissector and argon beam coagulator are not available then a careful decision has to be made concerning the option to pack the liver or to opt for resectional debridement. If the injury is extensive, if the injuries are multiple and if they extend close to either hepatic veins or into the porta hepatis then packing in the absence of specialist equipment will be the safer option. The decision should be guided by the goal of avoiding further injury, for example, lack of knowledge of segmental bile duct anatomy may result in injury to these structures. In contrast, a relatively peripheral injury allowing good access may lend itself to debridement and thus avoid the necessity for a second operation. Donovan and Berne[4] describe the use of the tip of a small sucker or a knife handle for teasing away hepatic tissue and exposing blood vessels and bile ducts. Vessels thus exposed can be clipped and to this end titanium clips are useful.

Ex-vivo surgery and liver transplantation for trauma

Ringe and Pichlmayr[49] reported a consecutive series of eight patients with severe liver trauma treated by total hepatectomy followed by liver transplantation. These patients had all undergone prior surgery for trauma which had been followed by severe complications – uncontrollable bleeding in four and massive necrosis in four. Where a donor liver was not immediately available a temporary portacaval shunt was used as a bridging procedure. There was a high mortality in this group with six of eight patients dying from multi-organ failure or sepsis. They conclude that total hepatectomy can be a potentially life-saving procedure in exceptional emergencies in patients with major liver injuries. Heparinised coated tubes such as the Gott shunt can be used to bridge caval defects if total hepatectomy and excision of a caval segment is required in order to obtain haemostasis.[50] The shunt acts as a temporary bridge during the anhepatic phase and has been reported to remain patent over an 18 h period.

Gall bladder and extrahepatic bile duct injury

Mechanism of injury

The extrahepatic bile duct can be injured in penetrating trauma. The management in such cases is often complicated by co-existing injury to other structures in the portal triad, liver, duodenum and pancreas. Extrahepatic bile duct injury due to blunt trauma can occur as a result of compression of the ductal system against the vertebral column.[4] Compromise of the blood supply to the duct may occur either at the time of the primary injury or may occur at operation during the Pringle manoeuvre. This may be a mechanism responsible for the development of late stricture.[51]

Awareness of injury

Extrahepatic bile duct injury is a relatively uncommon complication but as the current trend is towards non-operative management of a greater proportion of patients with liver trauma the clinician must maintain a high index of suspicion in order to detect these injuries at an early stage. Dawson et al.[52] reviewed the results of treatment of all patients with portal injuries presenting to a level 1 trauma centre in Seattle, USA over an 11-year period. A total of 21 patients (0.21% of 10 500 admissions) had injuries to the portal triad of whom 11 (52%) died. Isolated extrahepatic bile duct injury occurred in four of these patients. Injuries to the portal vein or hepatic artery whether in isolation or in association with extrahepatic bile duct injury were associated with the worst prognosis. Of note is the fact that in none of the 21 cases was the diagnosis of portal injury made preoperatively.

Burgess and Fulton[53] reported that over a 5-year period, 24 patients (13% of their total series) had extrahepatic bile duct or gall bladder injury as well as liver injury. They reported that this injury was often seen in severe hepatic trauma and in association with multiple organ injury.

If a non-operative course of management of liver injury is adopted, the suspicions of extrahepatic duct injury may be raised by CT scan evidence of a central liver injury involving the porta hepatis or the head of the pancreas, the presence on CT or ultrasound of fluid collections in the subhepatic space or CT evidence of periportal tracking of haematoma.[13] The diagnostic procedure of choice is ERCP and if a duct injury is present this can be treated by endoscopic stenting.[54] In Boone's series of 46 patients with liver trauma treated non-operatively one patient required operation at a later date for bile leak.[20]

Operative management

Injuries to the gall bladder are best treated by cholecystectomy. The principles of treating a patient with portal injury are to obtain haemostasis first. Although this may seem self-evident, the report of Dawson et al.[52] points out that these patients are at risk of exsanguinating on the operating table.

Conventional management of a partial transection of the common duct is by primary repair using absorbable sutures such as 4-0 polydioxanone over a latex T-tube inserted through a separate choledochotomy. However, there is a significant risk of stricture in this situation. In addition, in cases of traumatic injury to the extrahepatic bile duct there may be co-existent injury to the hepatic artery thus increasing the risk of ischaemic stricture. In gunshot injuries there may also be tissue loss involving part of the circumference of the bile duct making a primary repair unwise. As the published literature in this area is relatively limited the safest option is not conclusively established but is likely to be primary bilio-enteric anastomosis. This is in keeping with the advice of specialists in the field of iatrogenic bile duct injury for primary Roux-en-Y choledochojejunostomy or hepaticojejunostomy.[55]

Pancreatic injury

Mechanisms of injury

Deceleration injury is a major mechanism of blunt pancreatic injury with the region of the junction between the head and body being at risk of transection across the vertebral column. The deep location of the pancreas means that considerable force is needed to cause an injury and this level of force may often be sufficient to damage other organs.[56]

Diagnosis

Pancreatic injury should be suspected in any patient with penetrating trauma to the trunk, particularly if the entry site is between the nipples and the iliac crest and in any patient with blunt compression trauma of the upper abdomen.[56] Moretz et al.[57] found that there was no reliable correlation between a raised serum amylase and pancreatic injury. In blunt abdominal trauma a high index of clinical suspicion is required, in particular as the trend towards conservative management of liver injuries may mean that a concomitant pancreatic injury is missed or not appropriately treated.

Investigations

Contrast-enhanced CT scanning is the investigation of choice. The reported CT features of pancreatic injury include free intraperitoneal fluid, localised fluid in the lesser sac, retroperitoneal fluid, pancreatic oedema or swelling and changes in the peripancreatic fat.[58] The presence of fluid in the lesser sac between the pancreas and the splenic vein is reported by Lane et al.[58] to be a reliable sign in blunt pancreatic injury. However, Sivit and Eichelberger[59] reported that fluid separating the pancreas and the splenic vein is rarely the only abnormal CT finding in pancreatic injury.

Classification of pancreatic injury

Several classification schemes have been proposed. The scheme proposed by Lucas[60] allows appropriate treatment to be formulated according to the type of injury. This scheme divides pancreatic injuries into three groups: Grade I is a superficial contusion with minimal damage; Grade II is a deep laceration or transection of the left portion of the pancreas and Grade III is an injury of the pancreatic head. A more complex system of classification taking into account the frequent co-existence of duodenal and pancreatic injuries was proposed by Frey and Wardell.[61] This is summarised in Table 11.2. The most common site of injury is the junction of the neck and body of the pancreas. The relative frequency of pancreatic injuries reported in collected reviews is represented in Fig. 11.5.

Assessment of the integrity of the main pancreatic duct is central to the treatment of pancreatic injury. In an unstable patient this may be achieved by an intraoperative pancreatogram after first treating the cause of haemorrhage. In patients who are cardiovascularly stable, peroperative ERCP is indicated to assess major duct integrity.[62] In addition to being invaluable in diagnosing pancreatic duct injury, the major advantage of this procedure is that if an intact duct is demonstrated at ERCP it obviates the need for pancreatography at subsequent laparotomy. The limitation of ERCP is that it will not provide information about parenchymal pancreatic injury.[61]

Table 11.2 *Classification of pancreatic injury proposed by Frey and Wardell*[61]

Pancreatic injury

Class I	Capsule damage, minor gland damage (P_1)
Class II	Body or tail pancreatic duct transection, partial or complete (P_2)
Class III	Major duct injury involving the head of the pancreas or the intrapancreatic common bile duct (P_3)

Duodenal injury

Class I	Contusion, haematoma, or partial thickness injury (D_1)
Class II	Full thickness duodenal injury (D_2)
Class III	Full thickness duodenal injury with greater than 75% circumference injury; or full thickness duodenal injury with injury to the extrahepatic common bile duct (D_3)

Combined pancreaticoduodenal injuries

Type I	$P_1 D_1$, $P_2 D_1$ or $D_2 P_1$
Type II	$D_2 P_2$
Type III	$D_3 P_{1-2}$ or $P_3 D_{1-2}$
Type IV	$D_3 P_3$

Figure 11.5
Distribution of pancreatic injuries in the world literature. Note the preponderance of injuries in the junctional area of the neck of the gland.

From *Surgery of the pancreas.* Trede M, Carter DC (eds) Edinburgh: Churchill Livingstone, 1993.

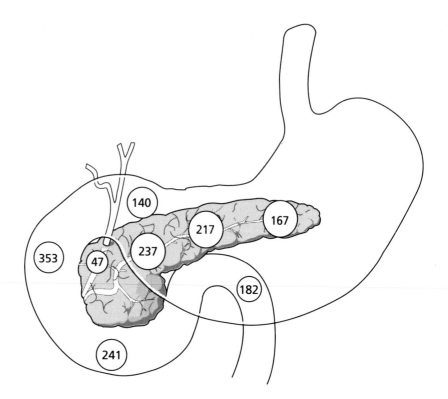

Operative management of pancreatic injury

In contrast to hepatic injury the mainstay of treatment remains operative. The important principles at laparotomy for pancreatic trauma are to gain good access to allow a thorough inspection of the gland. In order to do this it is necessary to gain access to the lesser sac to allow examination of the body of the pancreas. This is best done by creating a window in the gastrocolic omentum outside the gastroepiploic arcade. A Kocher manoeuvre is necessary to permit palpation of the head of the pancreas between thumb and fingers. The small bowel is withdrawn to permit a thorough inspection of the base of the transverse mesocolon. Injury to the pancreas is suspected if retroperitoneal haemorrhage can be seen through the base of the mesocolon or the lesser omentum. Absence of any sign of haemorrhage over the pancreas and duodenum makes injury very unlikely (with the exception being the possibility of injury to the posterior aspect of the duodenum).[61]

A recent report of a large series of patients with pancreatic injury from Durban recommended operative treatment for patients with penetrating or gunshot injury with signs of peritoneal irritation.[63] In this large series of 152 patients with pancreatic trauma presenting during a 5-year period, 63 patients had been shot, 66 stabbed and 23 had blunt trauma. The mainstay of treatment was exploratory laparotomy followed by drainage of the pancreatic injury site. Large bore soft silastic drains provide reliable drainage and minimise the risk of erosion into a major vessel. Drain effluent can be collected into a stoma bag to minimise skin excoriation from fluid which may be rich in pancreatic enzymes. The mortality rates in these groups were 8% after gunshot injury, 2% after stab wounds and 10% after blunt trauma. The majority of these deaths were attributed to injury to other organs. The proportion of patients developing pancreatic fistulae in the three groups was 14%, 9% and 13%, respectively. The conclusion that the authors drew was that 'conservative' surgical drainage was justified after pancreatic injury. This large contemporary report lends weight to the treatment plan proposed by Lucas for grade I injuries which consists of passive closed drainage using a wide bore drain, such as a chest drain. Madiba and Mokoena's[63] results would also suggest that patients with grade II injuries can be managed by drainage. If the distal pancreas is virtually transected the transection line can be converted into a distal pancreatectomy.

Injuries of the head of the pancreas (Lucas grade III) should be further assessed by means of intraoperative pancreaography. This can be a technically demanding procedure and Frey and Wardell[61] state that an 'experienced pancreatic surgeon' may elect to carry out pancreatography via a duodenotomy and retrograde cannulation of the papilla using a fine Fogarty catheter. If the pancreatic duct is intact, drainage alone is sufficient. If there is disruption of the duct it should be drained into a Roux-en-Y loop of jejunum. Transection of the pancreas at the junction of the head and body can be treated by drainage of the distal pancreas into a roux loop with the cut end of the proximal pancreatic head being oversewn. This avoids the risk of endocrine insufficiency that can occur after extended subtotal pancreatectomy.

A similar picture emerges from the report of Moncure and Goins from Washington DC.[64] They describe their experience with a consecutive series of 44 patients with pancreatic injury treated over a 6-year period. Penetrating abdominal trauma accounted for the majority of cases. Class I pancreatic injuries occurred in 55% of cases and the majority were managed by simple drainage. Grade II injuries occurred in 18% and grade III injuries in 21%. Co-existent duodenal injuries were treated by primary closure in 21% and more complex duodenal exclusion techniques were used in 20%. Their most frequent complication was intra-abdominal abscess which occurred in 31%. Pancreatic fistulae occurred in 16%. Craig and colleagues report similar results in a series of 13 patients with blunt pancreatic trauma treated over a 10-year period.[65] The smaller numbers in their series are perhaps more representative of the relative infrequency of this type of injury in many casualty departments in Europe.

Severe Lucas grade III injuries involving the head of the pancreas, duodenum and distal bile duct represent a major challenge but fortunately they are relatively rare, occurring in about 5% of all duodenal injuries.[66] The principles of treatment are to bear in mind that haemorrhage from concomitant injuries should be dealt with first as this is likely to be the major source of mortality.[67] Similarly a prolonged anaesthetic should be avoided in a potentially unstable patient. This type of injury requires the involvement of an experienced pancreatic surgeon. Duodenal injuries can be closed primarily or drained into a roux loop. Bile duct injuries may be repaired primarily over a T-tube or drained into a roux loop. The large variety of operative procedures described for these complex injuries suggests that treatment has to be tailored to the individual injury complex and that no single procedure is likely to be uniformly applicable or successful.

Complications and outcome

Complications of non-operative management of liver trauma

Complications after non-operative management of liver trauma can be considered in three main categories. First, it should be borne in mind that complications can arise as a result of inappropriate selection of a patient for conservative management. If a patient has continued bleeding this may present as episodes of hypotension requiring fluid and blood replacement, impaired renal function, impaired respiratory function (due to diaphragmatic splinting by intra-abdominal haematoma) and there may be evidence of coagulopathy. These features represent not so much a 'complication' as the natural progression of a patient with continued active intra-abdominal bleeding and in such a case the policy of non-operative intervention will require re-examination.

The second group of complications are those relating to co-existing injuries that have not been recognised at the time of initial presentation or to injuries such as damage to a bile duct which has become apparent after initial delay. A bile leak may manifest itself as biliary peritonitis or as a localised bile collection. Endoscopic retrograde cholangiography (ERCP) is useful in diagnosing the source of bile leaks in patients with liver trauma treated non-operatively and also in postoperative patients.[16] Treatment of this complication by ERCP and endoscopic sphincterotomy has been reported from Pennsylvania but in the UK a bile leak would be more likely to be treated by a period of endobiliary stenting without sphincterotomy.[68]

Another potential complication of non-operative treatment of liver injury in this second category is the risk of missing an associated non-hepatic injury. Injuries of the spleen and perforations of the intestine are at risk of being missed as the signs of abdominal tenderness may be attributed to intra-abdominal blood from the liver injury. The risk of missing this type of injury can be minimised by regular careful clinical observation and an intestinal perforation may become apparent on serial ultrasound or CT scanning by the presence of free intraperitoneal fluid or gas. In Sherman's series of patients with liver trauma treated non-operatively four of 30 (13%) patients initially treated without operation subsequently required laparotomy.[69] These were due to splenic injury in three patients and renal injury in one. Although the grade of injury to these organs is not specified in the author's paper in all cases the injuries became apparent after a period of clinical observation and thus the authors concluded that this risk of missed solid organ injury does not obviate the benefits of initial non-operative management.

The third category of complication relates to the late complications of liver injury. Liver injury may give rise to a transient elevation in liver transaminase enzymes and a rise in serum alanine transferase has been documented as commencing 15 min after injury.[70] Persisting elevation of these enzymes suggests significant liver injury. Septic complications such as intra-abdominal abscess and bile leak may present late. Haemobilia is another recognised late complication and the management of this complication is discussed in the section on postoperative complications.

Postoperative complications

Haemorrhage in the immediate postoperative period may be due to coagulopathy related to large volume transfusion and may require correction with fresh frozen plasma and platelet concentrates. If there is no evidence of a significant coagulopathy and bleeding continues to be a problem there have been reports of selective angiographic embolisation of the right or left hepatic artery (or more selected branches).[71] Bleeding in the later postoperative period may be due to haemobilia. Haemobilia or bleeding from the biliary tree into the gut is a relatively uncommon complication of liver trauma[72] and can be due to a pseudoaneurysm of the hepatic artery.[73] It has been reported to occur in 1.2% of patients with liver trauma.[73] The diagnosis of pseudoaneurysm can be confirmed by angiography and the risk of hepatic necrosis following angiographic embolisation should be minimal if a segmental artery is embolised selectively. Wagner's report cited three cases of hepatic necrosis after embolisation in a series of 61 patients (5%)[71] but in our experience significant hepatic necrosis is a rare complication of selective embolisation.

Postoperative sepsis may be due to infected collections of bile, blood or related to devitalised segments of liver parenchyma. Ultrasound and CT scanning are of value in the diagnosis and these modalities may be used to guide placement of drainage cannulae.

A biliary fistula occurring after surgery is a manifestation of an unrecognised bile duct injury. ERCP is of value in determining the precise location of the injury and as in bile leaks occurring in patients treated non-operatively, temporary stenting may encourage preferential drainage into the gut via the stent by bypassing the sphincter of Oddi.

Arteriovenous fistula is a not uncommon complication after injury in many sites of the body and can manifest after liver injury as an arterioportal fistula.[74] Large fistulae can result in portal hypertension.

Major haemorrhage as a late complication is rare. Berman et al.[75] found only one report of fatal late haemorrhage after blunt liver trauma in the world literature and concluded that this small risk was outweighed by the benefits of non-operative management. An uncommon postoperative complication related to packing is thrombosis of the inferior vena cava.[76] Hyperpyrexia occurs frequently after liver injury.[77] Cogbill *et al.*[77] reported that maximum daily temperatures exceeding 38°C were recorded in 64% of patients with severe liver trauma in the first three postoperative days. As this occurred in the absence of any infectious source the authors concluded that this was due to release of inflammatory mediators associated with severe liver injury. They also reported that as in patients with liver injury treated non-operatively there was a postoperative rise in biochemical liver function tests and in the serum bilirubin. The serum glutamic oxaloacetic transaminase (SGOT) and lactate dehydrogenase (LDH) peaked within 24 h of surgery and decreased rapidly over the subsequent 4 days. In contrast, serum bilirubin was maximal at 7 days. Hepatic enzyme elevations were reported to be more dramatic after blunt trauma – perhaps indicating greater parenchymal disruption.

Complications of pancreatic injury

Complications associated with injury to the pancreas include problems of sepsis such as pancreatic abscess and complications specific to pancreatic injury such as pancreatitis, pseudocyst, pancreatic fistula and pancreatic ascites. Madiba and Mokoena[63] reported an incidence of pancreatic fistula in 13% of their patients with penetrating trauma. The majority of these will close spontaneously with time with the exceptions being cases where there is untreated major duct injury.

In a series of 64 patients with pancreatic trauma pseudocysts developed in 15 patients (23%).[78] ERCP demonstrated duct injury in eight of these patients. Patients with pseudocysts related to distal duct injury were treated successfully by percutaneous aspiration. Three patients with duct injuries in the neck/body region underwent distal pancreatectomy. Pseudocysts related to ductal injury in the head of the pancreas were drained internally by Roux-en-Y cystjejunostomy. Lewis *et al.*[78] concluded that traumatic pancreatic pseudocysts associated with a peripheral duct injury may resolve spontaneously whereas those associated with injuries to the proximal duct require surgical intervention.

Moncure and Goins[64] reported that pancreatic abscess was the commonest complication after trauma in their series. The initial treatment was percutaneous drainage under either ultrasound or CT guidance.

Acute pancreatitis develops in up to 13% of patients after pancreatic trauma.[79]

Outcome after liver injury

The outcome after liver trauma is related not only to the severity of the injury but to the severity of associated injury. The large variation in case mix between different centres also makes comparison difficult. Feliciano *et al.*[2] reported that most of the mortality in patients with liver trauma was related to the severity of co-existent injuries. Injury severity assess-

Figure 11.6
*Outcome after liver
injury. Note that the
overall outcome will
be influenced by the
severity of co-
existing injuries.*

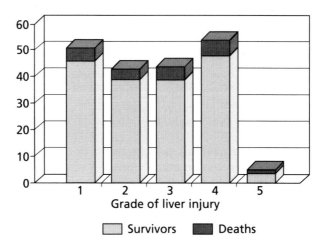

Figure 11.6
*Outcome after liver
injury. Note that the
overall outcome will
be influenced by the
severity of co-
existing injuries.*

ments such as the injury severity score can be used in an effort to standardise the outcomes reported from different centres.[80]

In a large series of 1000 cases of liver trauma from Houston, an overall mortality of 10.5% was reported.[2] A similar mortality rate was reported by White and Cleveland in their 1972 report with eight deaths occurring in a consecutive series of 126 patients (6.3%).[19] The series reported by Pachter *et al.*[51] examining significant trends in the treatment of hepatic trauma over the period 1977–1991 reported 30 deaths in 411 patients (7.3%). The outcome in Schweizer *et al.*'s[6] series from Berne is shown in graphic form in Fig. 11.6. This gives an impression of the outcome related to the grade of liver injury. The mortality rate was 11% for grade I injuries, 10% for grade II injuries, 13% for grade III and IV injuries and in the small number of grade V injuries 33%. The overall mortality was 12% (21 deaths in 175 patients).

An overall in-hospital mortality in the order of 10% is reported by units treating patients with liver trauma across the world[81-84] with the mortality being affected by the nature of injury and the frequency and severity of co-existent injury.

In conclusion, advances in diagnosis and management of liver injury together with an improved understanding of the pathophysiology of liver trauma have resulted in an improvement in outcome in these patients over the last 40 years. However, a paper by Hoyt *et al.*[85] dispels any tendency towards complacency in treating these patients. They examined the operating room records of eight American level I Trauma Centres to identify preventable causes of death. There were 537 operating room deaths from a total of 72 151 admissions. Abdominal injury was the major cause of death in 287 and 92 of these were liver-related. Delays in packing were highlighted as a preventable cause of death as was a need for better end-points for packing. The conclusion of this large survey was that the management of severe liver injuries remains a major technical challenge.

References

1. John TG, Greig JD, Johnstone AJ, Garden OJ. Liver trauma: a 10-year experience. Br J Surg 1992; 79: 1352–6.
2. Feliciano DV, Mattox KL, Jordan GL et al. Management of 1000 consecutive cases of hepatic trauma (1979–1984). Ann Surg 1986; 204: 438–42.
3. Feliciano DV. Abdominal trauma. In: Schwartz SI, Ellis H (eds) Maingot's abdominal operations, 9th edn. Connecticut: Appleton & Lange, 1990, pp. 457–512.
4. Donovan AJ, Berne TV. Liver and bile duct injury. In: Blumgart LH (ed.) Surgery of the liver and biliary tract, 2nd edn. Edinburgh: Churchill Livingstone, 1994, pp. 1221–42.
5. Moore EE, Shackford SR, Pachter HL et al. Organ injury scaling: spleen, liver and kidney. J Trauma 1989; 29: 1664–6.
6. Schweizer W, Tanner S, Baer HU et al. Management of traumatic liver injuries. Br J Surg 1993; 80: 86–8.
7. American College of Surgeons: Committee on Trauma. Advanced Life Support Course. Chicago, American College of Surgeons 1992.
8. Bickell WH, Wall MJ Jr, Pepe PE et al. Immediate versus delayed fluid resuscitation for hypotensive patients with penetrating torso injuries. N Engl J Med 1994; 331: 1105–9.
9. Attard AR, Corlett MJ, Kidner NJ et al. Safety of early pain relief for acute abdominal pain. Br Med J 1992; 305: 554–6.
10. Adam A, Roddie ME. Computed tomography of the liver and biliary tract. In: Blumgart LH (ed.) Surgery of the liver and biliary tract, 2nd edn. Edinburgh: Churchill Livingstone, 1994, pp. 243–70.
11. Croce MA, Fabian TC, Kudsk KA et al. AAST organ injury scale: correlation of CT graded liver injuries and operative findings. J Trauma 1991; 31: 806–12.
12. Goodman DA, Tiruchelvam V, Tabb DR et al. 3D CT reconstruction in the surgical management of hepatic injuries. Ann R Coll Surg Engl 1995; 77: 7–11.
13. Yokota J, Sugimoto T. Clinical significance of periportal tracking on computed tomographic scan in patients with blunt liver trauma. Am J Surg 1994; 168: 247–50.
14. Davis RA, Shayne JP et al. The use of computed axial tomography versus peritoneal lavage in the evaluation of blunt abdominal trauma: A prospective study. Surgery 1985; 98: 845–50.
15. Lujan JA, Robles R, Torralba et al. Laparoscopic surgery in the management of traumatic haemoperitoneum in stable patients. Br J Surg 1995; 82 suppl 1:84 (abstract).
16. Sugimoto K, Asari Y, Sakaguchi T, Owada T, Maekawa K. Endoscopic retrograde cholangiography in the non-surgical management of blunt liver injury. J Trauma 1993; 35: 192–9.
17. Vock P. Magnetic resonance imaging. In: Blumgart LH (ed.) Surgery of the liver and biliary tract, 2nd edn. Edinburgh: Churchill Livingstone, 1994, pp. 271–82.
18. Richie JP, Fonkalsrud EW. Subcapsular haematoma of the liver: non-operative management. Arch Surg 1972; 104: 780–4.
19. White P, Cleveland RJ. The surgical management of liver trauma. Arch Surg 1972; 104: 785–6.
20. Boone DC, Federle M, Billiar TR et al. Evolution of management of major hepatic trauma: identification of patterns of injury. J Trauma 1995; 39: 344–50.
21. Croce MA, Fabian TC, Menke PG et al. Nonoperative management of blunt hepatic trauma is the treatment of choice for hemodynamically stable patients. Results of a prospective trial. Ann Surg 1995; 221: 744–53.
22. Coburn MC, Pfeifer J, DeLuca FG. Nonoperative management of splenic and hepatic trauma in the multiply injured pediatric and adolescent patient. Arch Surg 1995; 130: 332–8.
23. Goff CD, Gilbert CM. Nonoperative management of blunt hepatic trauma. Am Surg 1995; 61: 66–8.
24. Clark DE, Cobean RA, Radke FR et al. Management of major hepatic trauma involving interhospital transfer. Am Surg 1994; 60: 881–5.
25. Meredith JW, Young JS, Bowling J et al. Nonoperative management of blunt liver trauma: the exception or the rule? J Trauma 1994; 36: 529–34.
26. Maione G, Tommasini Degna C, Baticci F et al. Les contusions du foie. Importance des lesions associeees chez les polytraumatises. J Chir (Paris) 1994; 131: 194–200.
27. Menegaux F, Langlois P, Chigot JP. Severe blunt trauma of the liver: study of mortality factors. J Trauma 1993; 35: 865–9.

28. Degiannis E, Levy RD, Velmahos GC *et al.* Gunshot injuries of the liver: the Baragwanath experience. Surgery 1995; 117: 359–64.

29. Calne RY, McMaster P, Pentlon BD. The treatment of major liver trauma by primary packing with transfer of the patient for definitive treatment. Br J Surg 1978; 66: 338–9.

30. Howdieshell TR, Purvis J, Bates WB *et al.* Biloma and biliary fistula following hepatorraphy for liver trauma: incidence, natural history and management. Am Surg 1995; 61: 165–8.

31. Krige JEJ, Bornman PC, Terblanche J. Therapeutic perihepatic packing in complex liver trauma. Br J Surg 1992; 79: 43–6.

32. Hannoun L, Borie D, Delva E *et al.* Liver resection with normothermic ischaemia exceeding 1 hour. Br J Surg 1993; 80: 1161–5.

33. Elias D, Desruennes E, Lasser P. Prolonged intermittent clamping of the portal triad during hepatectomy. Br J Surg 1991; 78: 42–4.

34. Launois B, Jamieson GG. General principles of liver surgery. In: Launois B, Jamieson GG (eds) Modern operative techniques in liver surgery. Edinburgh: Churchill Livingstone, 1993, pp. 23–37.

35. Bismuth H, Castaing D, Garden OJ. Major hepatic resection under total vascular exclusion. Ann Surg 1989; 210: 13–19.

36. Elias D, Lasser P, Debaene B *et al.* Intermittent vascular exclusion of the liver (without vena cava clamping) during major hepatectomy. Br J Surg 1995; 82: 1535–9.

37. Postema RR, Kate JW, Terpstra OT. Less hepatic tissue necrosis after argon beam coagulator than after conventional electrocoagulation. Surg Gynecol Obstet 1993; 176: 177–80.

38. Kram HB, Reuben BI, Fleming AW. Use of fibrin glue in hepatic trauma. J Trauma 1988; 28: 1195–201.

39. Rizk N, Champault G. Application of fibrin sealant in video surgery. Br J Surg 1995; 82 suppl 1:86 (abstract).

40. Feliciano DV, Pachter HL. Trauma to the liver vasculature, aneurysm and arteriovenous fistula. In: Blumgart LH (ed.) Surgery of the liver and biliary tract, 2nd edn. Edinburgh: Churchill Livingstone, 1994, pp. 1243–57.

41. Berguer R, Staerkel RL, Moore EE *et al.* Warning: fatal reaction to the use of fibrin glue in deep hepatic wounds. Case reports. J Trauma 1991; 31: 408–11.

42. Wood CB, Capperauld I, Blumgart LH. Bioplast fibrin buttons for liver biopsy and partial hepatic resection. Ann R Coll Surg Engl 1976; 58: 401–4.

43. Stone HH, Lamb JM. Use of pedicled omentum as an autogenous pack for control of hemorrhage in major injuries of the liver. Surg Gynecol Obstet 1975; 141: 92–4.

44. Brunet C, Sielezneff I, Thomas P *et al.* Treatment of hepatic trauma with perihepatic mesh: 35 cases. J Trauma 1994; 37: 200–4.

45. Reed RL, Merrell RC, Meyers WC, Fischer RP. Continuing evolution in the approach to severe liver trauma. Ann Surg 1992; 216: 524–38.

46. Mays ET. Hepatic trauma. Curr Probl Surg 1976; 13: 6–73.

47. Couinaud C. Surgical anatomy of the liver revisited. L'Imprimerie Maugein et Cie, Tulle 1989.

48. Chen RJ, Fang JF, Lin BC *et al.* Surgical management of juxtahepatic venous injuries in blunt hepatic trauma. J Trauma 1995; 38: 886–90.

49. Ringe B, Pichlmayr R. Total hepatectomy and liver transplantation: a life-saving procedure in patients with severe hepatic trauma. Br J Surg 1995; 82: 837–9.

50. Lin PJ, Jeng LB, Chen RJ *et al.* Femoro-arterial bypass using Gott shunt in liver transplantation following severe hepatic trauma. Int Surg 1993; 78: 295–7.

51. Pachter HL, Spencer FC, Hofstetter SR *et al.* Significant trends in the management of hepatic trauma: experience with 411 injuries. Ann Surg 1992; 215: 492–502.

52. Dawson DL, Johansen KH, Jurkovich GJ. Injuries to the portal triad. Am J Surg 1991; 161: 545–51.

53. Burgess P, Fulton RL. Gallbladder and extrahepatic biliary duct injury following abdominal trauma. Injury 1992; 23: 413–14.

54. Jenkins MA, Ponsky JL. Endoscopic retrograde cholangiopancreatography and endobiliary stenting in the treatment of biliary injury resulting from liver trauma. Surg Laparosc Endosc 1995; 5: 118–20.

55. Bismuth H, Franco D, Corlette MB. Long term results of Roux-en-Y hepaticojejunostomy. Surg Gynecol Obstet 1978; 146: 161–7.

56. Johnson CD. Pancreatic trauma. Br J Surg 1995; 82: 1153–4.

57. Moretz JA III, Campbell DP, Parker DE, William GR. Significance of serum amylase in evaluating pancreatic trauma. Am J Surg 1975; 130: 739–41.

58. Lane MJ, Mindelzun RE, Sandhu JS. CT diagnosis of blunt pancreatic trauma: importance of detecting fluid between the pancreas and the splenic vein. Am J Roentgenol 1994; 163: 833–5.

59. Sivit CJ, Eichelberger MR. CT diagnosis of pancreatic injury in children: significance of fluid separating the splenic vein and the pancreas. Am J Roentgenol 1995; 165: 921–4.

60. Lucas CE. Diagnosis and treatment of pancreatic and duodenal injury. Surg Clin North Am 1977; 57: 49–65.

61. Frey CF, Wardell JW. Injuries to the pancreas. In: Trede M, Carter DC (eds) Surgery of the pancreas. Edinburgh: Churchill Livingstone, 1993, pp. 565–89.

62. Hayward SR, Lucas CE, Sugawa C, Ledgerwood AM. Emergent endoscopic retrograde cholangiopancreatography: a highly specific test for acute pancreatic trauma. Arch Surg 1989; 124: 745–6.

63. Madiba TE, Mokoena TR. Favourable prognosis after surgical drainage of gunshot, stab or blunt trauma of the pancreas. Br J Surg 1995; 82: 1236–9.

64. Moncure M, Goins WA. Challenges in the management of pancreatic and duodenal injuries. JAMA 1993; 85: 767–72.

65. Craig MH, Talton DS, Hauser CJ, Poole GV. Pancreatic injuries from blunt trauma. Am Surg 1995; 61: 125–8.

66. Martin TD, Feliciano DV, Mattox KL, Jordan GL Jr. Severe duodenal injuries. Treatment with pyloric exclusion and gastrojejunostomy. Arch Surg 1983; 118: 631–5.

67. Feliciano DV, Martin TD, Cruse PA et al. Management of combined pancreatoduodenal injuries. Ann Surg 1987; 205: 673–80.

68. Scioscia PJ, Dillon PW, Cilley RE et al. Endoscopic sphincterotomy in the management of posttraumatic biliary fistula. J Pediatr Surg 1994; 29: 3–6.

69. Sherman HF, Savage BA, Jones LM et al. Nonoperative management of blunt hepatic injuries: safe at any grade? J Trauma 1994; 37: 616–21.

70. Hellstrom G. The activity of glutamic oxalacetic and glutamic-pyruvic transaminases (GOT and GPT), ornithine-carbamoyl transferase (OCT) and alkaline phosphatase (AP) in serum in closed liver injury. An experimental study. Acta Chir Scand 1966; 131: 476–84.

71. Wagner WW, Lundell CJ, Donovan AJ. Percutaneous angiographic embolisation for hepatic arterial hemorrhage. Arch Surg 1985; 120: 1241–9.

72. Maurel J, Aouad K, Martel B, Segol P, Gignoux M. Post-traumatic hemobilia. How to treat? Ann Chir 1994; 48: 572–5.

73. Croce MA, Fabian TC, Spiers JP, Kudsk KA. Traumatic pseudoaneurysm with hemobilia. Am J Surg 1994; 168: 235–8.

74. Oishi AJ, Nagorney DM, Cherry KJ. Portal hypertension, variceal bleeding and high output cardiac failure secondary to an intrahepatic arterioportal fistula. HPB Surg 1993; 7: 53–9.

75. Berman SS, Mooney EK, Weireter L Jr. Late fatal hemorrhage in pediatric liver trauma. J Pediatr Surg 1992; 27: 1546–8.

76. John TG, Chalmers N, Redhead DN, Kumar S, Garden OJ. Case report: inferior vena caval thrombosis following severe liver trauma and perihepatic packing – early detection by intraoperative ultrasound enabling treatment by percutaneous mechanical thrombectomy. Br J Radiol 1995; 68: 314–17.

77. Cogbill TH, Moore EE, Feliciano DV, Jurkovich GJ et al. Hepatic enzyme response and hyperpyrexia after severe liver injury. Am Surg 1992; 58: 395–9.

78. Lewis G, Krige JEJ, Bornman PC, Terblanche J. Traumatic pancreatic pseudocysts. Br J Surg 1993; 80: 89–93.

79. Stone HH, Fabian TC, Satiani B, Turkleson ML. Experience in the management of pancreatic trauma. J Trauma 1981; 21: 257–62.

80. Rowlands BJ. Management of abdominal trauma. In: Taylor I (ed.) Progress in surgery, Vol. 3. Edinburgh: Churchill Livingstone, 1989, pp. 101–16.

81. Cogbill TH, Moore EE, Jurkovitch GF et al. Severe hepatic trauma: a multi-center experience with 1,335 liver injuries. J Trauma 1988; 28: 1433–8.

82. Little JM, Fernandez A, Tait M. Liver trauma. Aust N Z J Surg 1986; 56: 613–19.

83. Durham RM, Buckley J, Keegan M et al. Management of blunt hepatic injuries. Am J Surg 1992; 164: 477–81.

84. Knudson MM, Lim RC, Olcott EW. Morbidity and mortality following major penetrating liver injuries. Arch Surg 1994; 129: 256–61.

85. Hoyt DB, Bulger EM, Knudson MM *et al*. Death in the operating room: an analysis of a multicenter experience. J Trauma 1994; 37: 426–38.

Index

Page numbers in *italic* refer to illustrations and tables; **bold** page numbers indicate a main discussion